Dyslexia

Edited by Jonathan Glazzard
and Samuel Stones

Published in London, United Kingdom

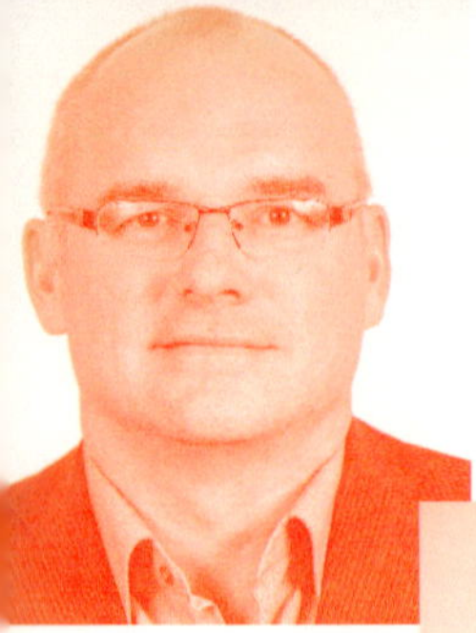
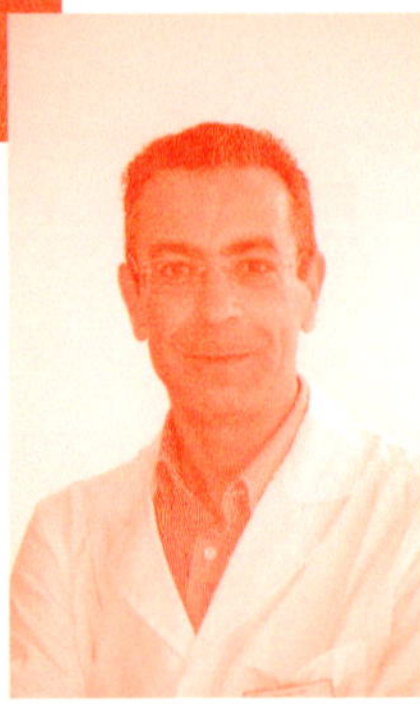
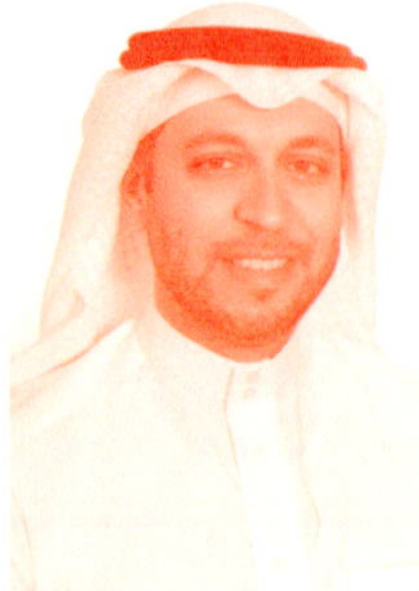
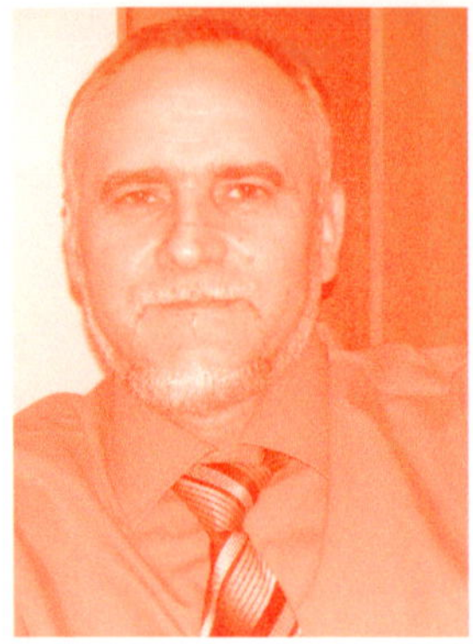
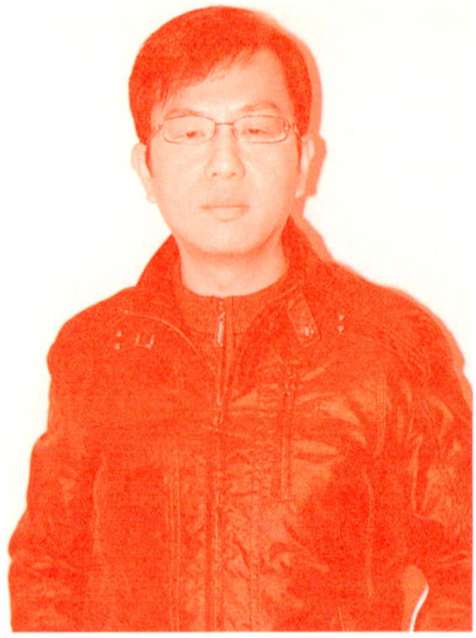
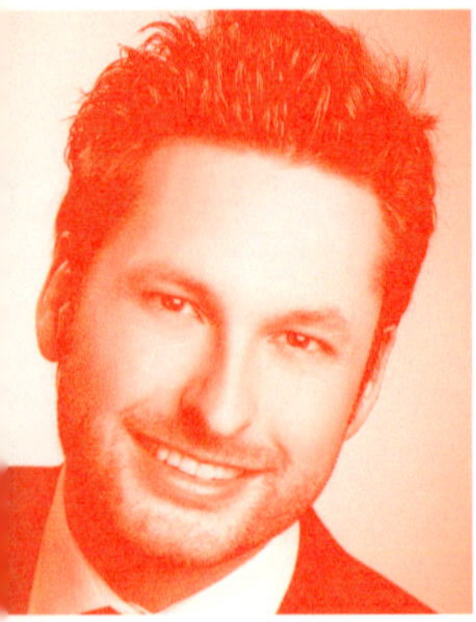
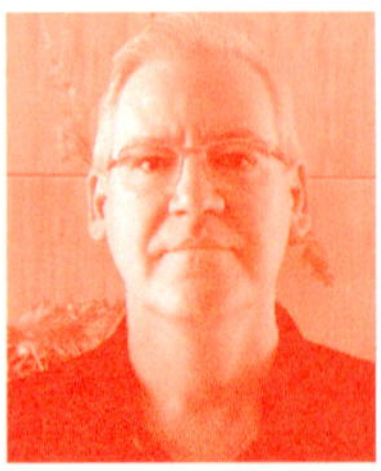

IntechOpen

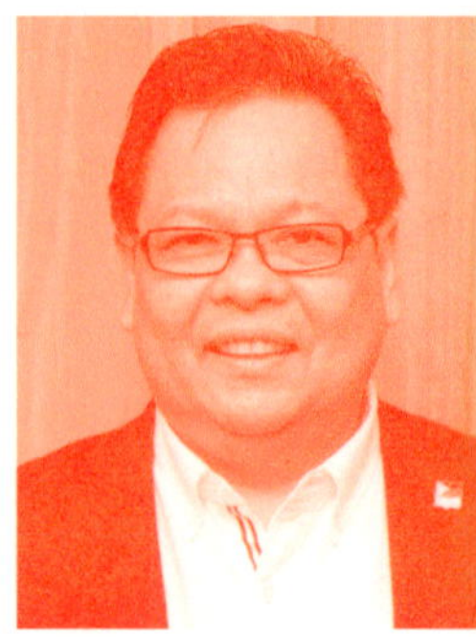
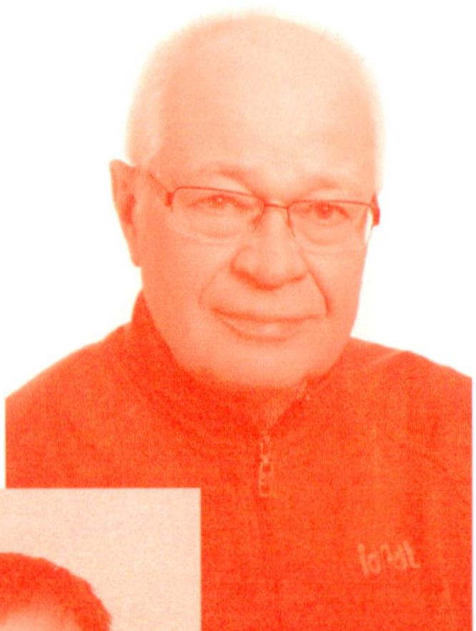
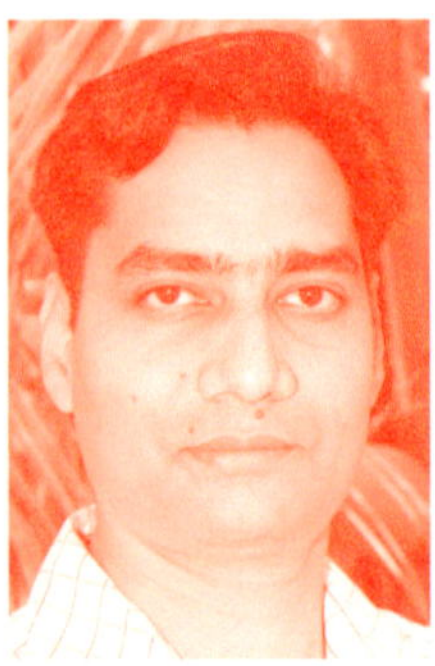
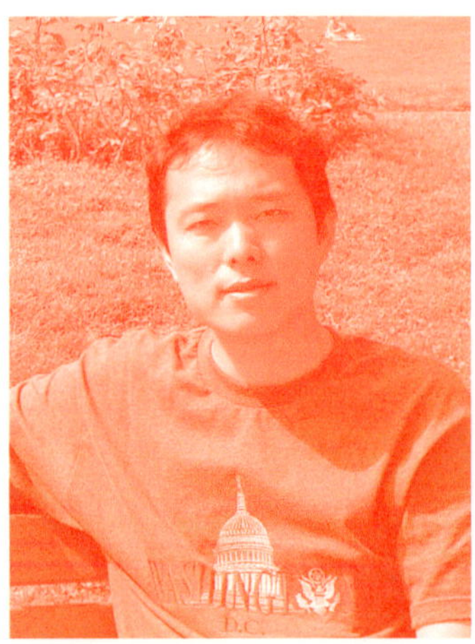
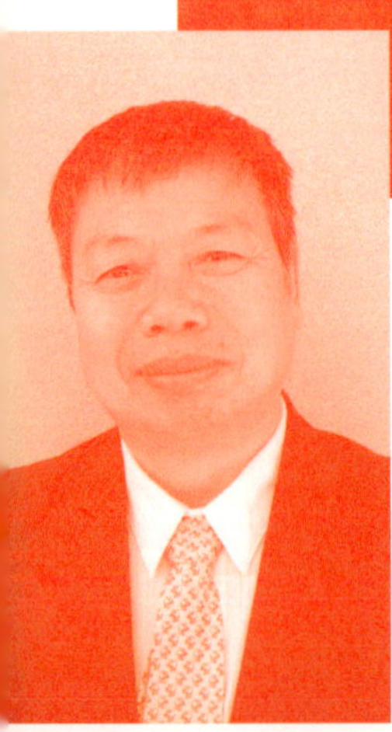
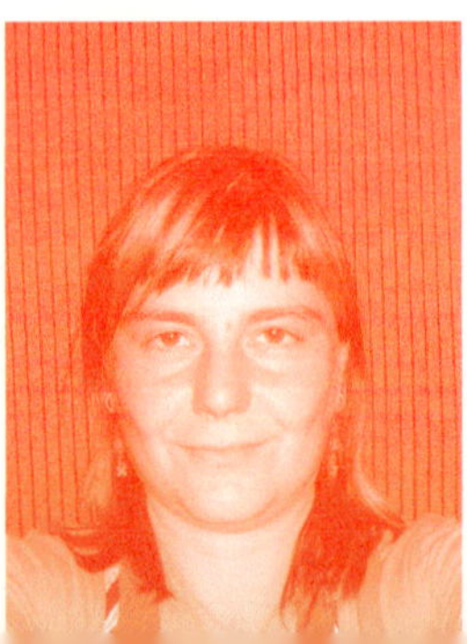

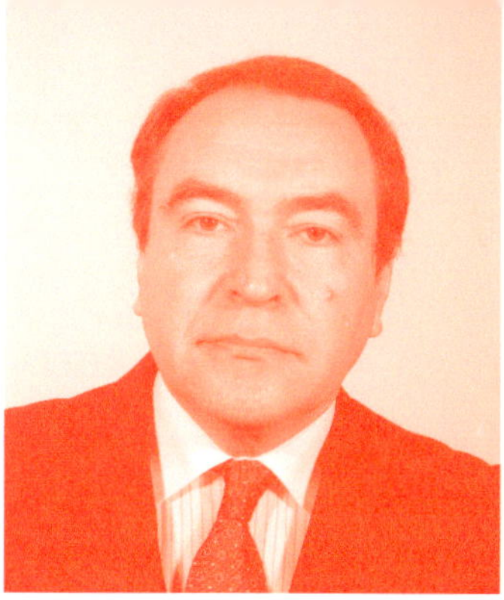
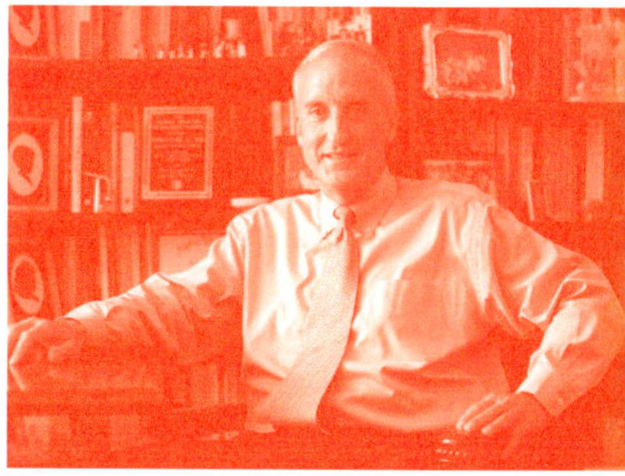
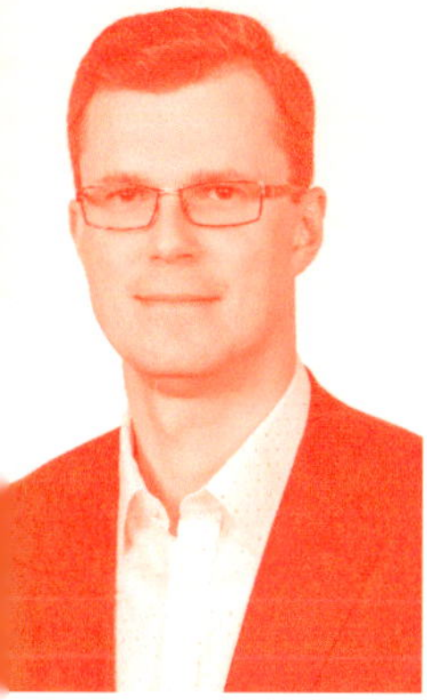
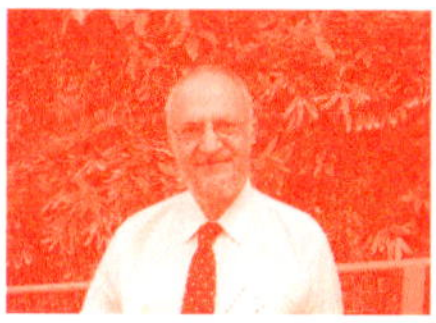
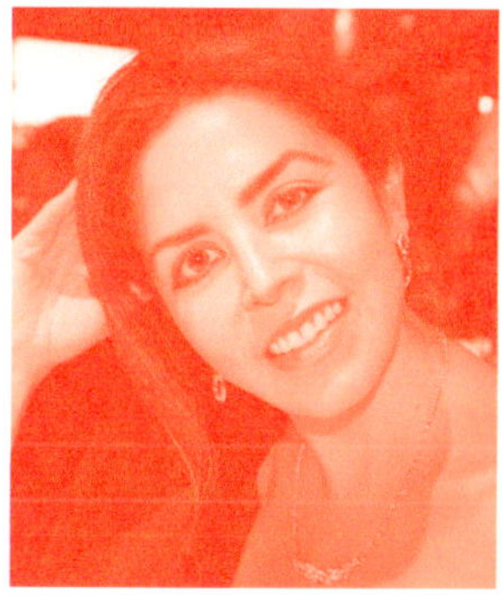

Supporting open minds since 2005

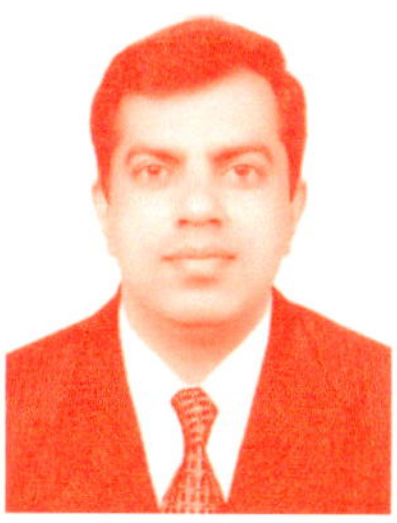
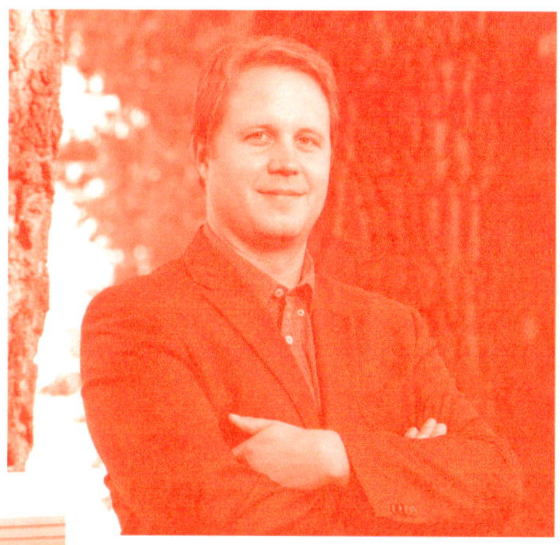
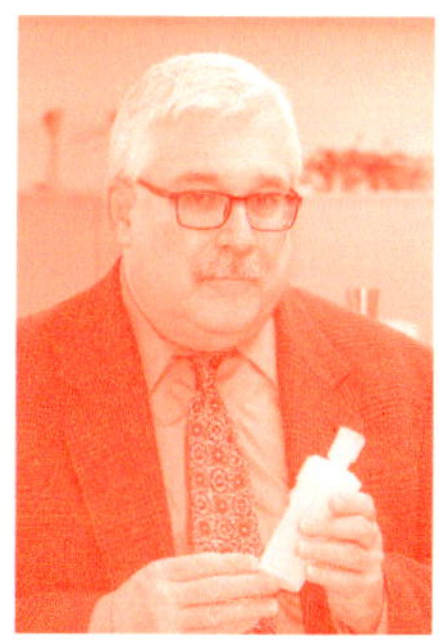
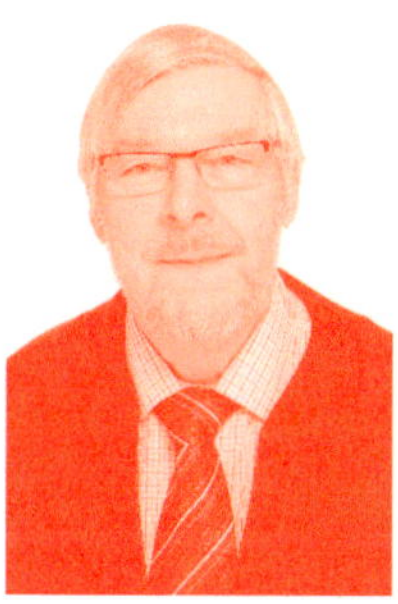
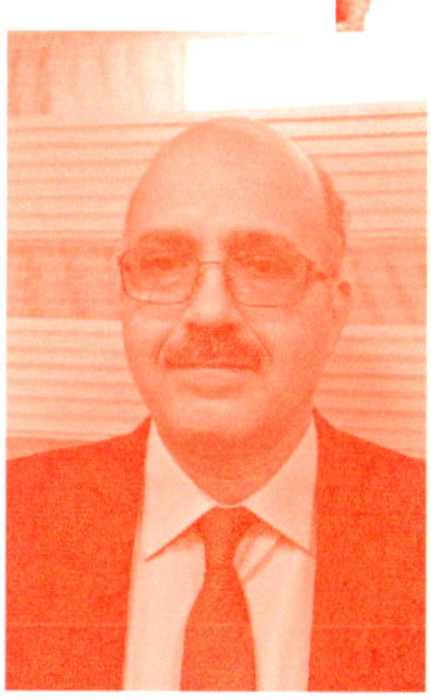
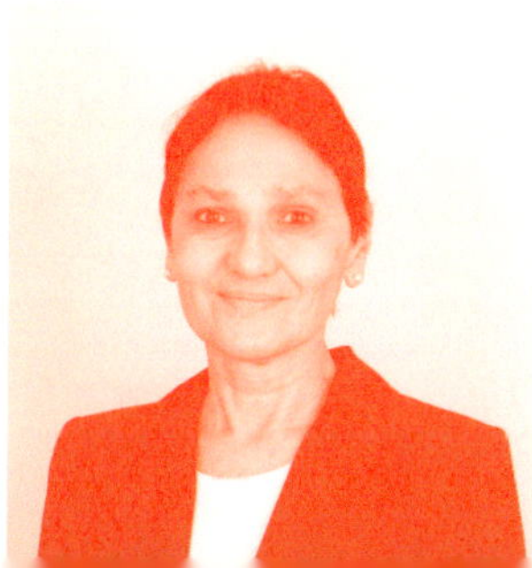
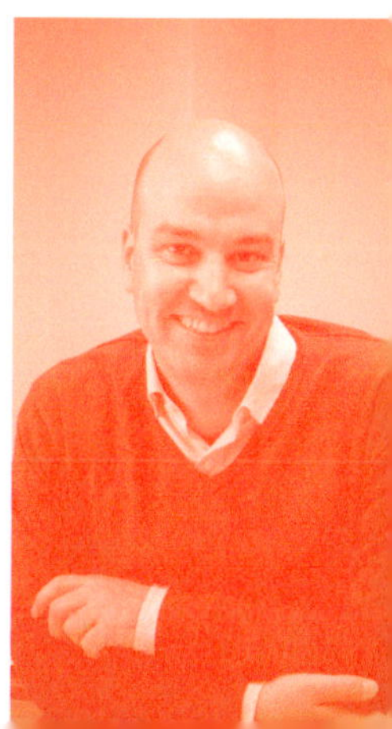

Dyslexia
http://dx.doi.org/10.5772/intechopen.91069
Edited by Jonathan Glazzard and Samuel Stones

Contributors
Trevor O'Brien, Suzan Cen-Yagiz, Berna Aytac, Ruth Falzon, Jane Roitsch, Helen Ross, Diane Montgomery, Maria Rontou, Simone Capellini, Larissa Sellin, Ilaria D'Angelo, Noemi Del Bianco, Catia Giaconi, Giseli Donadon Germano, Ying-Fang Sun, Pei-Shan Liao, Olga Malinovska, Jiri Jost, Zuzana Bilkova, Helena Havlisova, Martin Dobias, Jaromir Dolezal, Vratislav Fabian, Urs Ribary, Lawrence Ward, Nicolas Bedo, Dikla Ender-Fox, Janet Chow, Linda Siegel

First published in London, United Kingdom, 2021 by IntechOpen
IntechOpen is the global imprint of INTECHOPEN LIMITED, registered in England and Wales, registration number: 11086078, 5 Princes Gate Court, London, SW7 2QJ, United Kingdom
Printed in Croatia

British Library Cataloguing-in-Publication Data
A catalogue record for this book is available from the British Library

Additional hard and PDF copies can be obtained from orders@intechopen.com

Dyslexia
Edited by Jonathan Glazzard and Samuel Stones
p. cm.
Print ISBN 978-1-83881-966-8
Online ISBN 978-1-83881-967-5
eBook (PDF) ISBN 978-1-83881-968-2

Meet the editors

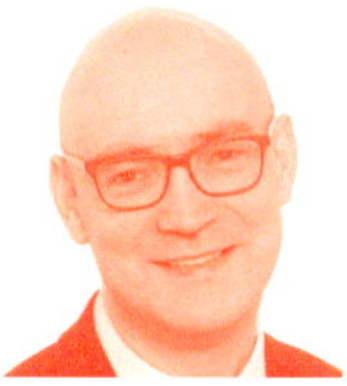

Professor Jonathan Glazzard's research focuses on mental health, well-being and inclusion in education. He is a qualitative researcher and uses a broad range of approaches, including narrative methodology, visual/participatory methods and more traditional interviews and focus groups. Jonathan's recent projects include exploration of head teacher resilience, teacher and child mental health and the experiences of teachers who identify as LGBTQ+. Jonathan is a co-convenor of the British Educational Research Association (BERA) Special Interest Group, Mental Health and Wellbeing in Education. He is also a member of the Excellence in International Transitions Research, which is led by Professor Divya Jindal-Snape. Jonathan is deeply committed to research that advances social justice. He has widely published on aspects of inclusion and social justice for marginalised groups and individuals, and he is deeply committed to research that improves the lives of individuals and research-informed teaching.

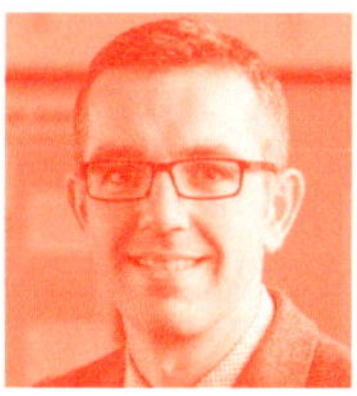

Samuel Stones is a Lecturer and Researcher at Leeds Beckett University as well as Assistant Headteacher at a secondary school and sixth form located in North Yorkshire, England. He also holds a national training role with a large multi-academy trust. Samuel's research outputs are linked with the Centre for LGBTQ+ Inclusion in Education and the Carnegie Centre of Excellence for Mental Health in Schools at Leeds Beckett University. His research explores the experiences of teachers who identify as Lesbian, Gay, Bisexual and Transgender, with specific emphasis on the impact of sexual orientation on teacher identity and mental health. Samuel's research explores issues of social justice and inclusion, particularly in relation to mental health, special educational needs, sexual orientation and gender identity.

Contents

Preface

This book explores different perspectives on dyslexia. We live in an ableist society where the ability to read and write is viewed as a sign of intelligence. However, we view dyslexia as a specific learning difference that is unrelated to intelligence. We also view dyslexia as a gift rather than as a difficulty. Many individuals with dyslexia are creative and skilled in lateral thinking. They are often verbally articulate and proficient in verbal reasoning.

We argue that the early identification of dyslexia is crucial so that children are not disadvantaged academically. The ability to read and write is critical to academic success. Reading is essential because it unlocks the door to the rest of the school curriculum. The gradual shift away from *learning to read* to *reading to learn* demonstrates the important role that reading plays in enabling children to access knowledge across the curriculum. Reading and writing are also critical skills that individuals need throughout their lives. We know that literacy skills can influence life chances. We only need to look at the extent of illiteracy in prisons and the wider criminal justice system to understand the relationship between reading and writing and long-term outcomes. However, skills in literacy should never be seen as an indicator of a person's intelligence, and it is for this reason that we have chosen to emphasise our preference that dyslexia should be viewed as a learning difference rather than a learning difficulty.

In our own research in this field, we have highlighted an association between dyslexia and self-esteem. Our data demonstrate that the experiences associated with having dyslexia can have a detrimental effect on a person's sense of self. We have also explored the experiences of dyslexic trainee teachers. Our data demonstrate the disconnect between pre-service teachers' experiences in university contexts and those in school contexts. In line with other researchers, we found that although dyslexic pre-service teachers often experience high levels of support within universities, this is often not matched by the level of support that they receive in schools. We found far too many examples of discrimination and prejudice, thus illustrating the ableist nature of the teaching profession. At the same time, we found that dyslexic pre-school teachers have numerous strengths. They are creative, empathetic and skilled in automatically adapting tasks to meet the needs of students with learning difficulties. Many were able to automatically break down tasks into smaller steps to enable students to achieve learning outcomes. It is these strengths that enable teachers with dyslexia to thrive in the teaching profession, and it is for these reasons that we emphasise dyslexia as a learning difference rather than a disability.

We recognize that the fundamental areas that dyslexics find more challenging lie in the areas of language processing and, even more specifically, phonological processing. We argue that many dyslexic children will benefit from a rich multi-sensory phonics programme that provides them with repeated opportunities to *overlearn* the skills of grapheme-phoneme correspondence, blending, segmenting and phoneme manipulation (including phoneme addition, deletion and substitution). We argue that although many dyslexics will eventually develop the skill of automaticity in word recognition, for many, the skills of spelling and transcription will remain lifelong challenges. Technological adaptations can support the writing process in classrooms and schools, and colleges and universities should invest in evidence-based technological adaptations that remove barriers to learning.

We emphasise the need for teachers to use a variety of approaches to enable students to record their learning in lessons and to explore the use of visual approaches, including *mind mapping* and *concept mapping*.

We hope you enjoy reading this book. There is no reason why students with dyslexia cannot thrive within educational environments. They should be viewed through a capability model rather than through a deficit lens.

Jonathan Glazzard and Samuel Stones
Leeds Beckett University,
United Kingdom

Chapter 1

Dyslexia and Academic Life

Ruth Falzon

Abstract

This chapter intends to discuss the experiences of university students with dyslexia and academic learning and assessment. It intends to challenge the traditional access to and production of examinations and to separate the ability to retrieve and produce verbal visual print from academic learning and performance in order to propose a model where educational systems join the fourth revolution. The intention is to address the brain drain that communities experience when students with Dyslexia are not able to show what they really know, due to possibly archaic access to and production of academic learning and assessment. The use of technology and independent access to printed material will also be discussed. The framework of this chapter is the Kannangara model of dyslexia: from Languishing to Thriving with Dyslexia. When reading this chapter, one also needs to remember that, whilst I refer to dyslexia, this profile more often than not co-occurs with other learning challenges and is often grouped with populations of Specific Learning Difficulties or Learning Disabilities in research and national data.

Keywords: academic success, access to academic learning, formal assessment, Dyslexia, Learning Disabilities, specific learning difficulties

1. Introduction

In April 2014 [1] Maltese educational psychologist Mr Juan Camilleri and I tabled a petition with the Parliament of Malta. We recommended the use of alternative access to and production of literacy for national academic examinations and throughout education. At the time, the Rector of the University of Malta (UM) refused to accept the petition, which is why we then tabled it with the Parliament of Malta. Since then, significant changes at the UM and the Ministry for Education and Employment indicate that Malta has started to embrace the rationale of this petition [2]. Notwithstanding, I think that there is still long way to go both locally and globally, particularly with reference to attitudes within the academic world. In spite of literature affirming that the ability to read and intelligence are not correlated [3, 4], people with dyslexia still experience being looked down upon by educators and fellow students due to their challenges with literacy (e.g., [5–7]). This chapter will discuss experiences of university students with dyslexia and suggest possible strategies that can be considered, also in the context of the present health situation. This chapter embraces Kannangara's [8] model From Languishing to Thriving Dyslexia.

To start, I will share the experience of an academic I heard speak during an international conference I attended in 2015. She used to work in a University in Europe. She had been working at this university for over 25 years and had always received positive feedback and evaluation reports about her lecturing, research, administration, co-ordination and research. She had never felt the need to disclose her profile of dyslexia. However, one day she mentioned her profile en passant during a meeting with University academic and administration. From that day on, the university started asking her to recheck her work, her work started to be supervised; and she was given the message that the university had concerns about her profile. The situation was so stressful for her that it became untenable and she actually had to leave her place of work. It seems that, after 25 years of sterling service to her university, the main focus became her profile rather than her actual sterling output and track record.

2. Personal worldview on literacy, dyslexia definition and intervention

At the outset, I would like to declare that one cannot diminish the extreme importance of reading and spelling skills and techniques. Globalisation is placing new demands on the kinds of literacies we need both in our work and in the daily demands of everyday life. A good quality basic education equips one with literacy skills for life and further learning. In most developed and developing countries, literacy skills are fundamental to daily living and affect the social, political, civic, economic and personal lives of citizens, directly affecting wellbeing [8]. Where literacy still does not have a fundamental function, oppression and poverty prevail [9–11]. Johnson and Kress [12] noted that "globalization is frequently thought about in economic terms alone, but there is equally a cultural globalization which is no less, maybe even more, potent in its shaping to the ways in which we communicate and represent meaning" (p. 5).

Literacy is regarded as a means to address poverty and oppression (e.g., [9, 13–15]). The post-war era has seen literacy on nations' educational, economic and political agendas (e.g., [15–17]). The United Nations' Educational, Scientific and Cultural Organisation (UNESCO) perceives literacy as a human right, a tool of personal empowerment, a means for social and human development, and at the heart of basic education for all [15]. The UNESCO Education for All (EFA) committee noted that eradicating poverty, reducing child mortality, addressing population growth, achieving gender equality and ensuring sustainable development, peace, democracy and empowerment are some of the good reasons why literacy is at EFA's core [15]. Indeed, since its foundation in 1946, UNESCO has been at the forefront of global literacy efforts and is dedicated to keeping literacy high on national, regional and international agendas [18].

2.1 Literacy?

Hirsch [19] proposed that failing to teach children what they must learn in order to be able to cope with further learning in school is the greatest form of injustice in education which can be prevented. What I challenge is what is regarded as a must to learn and how one defines literacy.

The literature is clear. Access to the printed text paves the way for learning and economic growth and justifies ensuring that young learners learn to read as early and as expediently as possible (e.g., [9, 20, 21]). The speed and effectiveness of this early literacy learning process affects success in learning and has a Matthew Effect (e.g., [22–24]). However, education needs to include those for whom learning to read is not so easy. Pedagogies need to embrace this and must use teaching strategies which include media other than the printed text to access learning, particularly in a context where technology is the reality of the day.

There is consensus that the ultimate purpose of reading printed text is to understand its meaning [25]. Research indicates that slow and effortful word-decoding/

word-recognition abilities limit reading comprehension abilities (e.g., [4, 26, 27]) and affect academic success [28], with success depending on the ability to read and write [29]. I simply want my dream to become a reality for all: "for whom reading and writing is not such an easy task or choice, alternatives for access to medium and expression of knowledge should be available so long as the aims and objectives of examinations are not compromised" ([1], p. 1).

Children and young people with dyslexia and other challenges are failing their national examinations due to access to medium and choice of medium of expression [30]. This is not only disheartening for the individual, but also a brain drain on communities, impacting the economy and wellbeing of families, communities and countries [31]. Education still needs to understand the need to teach all our children how to read and write, whilst at the same time addressing the need of access to learning without the use of the verbal visual [32, 33].

Literature clearly evidences the negative effects challenges with literacy have on the wellbeing of persons with dyslexia (e.g. [34–37]). Educational systems and educators must avoid unnecessary suffering by challenging their definition of learning and performance in examinations [30, 38]. Inasmuch as literacy must be given priority in education, for those with neurological challenges to access it, technology needs to be used as a compensatory strategy and a tool [39].

2.1.1 Reading comprehension

Reading comprehension is the ability to actively understand ideas and integrate them with prior knowledge to create efficient memory structures [28]. Since it is one of the most complex human activities, any reading theory must address underlying cognitive and linguistic processes involved in comprehension [40]. According to the Single View of Reading (SVR) model, linguistic comprehension contributes to reading comprehension [40] as does accurate and efficient word decoding/recognition [26]. Florit and Cain's [41] meta-analysis concluded that linguistic comprehension is a strong predictor of reading comprehension in transparent orthographies [e.g., Finnish) whilst word decoding skills were more influential in deep orthographies [e.g., English). Other researchers oppose this model, referring to more complexities.

For example, the Direct and Indirect Effects of Text Comprehension Model refers to relational pathway between lower- and higher-level skills involved in reading comprehension [42]. Lower-level skills include working memory, attention, vocabulary and grammatical knowledge, oral language [42] which are necessary to address higher-level skills such as inferences, perspective taking, comprehension monitoring, verbal working memory, and knowledge on text structures (e.g., [43–45]). Motivation, interest and purpose are then additional contributing factors [46].

My reflection on these two models' sets of skills needed for reading comprehension is that for all the skills required, effective and fluent word recognition are skills which can be replaced by technology, whilst the other skills can still be developed and addressed so that readers interact and involve themselves with written language to extract and construct new meaning.

2.1.2 Beyond traditional literacy

The theory of this chapter is that, wherever possible and so long as the academic learning and assessment objectives are retained, one should be allowed to choose whether, in light of their profile of abilities, skills and challenges, they would prefer to learn, study, access knowledge, develop skills and sit for their examinations orally, using the voice to produce printed material for examiners to read, in handwritten format or using the word processor/tablet. This should be regarded as a choice for all, rather than an examination access arrangement; in the same way that one chooses to sit for examinations using their prescriptive glasses or writing with blue or black pens.

Let us take the subject of History as an example. The aims and objectives of the History curricula and syllabi, as well as its content, never indicate that reading and writing per se are required. Why is it then such an issue and such a waste of human and financial resources for our system and for families to conclude whether candidates should sit for History orally, in typewritten format or handwritten format? One may query: but what about language examination? In my opinion, the same rationale can apply as the knowledge of knowing a language and being able to produce material for others to read is different from the ability to read and spell. Therefore, unless the examination objective is specifically the skills of decoding or encoding or the skill of producing written material through handwriting, the same rationale applies.

2.1.3 Writing (??) an essay

In dictionaries, an essay is usually defined as a "short literary composition on a particular theme or subject, usually in prose and generally analytic, speculative, or interpretative" ([47], para.1). No definition on the word essay includes that this task must have been written, typed, swiped or dictated. As such, it is perhaps about time that the ability to spin a yarn or present a thesis for others to read in another space and time is differentiated from the ability to spell, particularly in the context of modern technology. Essays can be produced using two (swiping), three (handwriting), ten (typing) fingers or no (voice-activated technology) fingers. This is not to diminish the importance of spelling, but simply to do justice to competencies required to produce essays. One would need a good speller to proofread documents. This is different from the ability to transform thoughts, creativity, theories, arguments and ideas into readable linguistic communication for others to access in another time and space. Does one ever question or reflect upon the spelling ability of great authors? Is the spelling of authors ever criticised or addressed when books/ articles/ scientific journals are published?

2.1.4 Technological support to literacy learning and proficiency

Research findings consistently conclude that early literacy learning affects success in learning (e.g. [22, 23, 48]). It is therefore of utmost importance that early education also includes the use of technology to access and present print for those struggling with literacy (e.g., [49–51]) as pupils are learning to break the code to literacy. Standard computers themselves already incorporate adaptations to address all aspects of literacy [52]. Free downloadable material (e.g., [53–55]) allows one to add applications. The market also has commercial affordable apparata which not only provide text-to-speech and speech-to-text but also present organisation features for general (e.g., [56–58]) or examination use [59, 60].

2.2 Dyslexia definition and intervention

Any research in this area is complicated by difficulties defining dyslexia. Most agree that dyslexia involves reading ability below age- and IQ-matched peers, which is not attributable to poor visual or auditory acuity or inadequate instruction; and where intellect is not affected by specific challenges attributed to this profile (e.g., [4, 61, 62]). Research findings, mostly quantitative, seem to indicate that dyslexia can be categorised into five challenged areas of brain function: phonological, visual, memory, semantic and kinaesthetic (e.g. [4, 61, 63]), where effects continue throughout lifetimes (e.g., [62, 64, 65]). However, there is still considerable debate in education and neuroscience literature regarding underlying causes, age distribution, diagnosis, identification, appropriate assessment methods and intervention (e.g., [66–68]).

The Guardian [69] lately presented a long article on whether dyslexia actually exists. Citing challenging literature that states that distinguishing between dyslexia and other reading difficulties results in children not being eligible for intervention [70]. Kale [69] referred to Yule's (1976) conclusion that:

> *The era of applying the label 'dyslexic' is rapidly drawing to a close. The label has served its function in drawing attention to children who have great difficulty in mastering the arts of reading, writing and spelling but its continued use invokes emotions which often prevent rational discussion and scientific investigation. (p. 166)*

Whilst I agree that (1) terminology and diagnostic conclusions should not deter access to intervention; (2) one should focus on behaviour, skills and abilities rather than labelling; (3) Intervention techniques designed for the dyslexia population are inclusive strategies and beneficial for all, I disagree with Yale. Ample research findings evidence this established neurological profile which, more often than not, co-occurs with other neurological profiles [71]. Apart from educational and psychological research on dyslexia, neuroscience research is leading to a deeper understanding of the identification, diagnosis and management of dyslexia. Such hard evidence provides for strong and persuasive lobbying for change [3, 4].

Snowling et al. [4] acknowledged challenges with co-occurrence and cut-offs and concluded that "Optimal outcomes for these children require us to embrace the dimensional nature of dyslexia and its associated complexities; to fail to do so is negligent and arguably morally indefensible" (p. 508). Lastly, knowledge about dyslexia may benefit all those who present challenges learning to read, whether they have a profile of dyslexia or not (e.g., [9, 20, 71]).

My views regarding learning and examination access arrangement as a choice-for-all rather than a concession for some, clearly presents that my framework and worldview is framed within principles of inclusion [72], diversity [73, 74] and otherness [75, 76]. This echoes Furedi's [77] resistance to the use of a diagnosis disability and pathologisation to justify allowances and additional support. Further, I frame dyslexia within Kannangara's [8] (2015) From Languishing to Thriving Dyslexia model, which lobbies for support, understanding and resilience.

3. Academic self-concept and academic success

Zeleke's [78] and Burden's [35] meta-analyses concluded that academic self-esteem and self-concept (ASC) are founded early and tend to be very stable and rather unaffected by later, more successful experiences. This then affects choices for further education, as is represented by data available regarding university students and research findings. Burden [35] reflected that values regarding, "how competent we think we are, ...how much in control of the outcomes we consider ourselves to be...[how] we react to disappointment and failure, the strategies that we have... effort we are prepared to invest in order to succeed,"(p. 20) affect ASC.

Therefore, it can be assumed that studies available on dyslexic university students would involve a particular dyslexic population which would have enough required abilities and skills to have enabled them to build ASC allowing them to remain resilient and motivated to learn and who, perhaps, were in supportive home environments and school systems [8, 30]. The question that lingers is: what brain drain are our communities experiencing because school environments lead students to low ASC?

Research findings consistently suggest that teachers and lecturers fail to understand the complexities related to dyslexia and other learning challenges (e.g., [79–81]). They tend to perceive dyslexia as similar to other learning difficulties [82] and are less likely to account for students' abilities [81]. Lack of understanding and adequate appropriate support may lead to students not completing their studies or graduating with inferior degree classifications than deserved. Caskey's [83] Australian research identified that adult dyslexics tend to live in a "dual world, one that is related to the Medical versus Social Model of Disability. Despite the research on 'ableism' ...adult students diagnosed with dyslexia were navigating through the system barriers searching for support, between the inclusion and exclusion zones" (p. 264). However, when "advocate, support and services were provided...in the form of advocacy, success can occur" ([83], p. 266).

Kannangara [8] concluded that experiences can present a model where one can either languish or thrive with a profile of dyslexia. She reported that, a thriving dyslexic presents positive acceptance towards challenges, embraces difficulties, uses signature strengths to address obstacles, learns from criticisms, perseveres, withstands, and finds alternative approaches to address failures. Unfortunately, a 2019 report [84] by the British Dyslexia Association (BDA) evidenced that parents reported the following effects of a profile of dyslexia on their children: 82% try to hide their struggles; 88% experience poor self-esteem, 84% suffer from anxiety; 52% try to avoid school; 78% feel embarrassed; 48% had been bullied, 95% experience frustration, 58% avoid discussing their dyslexia, and 82% try to hide their difficulties relating to dyslexia.

BDA [84] concluded that "children and young people are uncomfortable, and experience negative emotions linked to their dyslexia ...our data may demonstrate an association between dyslexia and mental health difficulties" (p. 19).

Studies exploring school experiences through interviews offer an overall experience of strong, negative emotions (e.g., [34, 85, 86]). Studies exploring how dyslexic people make sense of their positive and negative emotions in relation to school experiences have also presented positive experience (e.g., [8, 87, 88]). One needs to, however, take into consideration that some of the participants of such studies were students attending specialised schools (e.g. [35, 88, 89]). Hellendoorn and Ruijssenaars [90] interviewed 27 dyslexic adults, 8 of whom had negative, 11 mixed and 8 positive experiences. Hughes and Dawson [86] interviewed 54 dyslexic adults. Just over half said they mostly disliked school. Riddick et al. [91] interviewed 16 dyslexic students in higher education, of whom only three reported overall positive experiences. Though none of these studies claim to be representative of the whole population of dyslexic people, they suggest that from one third to one half of dyslexic adults may remember school in primarily negative terms.

4. The highest echelon of university assessment

Currently, the highest level of global academic examination is Doctorate of Philosophy (PhD), for which most university use oral examination (viva voce) (e.g. [92–94]). Doctorate examination boards do not question, query, consider or ask for verification whether the verbal-visual 80,000–120,000 word PhD document has been handwritten, typewritten, dictated to a secretary, or produced through assisted technology. The Board of Examiners simply accepts the PhD Document, as this would still the candidate's work irrespective of the process of the medium of expression. On the other hand, examiners may choose to read the work in the traditional format or use assisted technology to listen to the document. The conundrum is: why it is then not so easy for students in compulsory or university education to be given such choices? Rather an oxymoron!

Examinations at critical stages in students' education are becoming increasingly more high stakes [38, 95]. They provide students with necessary qualifications for further education or employment [96]. They therefore have a significant impact on students' life chances and opportunities [97], thus dominating students' lives and school experiences, further influencing future plans affecting life styles (e.g., no time for extracurricular activities) due to the constant pressure to do well [96, 97]. This of course applies to all students but may be more stressful for those with a profile of dyslexia (e.g., [8, 34, 89]).

5. The examination experience

Research findings clearly indicate that examinations have an impact on all students' lives (e.g., [98–100]). However, "the effects of examinations may be magnified for those who enter the process already labouring under a disadvantage" ([101] p. 8). Research findings consistently conclude that dyslexic students experience greater challenges than non-dyslexic students when sitting for examinations. These challenges include reading fluency and accuracy, auditory sequential short-term memory, sequencing, and organisation of ideas that all impact on the performance of students in examinations (e.g., [102–104]).

The lack of scientific consensus about what dyslexia really is leads examination boards to query this profile [4]. Crisp et al. [102] lamented that assessment communities have continued to persist that difficulties and challenges students with dyslexia face are similar to students with weak reading abilities or lower cognitive skills. Chetcuti et al. [38] presented the voices of young people with dyslexia and concluded that the participants shared their "frustrations, anxieties and hopes for a fairer examinations system" (p. 445). To address equity, fair play and wellbeing, dyslexic youth in the Chetcuti et al. [39] research perceived a need for radical transformations of examination systems and implored for participatory justice [105, 106], where they should "participate meaningfully throughout the decision-making processes" ([107], p. 346). Hence, my argument to switch to choice rather than examination concessions.

6. University students with dyslexia - crunching numbers

Whilst it is generally accepted that dyslexia affects 10–15% of the general population (e.g., [3, 108, 109]), research evidences underrepresentation at universities. For example, Richardson and Wydell [110] reported 0.48% British-based; and Stampoltzis and Polychronopoulou [111] 0.16% Greek University Students noting reading difficulties. Further, during academic year 2019–2020, out of 11,117 students attending the UM, only 201 (1.18%) students registered with its Access Disability Support Unit (ADSU). Of these, seven (0.06%) described themselves as Specific Learning Difficulties/Learning Difficulties, six as dyscalculic (0.05%) and 36 (0.33%) as dyslexic.[1]

[1] September 2020 e-mails' correspondence with ADSU official Ms Marchita Mangiafico and ADSU chair Dr Anne-Marie Callus.

Richardson and Wydell [110] reported that their analysis of databases of students in British higher education evidenced 0.46% in 1995–1996 and 1.51% by 2000-to 2001. Mortimore and Crozier' [112] reported that between 1999 and 2010, British University students with dyslexia or Specific Learning Difficulties almost quadrupled: from 8370 to 32,655. Richardson [113] reported that the situation continued to improve, as in 2013–2014, 37,710 students with dyslexia or other specific learning difficulties (4.97% of all freshers) were admitted to their first year of study. Likewise, UM reported an increase of students requesting examination access arrangements for national examinations: from 1.6% in 2004 to 10.9% in 2019 [114]. This may mean that most Maltese University Students do not inform UM of their profile and do not utilise any possible learning and examination arrangements. This needs further research.

Richardson [113] reflected that "the increase in the prevalence of dyslexia amongst students in UK higher education may reflect changes in diagnostic procedures, public awareness and admissions policies" (p. 325) and the need for more flexible admission policies by institutions of higher education. Likewise, Olofsson et al. [115] reported that "there are now more students with dyslexia in [Swedish] university courses, in both actual and proportional numbers, from 3634 (1.2%) in 2009 to 5457 (about 1.9%) in 2013" (p. 338). They attributed this increase to four factors: (1) earlier identification and provision; (2) financial and other support in higher education; (3) wider access for older students, thus including those who had performed poorly at school because of undetected dyslexia; and (4) the adoption of more flexible university admissions policies.

6.1 Higher education success

Although the literature is limited, studies seem to indicate that success in higher education is "not impossible for students with dyslexia but may be more difficult" ([116], p. 3). Olofsson et al. [115] reported that around 20% Swedish university students with dyslexia required additional time to complete their degrees, whilst others were able to progress at a normal pace. Richardson and Wydell [110] reported that approximately 40% UK dyslexic graduates obtained first-class or upper second-class honours. This was, however, lower than the 50% rate for graduates with no reported disabilities. Mortimore and Crozier's [112] study across 17 higher education institutions also concluded challenges with academic skills, higher risk of either discontinuing or acquiring inferior degrees due to a lack of appropriate support. Byrne [117] further noted that, whilst the proportion of British university dyslexic students has lately increased to around 5%, a significant attainment gap remains, as only "around 40% of dyslexic students achieve a 2.1 or above, compared to 52% of non-dyslexic students" (para. 2). Richardson and Wydell [110] used a 1995–1996 British higher education database and discovered that it was more common among students with dyslexia than among other students to either abandon their studies in the first year of study or not finish their study programmes.

This is happening in spite of enshrined university legislations stressing that educational access is moral and humanitarian imperative (e.g., [2, 118, 119]). One also needs to take into considerations that such statistics include students who declare and know that they have such a profile. One then wonders how many more may be university students without awareness of, or fear of disclosing, their profile of dyslexia. Notwithstanding, we still need to take heed of these data as it is "important to identify factors that could contribute to poor representation and experiences of dyslexic students in higher education and seek appropriate solutions" ([116], p. 3).

Despite vast knowledge and conclusive findings, this population continues to struggle to achieve and maintain success. While enrolment in post-secondary institutions has increased [120], the dropout rate, unemployment rate, more placement in lower prestige jobs, lower income and poverty remain high [121].

7. The university experience

Research on dyslexia and university students also presents challenging experiences. For example, Denhart [5] reported that her participants' "three [main] findings [were] inextricably bound with the reluctance to ask for accommodations: (a) an overwhelming workload that is (b) unrecognized and (c) yields products incommensurate with the effort (p. 493)". Additionally, Lock and Layton's [6] participants and Rodis et al.'s [7] autobiographical accounts presented experiences where lecturers perceived dyslexic university students as lazy or lacking effort, also because lecturers were not aware of students' profiles [122]. Rodis et al. [7] and Greenbaum et al. [123] reported that their participants' fear of stigma was worse than others' perceptions of laziness or lack of motivation, even if this led to exhaustion and illness. Further, these participants also regarded the use of accommodations as a failure. This highlights that "the finest accommodations based on the most sophisticated science will have no value if intolerance denies their use" [5], p. 495.

Most research on dyslexia and higher education addresses diagnosis, cognitive abilities, compensation strategies and study techniques (e.g., [124–126]). Less research has been directed towards students' own experiences of inclusion in higher education [38, 127]. Olofsson et al. [115] reported that in 2011, Swedish researcher Eriksson Gustavsson carried out a study with 186 students with dyslexia attending six Swedish higher education six institutions. Gustavsson reported that the rate of study of most students was lower than expected, but only few had an extremely slow rate of study. Further, limited achievements had occurred early on in their studies.

Olofsson et al. [115] carried out a study with 50 Swedish students with dyslexia using semi-structured interviews and a self-report scale. Their participants reported that reading course books in English (not their mother tongue) and taking notes during lessons were the two most challenging tasks. They felt less challenges when textbooks were in Swedish, and with spelling and written assignments. Half rated themselves as good and slightly more than 10% as particularly good with regard to reading and understanding textbooks in Swedish, whilst their confidence in spelling was less good. On the other hand, 90% rated their ability to find information on Google or other sites on the Internet as good (46%) or very good (44%), whilst 88%, rated their ability to find what they look for on the Internet as good (52%) or very good (36%). Regarding the continuation and completing of a university degree, Olofsson et al. [115] reported that this depended on the students' rate of study. They concluded that about half:

> *Manage[d] pretty well despite their reading and writing problems. The mean rate of study for the dyslexic students in the present study was just below the national baseline. However, it should be noted that one-fifth of the dyslexic students have a very low rate of study and will thus need special attention from their teachers. The dyslexic students' mistrust in their own abilities in reading course books and articles in English and in taking notes should be taken into consideration in the development of support systems for students with dyslexia. (p. 347)*

7.1 Successful graduates

British and Maltese bachelor's degrees are classified as first, second-upper, second-lower or third class. A first-class or second-upper class is often described as a good degree. Richardson and Wydell [110] found that 53.6% of students with no disability and 43.9% of students with dyslexia were awarded good degrees. The difference in these proportions was rated highly significant, even when possible effects of demographic and programme-related variables were considered. However, data on detailed accounts of students with dyslexia's higher education academic attainment are difficult because national statistics are not collected about other academic outcomes, since many do not disclose their profile, because of description of profile, and due to co-occurrence.

Pino and Mortari's [127] systematic review of published studies on inclusion of students with dyslexia in higher education identified 15, mostly qualitative, studies. They concluded that, whilst valuable information for support services was presented, there was no evidence on attainment. Richardson and Wydell [110] reported that whilst they were aware that the British Open University is known for attracting students with dyslexia, perhaps due to its option for distance learning, they unfortunately had to exclude Open University students from a more detailed analysis because many had been omitted from the database. Richardson and Wydell [110] had concluded that students with dyslexia who had taken undergraduate modules in 2003 with the British Open University were as likely as were nondisabled students to complete their modules. However, they were more likely to obtain poorer grades. A problem with the study was that they were concerned only with students with dyslexia and no other disabilities. They in fact omitted students with dyslexia and additional disabilities from their sample. This is problematic, especially with the conclusion that co-occurrence with other profiles is now considered the norm, exception [71].

7.2 Cognitive skills and university learning and performance

Further to the context of co-occurrence [71], one needs to consider that a profile of dyslexia does not merely involve challenges to access literacy. Such a profile may also include difficulties organising essays, timekeeping, expressing ideas verbally, concentrating and using short-term memory, listening and organisation (e.g., [4, 112, 115]). For example, Simmons and Singleton [128] concluded that dyslexic university students experience challenges drawing inferences from complex texts. They, however, did not specify if alternative access to verbal visual print would have affected such results. This is supported by conclusions that reading characteristics vary widely between students [129].

Studies on writing skills conclude that dyslexic university students present particular challenges with spelling (e.g., [124, 130, 131]), overall written text quality [130, 131], number of words written [132], organisation [112], and vocabulary chosen [132]. On the other hand, comparative differences between university students with or without dyslexia indicate no significant differences in sentence structure, length of sentences [132], expression of ideas or other higher order skills [130]. These findings indicate that such students can cope with university learning, if given the chance, the appropriate support, and with training for university academic [83, 117]. As one youth shared: "I wonder how many great minds were lost simply because the type of intelligence [, access,] and ideas they had were not the the examiners wanted" ([38], p. 439).

Often, these studies refer to challenges experienced using traditional access and presentation of verbal visual print. Therefore, there is a dearth in the literature for one to conclude whether one would experience such challenges if technology were to be used. This is similar to literature available regarding foreign language learning. For example, the British Dyslexia Association (BDA) promotes [133] that "dyslexic children should be given the opportunity to learn a foreign language. Many ...will enjoy the multi-sensory methods of language teaching ...Learning a foreign language broadens pupils' horizons as their awareness of other cultures develops" ([133], para. 1). However, BDA also seems to be chained by traditional access to literacy and pedagogy for foreign language teaching, as it suggests that, "Some languages may be more problematic for dyslexic learners. Languages such as French and English are less transparent than other languages" ([133], para. 2). In a context where (a) the literature clearly concludes that foreign language learning and bilingualism has a positive effect on general cognitive development (e.g., [134–136]); and (b) the EU requires all its citizens to be tri-lingual [137], there seems to be the practice to discourage persons with dyslexia to learn a foreign language. Contrastingly, I have to date not found any literature (written in Maltese, English or Italian) to support this myth.

8. The lived experience

Literature addressing day-to-day experiences of university students with dyslexia is dearth. Whilst there is a considerable body of literature exploring overall university experiences of students with a broad range of disabilities, including students with dyslexia (e.g., [138–140]), such studies tend to focus on physical access, social stigma, reasonable adjustments (e.g., [138, 141, 142]). Further, findings regarding dyslexic students are difficult to differentiate from other findings of these studies.

Research available addressing experiences (e.g. [115, 116, 127]) evidences challenges, difficulties and frustration. Participants reported difficulties with notetaking, reading journal articles and course books, technology, accessibility and adjustments. These studies seem to indicate that some students, "will overcome these difficulties, [but] the additional effort may lead to greater frustration and lower completion rates than might otherwise be expected" ([116], p. 16). Further, MacCullagh et al. [116] rightly acknowledged that disadvantages may include, "insufficient time to research topics broadly, difficulty balancing paid work and other responsibilities, mental health risks of overwork and less time to participate in social, sporting, artistic and other extra-curricular activities" (p. 16).

Pino and Mortari [127] conducted a systematic review of published research on the university experiences of students with dyslexia and reported finding 15 relevant studies. They synthesised the findings in five key themes: (1) Coping strategies (Study skills and Compensatory Strategies); (2) Profile identification; (3) Interaction with academic staff; (4) Accessibility and adjustments to learning and assessment; and (5) Use of technologies.

Helpful study skills included making notes from books, accessing materials in multiple formats, colour coding, concept mapping and discussing ideas verbally. Compensatory strategies included downloading slides prior to lectures, obtaining copies of lecture notes, lecture recordings help from family and friends, metacognitive skills included time planning, graphic organisation of information and meta-affective skills.

Notwithstanding, Pino and Mortari [127] concluded gaps in the literature, particularly regarding strategies for improvement. The available research findings also report difficulties identifying main ideas in text, preparing for tests [126], reading course books and taking notes [143]. Again, one needs further exploration regarding the use of technology as such studies sometimes do not differentiate between traditional reading and reading using technology. For example, Olofsson et al. [143] reported additional information from the internet as a key compensatory strategy; whilst Kirby et al. [126] reported study aids, time management strategies and deep learning approaches as key compensatory strategies. More research exploring study practices and opportunities for support is needed.

MacCullagh et al.'s [116] semi-structured interviews based on best practice methodologies yielded similar data to literature (e.g., [115, 126, 127]). Findings concluded positive themes such as appreciation for engaging speaking style, flexible lecture formats, deep engagement with learning tasks and self-directed learning. Further, students with dyslexia "reported spending a great deal of effort on learning tasks. Participants with dyslexia described engaging with learning tasks intensively and frequently, using multiple strategies. Possible advantages of this effort could include deeper learning and development of creative problem-solving skills" ([116], p. 16). It is interesting that such behaviours [144] are highly sought after in workplaces (e.g. [145–147]). Further, such characteristics are also helpful for all students (e.g. [148–150]).

Disadvantages also include insufficient time to research topics broadly, difficulty balancing paid work and other responsibilities, mental health risks of overwork, and less time to participate in extra-curricular and social activities. These findings add to moral and legal justifications for understanding rather than judging profile of university students with dyslexia. Future research in this area could focus on number of hours per week spent on learning tasks. MacCullagh et al. [116] also discussed that the very coping learning strategy these individuals use are strategies which actually lead to deeper learning and memory. One also needs to consider that such individuals would probably be more highly motivated to be university students, given that they keep striving despite challenges. Additionally, they would most probably have the necessary support system which led them to thrive in, rather than languish for, higher education [8].

Also noteworthy was the strong appreciation among students with dyslexia for face-to-face lectures and for recorded lectures that included a video of the lecturer's face. This is particularly important considering recent trends in the higher education sector towards partially and wholly online courses. Such changes must be critically appraised to prevent compounding disadvantages for students with dyslexia. It may be important to continue offering some face-to-face lectures, and to ensure that recorded lectures include a video of the lecturer talking. This is extremely relevant and important in the current health challenges humans are experiencing. The question would be: how can we find a technological alternative to address the participants' recommended face-to-face intervention?

9. University support services

Studies addressing use of services indicate a strong uptake for resources such as additional time in examinations, dyslexia-support tutors and information technology assistance [112, 143]. Other services include appropriately skilled note-takers, lecture slides in advance, support with organisation and support with academic writing (e.g., [38, 112, 143]).

However, international data consistently reports poor uptake of support services by students with dyslexia. Reasons include poor awareness of services, poor suitability of services and non-disclosure. Most services seem to be designed for people with low vision, illiteracy, general learning disabilities or physical disabilities, rather than students with dyslexia per se. New services may therefore need to be designed specifically for students with dyslexia or existing services tailored to specific needs as identified by students themselves. For example, students suggest dyslexia-specific tutoring and tailored note-taking services (e.g., [112, 143, 151]).

Research findings on appropriate, satisfying and effective support and strategies are consistent with current best practices on inclusive design and accessibility standards [152]. For example, findings of appreciation for videos, images and face-to-face teaching support the efficacy of multi-modal or multi-sensory teaching for dyslexic learners. This reflects current research and best practice where all learners generally benefit from having information presented in auditory, tactile and visual modalities [151]. Further, all students learn better from lectures presented in shorter 5–20 minute segments rather than longer 60–120 minute sessions [153]. This is in keeping with recent educational trends towards the flipped classroom model, in which lectures are broken into smaller chunks and interspersed with other activities [154].

Research also indicates that dyslexic students mostly manage their own difficulties on an individual level with minimal access to or assistance from each other. Participants reported developing a unique set of compensatory strategies in isolation from others and without any sharing or supporting each other, support groups or dyslexia associations and agencies (e.g. [115, 116, 127]). In the context of the broader disability and social inclusion literature [155, 156] moving towards a more collectivist community approach is optimal, as students would benefit from collaborating and sharing their ideas, strategies, experiences and insights. For example, MacCullagh et al.'s [116] participants noted that university students with dyslexia not only face considerable learning and assessment challenges but also exhibit strengths. They reported helpful and effective strategies at individual and institutional levels, study techniques, adjustments to course materials, variety of teaching and assessment formats, and specific staff and student training. These were considered as effective measures towards university success for students with dyslexia.

MacCullagh et al. [116] linked appropriate and effective learning experiences to university legislation on equity and opportunity, and notes that research findings, "add to moral and legal justifications for provision of accommodations for university students with dyslexia" (p. 16). Likewise, when focusing on post-secondary assessment, Chetcuti et al. [38] implore for more fair play and feedback from young people with dyslexia themselves as the main stakeholders.

10. Knowledge, attitudes and stigma

Studies addressing issues of shame and humiliation cannot just address the university experience, but need to also understand the whole school experience. Many share stories of humiliation, mostly due to being made to read aloud in class or taking longer and/or being punished for taking longer to complete work (e.g. [90, 157, 158]). Participants in such studies narrate that the humiliation was not only due to public exposure of their reading and writing difficulties, but also ridicule from teachers. Such negative experiences affect so deeply, they linger throughout one's lifetime as a traumatic and permanent experience (e.g. [38, 85, 157]) or what Khan [159] termed as cumulative trauma.

Persons with covert challenges tend to report more negative experiences that those with overt challenges [160]. Barga [161] explored the experiences of nine university students with dyslexia and evidenced experiences of labelling and stigma as barriers to learning. Six participants deliberately did not disclose for fear of rejection, ridicule and stigmatisation. Likewise, Rao [162] reported non-disclosure to avoid negative social repercussion, even though participants were aware that this may have hinder their academic progress and success. Further, the literature continues to evidence stigma towards such a population as being intellectually inferior (e.g., [5, 30, 157]). Dyslexic university students' preference to manage their own difficulties with minimal access to assistance (e.g. [112, 151, 153]) supports research findings indicating shame, embarrassment (e.g. [84, 163, 164]) and complex decision-making processes regarding disclosure [164]. One needs to dream of better inclusive societal approaches and attitudes (e.g., [34, 155, 156]).

Mortimer and Crozier [112, 165] reported that students in their studies expressed frustration at "the lack of communication between the [support] unit and the academic departments. Academic tutors frequently had little knowledge about dyslexia" [112, p, 248]. One of their participants shared how she was publicly Chastised: "In my exam, the lecturer didn't realise I had extra time. In the hall, in public, he said, 'Put your bloody pen down'. I had to say 'I'm sorry I'm dyslexic'. It made me feel like a total leper. There is a lack of communication between departments, some know, some don't (p. 248)." Mortimer and Crozier [112] reported that:

> *Although students were unanimous in their appreciation of the staff in support units, they did express criticisms of the lack of staff available, overworked members of staff, a dearth of equipment, limited opening hours and difficulty of access—several students reported that initially they did not know where to go or could not find the unit. Others expressed concern about the stigma of entering a unit labelled 'Disability'. (p. 248)*

10.1 Educators' perceptions

Regarding labelling and teachers' perceptions, strategies and actions, research presents various scenarios. These include difficulties to teach, less intelligence, and feeling sorry for the students (e.g., [166–168]). Frymier and Wanzer [169] also noted that such perceptions often stem from the issue of hidden challenges and negotiations regarding fair accommodations, also in respect to other students. This strengthens my thesis that such accommodation should be a choice-for-all rather than an accommodation. Lock and Layton [6] concluded that lecturers in their study believed that such a label was to get out of doing work, out of laziness, or not trying hard enough. This belief was reaffirmed even when these lecturers were presented with studies that such a population tends to work itself to illness and exhaustion to achieve levels expected from their peers (e.g., [5, 38, 170]).

The literature indicates several reasons for such stigma. These include lack of knowledge [171], invisibility of profile [172], accommodation perceived as cheating by teachers and peers [173], self-fulfilling prophecies leading to underperformance and even criminality [174, 175], confirmation of bias with beliefs, ignoring individual characteristics (e.g., [176–178]) and generation of negative expectations [179].

Labelling, however, also has positive effects as willing teachers may be able to interpret behaviours better to then provide appropriate teaching strategies (e.g., [34, 180, 181]). Further, the label also helps one's understanding of one's own behaviour (e.g., [158, 166, 182]).

11. Demographics and effects on lecturers

One cannot underestimate that dyslexia presents challenges to university lecturers (e.g., [122, 183, 184]). This population has not been visible, although it has always existed (e.g., [112, 165, 185]). Since the challenges are invisible, teaching adaptations for such a population have perhaps been neglected. Widened access to university studies for students with functional disorders, such as dyslexia, have led to this neglect being made visible [143].

Teachers are undoubtedly important people in the lives of dyslexic schoolchildren and teachers who help or hinder play a part in dyslexic people's lives. Teachers remembered most negatively were those who humiliated dyslexic pupils in front of their peers. Many report negative teachers' attitudes towards dyslexic-type difficulties, and lack of knowledge about dyslexia and intervention for dyslexic difficulties. However, pupils who had attended specialist schools were more likely to report positive experiences [88].

Riddick et al. [91] reported that three dyslexic student-participants in higher education experienced positive school experiences and stated that their lecturers had acknowledged their profile, were sensitive to their needs and had provided helpful intervention. A participant from Hellendoorn and Ruijssenaars' [90] study reported that "I will never forget Mr X. When he came in my life, something changed, because he really understood. He at least gave me credit for the hard work I did, even though I still could not read" (p. 233). In contrast, others speak of teachers who treated them as if they were unintelligent and/or lazy, refused to accept that students were dyslexic and/or provide any accommodation and/or taught them inappropriately (e.g., [90, 91, 167]).

Students with dyslexia judged support received from specialists, teachers from special schools, licenced remedial teachers, speech therapists and psychomotor therapists favourably (e.g. [90, 91, 186]). Burden [88] reported that out of 50 dyslexic boys, 62% explained that mainstream teachers had not understood their feelings, whereas at their specialist school only 4% felt the teachers did not understand their profiles. These findings suggest a need for additional training [9].

12. Post Covid-19 and technology - compensatory strategies to academic success

Technology has improved so much [187], that schools [188, 189]must consider its use to access and create print (e.g., [189–191]). Technology is regarded as the "fourth revolution in the means of production of knowledge following language, writing and print" ([190], p. 39). Warschauer and Matuchniak [192] reported a broad consensus among educators, communciation scholars, sociologists and economists that, "information and communication technolgoies (ICT)...bridge the interactive features of speech and archival characterists of writing" (p. 179). Gutenberg's printing press (c. 1440) started the third revolution - printing. However, it took centuries for printing to truly infiltrate and affect society with the advent of industrial Revolution (c. 1760). The transition between the third (Print) and fourth (Technology) revolution was faster. We have transitioned from an industrial to an informative economy in mere decades [193, 194].

Given the present global health situation, such research is now even more important. Current social distancing has necessitated more independent learning and further use of technology [195]. This may prove more beneficial if the necessary skills are addressed. An Economist's [196] weekly editorial dedicated to the absent university student reported that:

> *COVID-19 is catalysing innovation ...offering ...students the opportunity to take online courses...huge scope for using digital technology to improve education. University are rightly proud of their centuries-old traditions, but their ancient pedigrees have too often been used as an excuse for resisting change. If COVID-19 shakes them out of their complacency, some good may yet come from this disaster.* (p. 7)

One also needs to be cautious and not conclude that millennials and younger generations are automatically technology experts or comfortable with all computer usage. For example, Prensky [197] reported that, with regard to reading materials, approximately half of the students in their study (average age 23.7 years), both dyslexic (7 of 13) and non-dyslexic (11 of 20), expressed difficulty reading text online and using learning technologies. This contradicts assertions that the 'net generation' is all 'digital natives' and can be expected to use educational technology with ease and proficiency. Rather, the data from this study support Kennedy, et al.'s [198] conclusion that students in the 'net generation' are not necessarily technology experts and may require explicit technology training. This may also be due to their school experiences regarding Access to literacy and learning.

13. Final thought

UNESCO [199] reports that "at least 750 million youth and adults still cannot read and write and 250 million children are failing to acquire basic literacy skills" [para. 3], thus excluding excludes them from "full participation in their communities and societies" [para.3]. Clinton's [200] International Literacy Day message implored that:

> *If our world is to meet the challenges of the twenty-first century, we must harness the energy and creativity of all our citizens. Nearly half of American adults lack many of the basic literacy skills so essential to success in today's complex and ever-changing world. Literacy is not a luxury; it is a right and a responsibility. And in an international community increasingly dedicated to the principles of equality and opportunity, illiteracy is unacceptable. (p. 1713)*

In this chapter, I endeavoured to reflect on what should be considered as literacy in the 21st century and how our communities need to ensure that all who want to pursue further academic education may do so easily and with dignity. The aim was to help highlight what literacy means in the 21st century and what competencies relate to intelligence and academic success, or otherwise. In human's fourth revolution of knowledge, transmission and sharing [190], whilst we need to appropriately train educators to ensure that all become proficient in all literacies as early as possible (e.g. [9, 20, 21]), we must also consider that traditional skills of reading and writing cannot continue to remain obstacles [201] for whom such skills are not so easy to learn and become proficient in. As Leonardi da Vinci noted: "I would rather have a scientific mind without literary skills, than a literary person without a scientific mind"[2].

Acknowledgements

I would like to thank my colleagues, Dr Anne Marie Callus and Marchita Mangiafico for providing me with the data regarding University of Malta students. I would also like to thank all those children and young people with dyslexia whose experiences and wisdom have enriched my life, including my son.

Conflict of interest

The author declares no conflict of interest.

[2] Sentence often attributed to Leonardo da Vinci (e.g. azquotes, quotefancy, quotemaster). I continue to search for the original source in his writings.

Author details

Ruth Falzon[1,2,3,4,5,6]

1 University of Malta, Tal-Qroqq L-Imsida, Malta EU MSD2080

2 Elected Board Member and Secretary of the Malta Dyslexia Association (MDA)

3 Elected Board Director and Treasurer of the European Dyslexia Association (EDA)

4 Elected Council Member/Vice-Secretary of the Malta Association for the Counselling Profession (MACP)

5 Membership Chair of the International Association for Counselling (IAC)

6 Elected Council member and Treasurer of The International Society for Policy Research and Evaluation in School-Based Counseling (ISPRESC)

*Address all correspondence to: ruth.falzon@um.edu.mt

References

[1] Falzon, R. & Camilleri J. (2014) Request for oral examinations at the SEC and MATSEC levels. National petition presented to the Maltese Parliament. https://www.change.org/p/ministry-for-education-and-employment-give-the-option-to-students-to-do-their-examinations-in-writing-orally-or-using-a-word-processor

[2] University of Malta (2018). The University of Malta Access Arrangements. Available from https://www.um.edu.mt/__data/assets/pdf_file/0004/378481/UMGuidelinescomplete2018.pdf

[3] Shaywitz, S. E., & Shaywitz, B. A. (2003). Dyslexia (specific reading disability). *Pediatrics in Review*, *24*(5), 147-153. http://citeseerx.ist.psu.edu/viewdoc/download? doi=10.1.1.840.6505&rep=rep1&type=pdf

[4] Snowling, M., Hulme, C. & Nation, K. (2020). Defining and understanding dyslexia: past, present and future, *Oxford Review of Education*, 46:4, 501-513, https://doi.org/10.1080/03054985.2020.1765756

[5] Denhart, H. (2008). Deconstructing barriers: Perceptions of students labeled with learning disabilities in higher education. *Journal of learning disabilities*, *41*(6), 483-497. https://doi.org/10.1177/0022219408321151

[6] Lock, R. H., & Layton, C. A. (2001). Succeeding in Postsecondary Ed through Self-Advocacy. *Teaching Exceptional Children*, 34, 66-71. https://doi.org/10.1177/004005990103400210

[7] Rodis, P., Garrod, A., & Boscardin, M. L. (2001). Learning disabilities and life stories. Allyn & Bacon.

[8] Kannangara, C. S. (2015). From languishing dyslexia to thriving dyslexia: developing a new conceptual approach to working with people with dyslexia. *Frontiers in psychology*, 6, 1976. https://doi.org/10.3389/fpsyg.2015.01976

[9] Falzon, R. (2012). *Early educators' awareness and knowledge of structured multisensory literary instruction* (Doctoral dissertation, Northumbria University). http://nrl.northumbria.ac.uk/ id/eprint/10837/1/falzon.ruth_phd.pdf

[10] Freire, P. (1970). *The pedagogy of the oppressed*. Harper and Harper

[11] Freire, P. (1985). *The politics of education: Culture, power, and liberation*. Greenwood Publishing Group

[12] Johnson, D., & Kress, G. (2003). Globalisation, literacy and society: Redesigning pedagogy and assessment. *Assessment in Education: Principles, Policy & Practice*, *10*(1), 5-14. https:doi.org/10.1080/09695940301697

[13] Adams, M.J. (1990). *Beginning to read: thinking and learning about print*. MIT Press.

[14] Adams, M. J. (2011). The relation between alphabetic basics, word recognition, and reading. *What research has to say about reading instruction*, 4-24. Available from https://www. researchgate.net/profile/Marilyn_Adams3/publication/294428324_

[15] UNESCO (2005) Education for All Global Monitoring Report - Education for all: 2006 Literacy for life. Paris France: UNESCO. Available from http://unesdoc. unesco.org/ images/0014/001416/141639e.pdf

[16] Cameron, D. (2011). David Cameron's Thursday 11th Aug 2011 address to parliament. https:// www.telegraph.co.uk/news/uknews/

crime/8695272/UK-riots-text-of-David-Camerons-address-to-Commons.html

[17] Clinton W.J. (1997). State of the Union Address. https://clintonwhitehouse2.archives.gov/WH/SOU97

[18] Al Nasser, N. A (2012). Celebrating International Literacy Day. Rethinking Literacy: How Far Have We Gone in Reaching the Literacy Goal? http://www.un.org/en/ga/president/66/International-Literacy-Day%20 Brochure-Modified.pdf

[19] Hirsch, E.D. Jnr. (1996). The schools we need and why we don't have them. (2nd Ed.). Anchor Books, Doubleday.

[20] Moats, L. C. (2009). Still wanted: Teachers with knowledge of language. *Journal of Learning Disabilities, 42 (5),* 387-391. https://doi.org/10.1177/0022219409338735

[21] Stanovich, K. E. (2009). Matthew effects in reading: Some consequences of individual differences in the acquisition of literacy. *Journal of education*, *189*(1-2), 23-55. https://doi.org/10.1177/0022057409189001-204

[22] Ehri, L. C. (2020). The science of learning to read words: A case for systematic phonics instruction. *Reading Research Quarterly*. 55 (S1) S45-S60. https://doi-org.ejournals. um.edu. mt /10.1002/rrq.334

[23] Rigney, D. (2010). *The Matthew effect: How advantage begets further advantage.* University Press.

[24] Stanovich, K. E. (1986). Matthew Effects in Reading: Some Consequences of Individual Differences in the Acquisition of Literacy. *Reading Research Quarterly, 21 (4),* 360-407. https://doi.org/10.1598/RRQ.21.4.1

[25] Tannenbaum, K. R., Torgesen, J. K., & Wagner, R. K. (2006). Relationships between word knowledge and reading comprehension in third-grade children. *Scientific Studies of Reading*, 10(4), 381-398. https://doi.org/10.1207/s1532799xssr1004_3

[26] Cain, K. (2016). Reading comprehension development and difficulties: An overview. *Perspectives on Language and Literacy,* 42(2), 9-16. https://mydigitalpublication.com/publication/?m=13959

[27] Paris, S. G. (2005). Reinterpreting the development of reading skills. *Reading Research Quarterly*, 40(2), 184-202. https://doi.org/10.1598/RRQ.40.2.3

[28] Wijekumar, K. (2020). The 'GIST' of the reading comprehension problem in grades 4 and 5. *Dyslexia*, 1-18. https://doi.org/10.1002/dys.1647

[29] Mendes, G. G., & Barrera, S. D. (2017). Phonological Processing and Reading and Writing Skills in Literacy. *Paidéia (Ribeirão Preto)*, *27*(68), 298-305. https://doi.org/10.1590/1982-43272768201707

[30] Chetcuti, D., Falzon, R., & Camilleri S. (2016). *D pebble in my shoe: Teenagers' experiences of dyslexia and examinations.* Published by the authors (Erasmus+ programme) 978-99957-0-999-0

[31] Macdonald, S. J., & Deacon, L. (2019). Twice upon a time: Examining the effect socio-economic status has on the experience of dyslexia in the United Kingdom. *Dyslexia*, *25*(1), 3-19. https://doi.org/10.1002/dys.1606

[32] Daily, S. M., Mann, M. J., Lilly, C. L., Dyer, A. M., Smith, M. L., & Kristjansson, A. L. (2020). School Climate as an Intervention to Reduce Academic Failure and Educate the Whole Child: A Longitudinal Study. *Journal of School Health*, *90*(3), 182-193. https://doi.org/10.1111/josh.12863

[33] Nickerson, R. S. (2020). Technology in education in 2020: Thinking about the not-distant future. In R.S. Nickerson & Zodhiates, P.P. (Eds.) *Technology in education: Looking toward 2020,* (pp. 1-9). Routledge

[34] Antonelli, L., Bilocca, S., Borg, D., Borg, S., Boxall, M., Briffa, L. Debono, C., Falzon, R., Farrugia, V., Gatt, L., Formosa, M., Mifsud, D., Mizzi, K., Scurfield, L., Scurfield, M. & Vella, G.L. (2014). Drama, performance ethnography, and self-esteem: Listening to youngsters with dyslexia and their parents. *SAGE Open*, *4*(2), https://doi.org/10.1177/2158244014534696

[35] Burden, R. (2008). Dyslexia and self-concept: A review of past research with implications for future action. In G. Reid., A. J. Fawcett, F. Manis, L.S. Siegel, *The Sage handbook of dyslexia*, 395-410. Sage Publications Ltd

[36] Humphrey, N., & Mullins, P. M. (2002). Research section: Personal constructs and attribution for academic success and failure in dyslexia. *British Journal of Special Education*, *29*(4), 196-203. https://doi.org/10.1111/1467-8527.00269

[37] Humphrey, N., & Mullins, P. M. (2002). Self-concept and self-esteem in developmental dyslexia. *Journal of Research in Special Educational Needs*, *2*(2). https://doi.org/10.1111/j.1471-3802.2002.00163.x

[38] Chetcuti, D., Falzon, R. & Camilleri S. (2019) 'The Pebble in my shoe': Dyslexic students and their views of examinations. In C. Bezzina & S. Caruana (Eds.) *Teacher Education Matters: Transforming*, 433-447. University of Malta

[39] Falzon, R. (2019). Literacy and Wellbeing. In S. Vella, R. Falzon & A. Azzopardi (Eds), *Perspectives on Wellbeing - A Reader* (pp. 79-95). Brill Sense.

[40] Kendeou, P., McMaster, K. L., & Christ, T. J. (2016). Reading comprehension: Core components and processes. *Policy Insights from the Behavioral and Brain Sciences*, *3*(1), 62-69. https://doi.org/10.1177/2372732215624707

[41] Florit, E., & Cain, K. (2011). The simple view of reading: Is it valid for different types of alphabetic orthographies?. *Educational Psychology Review*, *23*(4), 553-576. https://doi.org/10.1007/ s10648-011-9175-6

[42] Aarnoutse, C., van Leeuwe, J., & Verhoeven, L. (2005). Early literacy from a longitudinal perspective. *Educational Research and Evaluation*, *11*(3), 253-275. https://doi.org/10.1080/08993400500101054

[43] Kim, Y. S. G. (2017). Why the simple view of reading is not simplistic: Unpacking component skills of reading using a direct and indirect effect model of reading (DIER). *Scientific Studies of Reading*, *21*(4), 310-333. https://doi.org/10.1080/10888438.2017.1291643

[44] Cain, K., Oakhill, J., & Bryant, P. (2004). Children's reading comprehension ability: Concurrent prediction by working memory, verbal ability, and component skills. *Journal of educational psychology*, *96*(1), 31-42. https://doi.org/10.1037/0022-0663.96.1.31

[45] Oakhill, J. V., & Cain, K. (2012). The precursors of reading ability in young readers: Evidence from a four-year longitudinal study. *Scientific studies of reading*, *16*(2), 91-121. https://doi.org/10.1080/10888438.2010.529219

[46] Abadiano, H. R., & Turner, J. (2005). Reading fluency: The road to developing efficient and effective readers. *New England Reading Association Journal*, *41*(1), 50-56. https://pdfs.semanticscholar.org/21dd/7d8c43c1a3e5d39adb90d21b76db45db98ca.pdf

[47] *Essay* (n.d.). Dictionary.com .Available from http://dictionary. reference. com/browse/essay. [Accessed 2020-09-11]

[48] Stanovich, K. E. (2000). *Progress in Understanding Reading: Scientific Foundations and New Frontiers*. Guilford Press.

[49] Gotesman, E., & Goldfus, C. (2010). The impact of assistive technologies on the reading outcomes of college students with disabilities. *Educational Technology*, *50*(3), 21-25. http://telem-pub.openu.ac.il/uscrs/chais/2009/noon/2_2.pdf

[50] Higgins, E. L., & Raskind, M. H. (2004). Speech recognition-based and automaticity programs to help students with severe reading and spelling problems. *Annals of Dyslexia*, *54*(2), 365-388. https://doi.org/10.1007/s11881-004-0017-9

[51] Meridith, L., & Linda, P. (2009). Commercial software programs approved for teaching reading and writing in the primary grades: Another sobering reality. *Journal of Research on Technology in Education*, *42*(2), 197-216. https://doi.org/10.1080/15391523.2009.10782547

[52] AbilityNet (2015). Factsheet - Dyslexia and computing. https://www.abilitynet.org.uk/sites/abilitynet.

[53] Microsoft 365 (n.d.) Introducing Microsoft 365. Available from https:// www. microsoft.com /en/microsoft-365 [Accessed 2020-09-11]

[54] My Computer My Way (n.d.) My Computer My Way: Help making your device easier to use Available from https://mcmw.abilitynet.org.uk/[Accessed 2020-09-11]

[55] Natural Reader (n.d.) Available from https://www.naturalreaders.com/[Accessed 2020-09-11]

[56] C-Pen® (n.d.) A reading pen from C-PEN®. Available from https://cpen.com/ product/ readerpen/ [Accessed 2020-09-11]

[57] Scanmarker (n.d.). The Digital Highlighter. Available from https://scanmarker.com/[Accessed 2020-09-12]

[58] Scanning Pens (n.d.). Reader pen - a major technological breakthrough. Available from https://www.scanningpens.co.uk/[Accessed 2020-09-12]

[59] C-Pen® ExamReader™ (n.d.). ExamReader™. Available from https://cpen.com/ product/examreader/ [Accessed 2020-09-11]

[60] Exam reader (n.d.) Exam reader powered by Scanning Pens. Available from https://www.scanningpens.com/ExamReaderUS/ [Accessed 2020-09-11]

[61] Lyon, G. R., Shaywitz, S. E., & Shaywitz, B. A. (2003). A definition of dyslexia. *Annals of Dyslexia*, *53*(1), 1-14. https://doi.org/10.1007/s11881-003-0001-9

[62] Tunmer, W., & Greaney, K. (2010). Defining dyslexia. *Journal of Learning Disabilities*, 43(3), 229-243. https://doi.org/10.1177/0022219409345009

[63] Stanovich, K. (1999). The sociopsychometrics of learning disabilities. *Journal of Learning Disabilities, 32*(No. 4 July/August), 350-361. http://www.keithstanovich.com/Site/Research_on_Reading_files/JLD99.pdf

[64] Bell, S. (2010). Inclusion for adults with dyslexia: Examining the transition periods of a group of adults in England: 'Clever is when you come to a brick wall and you have got to get over it without a ladder'. *Journal of Research in Special Education Needs*, 10(3), 216-226. https://doi.org/10.1111/j.1471-3802.2010.01167.x

[65] McLoughlin, D., & Leather, C. (2013). *The dyslexic adult: Interventions and outcomes – an evidence-based approach* (2nd Ed/). John Wiley & Sons.

[66] Riddell, S., & Weedon, E. (2006). What counts as reasonable adjustment? Dyslexic students and the concept of fair assessment. *International Studies in Sociology of Education, 16*(1), 57-73. https://doi.org/10.1080/19620210600804301

[67] Su, M., Zhao, J., de Schotten, M. T., Zhou, W., Gong, G., Ramus, F., & Shu, H. (2018). Alterations in white matter pathways underlying phonological and morphological processing in Chinese developmental dyslexia. *Developmental cognitive neuroscience*, *31*, 11-19. https://doi.org/10.1016/j.dcn.2018.04.002

[68] Zoccolotti, P., & Friedmann, N. (2010). From dyslexia to dyslexias, from dysgraphia to dysgraphias, from a cause to causes: a look at current research on developmental dyslexia and dysgraphia. https://doi.org/0.1016/j.cortex.2010.09.003

[69] Kale, S. (2020, September 17). *The Long Read: The Battle over Dyslexia.* https://www. theguardian.com/news/2020/sep/17/battle-over-dyslexia-warwickshire-staffordshire

[70] Elliot, J. G., & Grigorkenko, E. L. (2014). *The dyslexia debate*. Cambridge University Press.

[71] American Psychiatric Association. (2013). *Diagnostic and statistical manual of mental disorders (DSM-5)*. American Psychiatric Publishing.

[72] Mitchell, D., & Sutherland, D. (2020). *What really works in special and inclusive education: Using evidence-based teaching strategies*. Routledge.

[73] Mackelprang, R. W., & Salsgiver, R. O. (2016). *Disability: A diversity model approach in human service practice*. Oxford University Press.

[74] Skarstad, K. (2018). Human rights through the lens of disability. *Netherlands Quarterly of Human Rights*, *36*(1), 24-42. https://doi.org/10.1177/0924051917753251

[75] Corcodel, V. (2019). *Modern law and otherness: the dynamics of inclusion and exclusion in comparative legal thought*. Edward Elgar Publishing.

[76] Hallam, E., & Street, B. (Eds.). (2013). *Cultural encounters: Representing otherness*. Routledge.

[77] Furedi, F. (2004). *Therapy culture: cultivating vulnerability in an uncertain age*, Routledge.

[78] Zeleke, S. (2004). Self-concepts of students with learning disabilities and their normally achieving peers: a review. European Journal of Special Needs Education, 19(2), 45-170. https://doi.org/10.1080/08856250410001678469

[79] Jobling, A., & Moni, K. (2004). 'I never imagined I'd have to teach these children': providing authentic learning experiences for secondary pre-service teachers in teaching students with special needs. *Asia-Pacific Journal of Teacher Education, 32*(1), 6-22. https://doi.org/ 10.1080/1359866042000206026

[80] Marshall, J., Ralph, S., & Palmer, S. (2002). 'I wasn't trained to work with them': mainstream teachers' attitudes to children with speech and language difficulties. *International Journal of Inclusive Education, 6*(3), 199-215. https://doi.org/10.1080/13603110110067208

[81] Tanner, K. (2010). *The Lived Experience of Adults with Dyslexia: An Exploration of the Perceptions of Their Educational Experiences.* (Doctor of Philosophy), Murdoch University, Perth. https://researchrepository.murdoch.edu.au/id/eprint/4128/

[82] Reid Lyon, G., & Weiser, B. (2009). Teacher knowledge, instructional

expertise and the development of reading proficiency. *Journal of Learning Disabilities, 42 (5),* 475-480. https://doi.org/10.1177/0022219409338741

[83] Caskey, J. (2017). When Educational Support Is Just Not Enough: Adult Students Diagnosed with Dyslexia in Technical and Further Education (TAFE). *Doctor of Philosophy dissertation University of the Sunshine Coast.* https://www. google.com/search?q=Caskey%2C+J.+(2017). +When+Educational+Support+Is+Just+Not+Enough

[84] British Dyslexia Association (2019). *The human cost of dyslexia The emotional and psychological impact of poorly supported dyslexia. Report from the All-Party Parliamentary Group for Dyslexia and other SpLDs April 2019.* https://cdn.bdadyslexia.org.uk/documents/Final-APPG-for-Human-cost-of-dyslexia-appg-report.pdf

[85] Edwards, J. (1994). *The scars of dyslexia.* Cassell.

[86] Hughes, W. & Dawson, R. (1995) Memories of school: Adult dyslexics recall their school days. *Support for Learning,* 10(4), 181-184. https://doi.org/10.1111/j.1467-9604.1995.tb00037.x

[87] Armstrong, D. & Humphrey, N. (2009) Reactions to a diagnosis of dyslexia among students entering further education: Development of the 'resistance-accommodation' model. *British Journal of Special Education,* 36(2), 95-102. https://doi.org/10.1111/j.1467-8578.2008.00408.x

[88] Burden, R. (2005). Dyslexia & Self-concept. Seeking a Dyslexic Identity. Whurr Publishers Ltd.

[89] Burden, R., & Burdett, J. (2005). Factors associated with successful learning in pupils with dyslexia: a motivational analysis. *British Journal of special education*, *32*(2), 100-104. https://doi.org/10.1111/j.0952-3383.2005.00378.x

[90] Hellendoorn, J. & Ruijssenaars, W. (2000) Personal experiences and adjustment of dutch adults with dyslexia. *Remedial and Special Education,* 21(4), 227-239. https://doi.org/10.1177/074193250002100405

[91] Riddick, B., Sterling, C., Farmer, M. & Morgan, S. (1999) Self-esteem and anxiety in the educational histories of adult dyslexic students. *DYSLEXIA,* 5, 227-248. https://doi.org/10.1002/(SICI)1099-0909(199912)5:4<227::AID-DYS146>3.0.CO;2-6

[92] Bernstein, B. L., Evans, B., Fyffe, J., Halai, N., Hall, F. L., Jensen, H. S. & Ortega, S. (2014). In *Globalization and its impacts on the quality of PhD education* (pp. 5-30). Brill Sense.

[93] Park, C. (2005). New variant PhD: The changing nature of the doctorate in the UK. *Journal of higher education policy and management*, *27*(2), 189-207. https://doi.org/10.1080/13600800500120068

[94] Tinkler, P., & Jackson, C. (2000). Examining the doctorate: institutional policy and the PhD examination process in Britain. *Studies in higher education*, *25*(2), 167-180. https://doi.org/10.1080/713696136

[95] Hopfenbeck, T. (2017). Balancing the challenges of high-stakes testing, accountability and students' well-being. *Assessment in Education: Principles, Policy & Practice, 24*(1), 1-3. https://doi.org/10.1080/0969594X.2016.1277068

[96] Elwood, J. (2012). Qualifications, examinations and assessment: views and perspectives of students in the 14-19 phase on policy and practice. *Cambridge Journal of Education, 42*(4), 497-512. https://doi.org/10.1080/0305764X.2012.733347

[97] Elwood, J., Hopfenbeck, T., & Baird, J. (2017). Predictability in high-stakes examinations: students' perspectives on a perennnial assessment dilemma. *Research Papers in Education, 32*(1), 1-17. https://doi.org/10.1080/02671522.2015.1086015

[98] Costarelli, V., & Patsai, A. (2012). Academic examination stress increases disordered eating symptomatology in female university students. *Eating and Weight Disorders-Studies on Anorexia, Bulimia and Obesity*, *17*(3), e164-e169. https://doi.org/10.1007/BF03325343

[99] Oaten, M., & Cheng, K. (2005). Academic examination stress impairs self–control. *Journal of social and clinical psychology*, *24*(2), 254-279. https://doi.org/10.1521/jscp.24.2.254.62276

[100] Xiang, Z., Tan, S., Kang, Q., Zhang, B., & Zhu, L. (2019). Longitudinal effects of examination stress on psychological well-being and a possible mediating role of self-esteem in Chinese high school students. *Journal of Happiness Studies*, *20*(1), 283-305. https://doi.org/10.1007/s10902-017-9948-9

[101] Gardner, J., Holmes, B., & Leitch, R. (2009). *Assessment and Social Justice: a Futurelab literature review, Report 16.* Bristol: Futurelab. https://www.researchgate.net/publication/322896490_Assessment_and_Social_Justice

[102] Crisp, V., Johnson, M., & Novacovic, N. (2012). The effects of features of examination questions on the performance of students with dyslexia. *British Educational Research Journal, 38*(5), 813-839. DOI: https://doi.org/10.1080/01411926.2011.584964

[103] Falzon, R. & Camilleri J. (2014) Request for oral examinations at the SEC and MATSEC levels. National petition presented to the Maltese Parliament. https://www.change.org/p/ministry-for-education-and-employment-give-the-option-to-students-to-do-their-examinations-in-writing-orally-or-using-a-word-processor

[104] Lerner, J. W., & Johns, B. (2011). *Learning disabilities and related mild disabilities*. Cengage Learning.

[105] Cribb, A., & Gerwitz, S. (2003). Towards a sociology of just practices: an analysis of plural conceptions of justice. In C. Vincent (Ed.). *Social Justice in Education* (pp. 15-29). Routledge, Falmer.

[106] Klenowski, V. (2009). Australian indigenous students: addressing equity issues in assessment. *Teaching Education, 20*(1), 77-93. https://doi.org/10.1080/10476210802681741

[107] Elwood, J., & Lundy, L. (2010). Revisioning assessment though a children's rights approach: implications for policy, process and practice. *Research Papers in Education, 25*(3), 335-353. https://doi.org/10.1080/02671522.2010.498150

[108] Katusic, S. K., Colligan, R. C., Barbaresi, W. J., Schaid, D. J., & Jacobsen, S. J. (2001). Incidence of reading disability in a population-based birth cohort, 1976-1982, Rochester, Minn. *Mayo Clin Proc*, 76, 1081-1092. https://doi.org/10.4065/76.11.1081

[109] Rao, S., Raj, A., Ramanathan, V., Sharma, A., Dhar, M., Thatkar, P. V., & Pal, R. (2017). Prevalence of dyslexia among school children in Mysore. *International Journal of Medical Science and Public Health*, 6(1), 159-164. https://www.researchgate.net/profile/Murali_Dhar4/publication/311715972_Prevalence_of_dyslexia_among_school_children_in_Mysore/links/585788ff08aeff086bfcaf8f/Prevalence-of-dyslexia-among-school-children-in-Mysore.pdf

[110] Richardson, J. T. E., & Wydell, T. N. (2003). The representation and attainment of students with dyslexia in UK higher education. *Reading and Writing: An Interdisciplinary Journal*, 16, 475-503. https://doi.org/10.1023/A:1024261927214

[111] Stampoltzis, A., & Polychronopoulou, S. (2008). Dyslexia in Greek higher education: A study of incidence, policy and provision. *Journal of Research in Special Education Needs*, 8(1), 37-46. https://doi.org/10.1111/j.1471-3802.2008.00100.x

[112] Mortimore, T., & Crozier, W. R. (2006). Dyslexia and difficulties with study skills in higher education. *Studies in higher education*, *31*(2), 235-251. https://doi.org/10.1080/03075070600572173

[113] Richardson, J. T. (2015). Academic attainment in students with dyslexia in distance education. *Dyslexia*, *21*(4), 323-337. https://doi.org/10.1002/dys.1502

[114] University of Malta (2020). *Statistical report secondary education certificate examinations 2019*. https://www.um.edu.mt/__data/assets/pdf_file/0007/438694/ SECStatReport 2019FINAL.pdf

[115] Olofsson, A., Taube, K., & Ahl, A. (2015). Academic achievement of university students with dyslexia. *Dyslexia*, 21, 338-349. https://doi.org/10.1002/dys.1517

[116] MacCullagh, L., Bosanquet, A., & Badcock, N. A. (2017). University students with dyslexia: A qualitative exploratory study of learning practices, challenges and strategies. Dyslexia, 23(1), 3-23. https://doi.org/10.1002/dys.1544

[117] Byrne, C. (2018) *Why do dyslexic students do worse at university?* The Guardian. https://www. theguardian.com/education/2018/dec/06/why-do-dyslexic-students-do-worse-at-university

[118] Hall, L. M., & Belch, H. A. (2000). Setting the context: Reconsidering the principles of full participation and meaningful access for students with disabilities. *New Directions for Student Services*, 91, 5-17. https://doi.org/10.1002/ss.9101

[119] University of Oxford (n.d.) *Guidance for disabled applicants*. Available from https://www.ox.ac.uk/admissions/undergraduate/applying-to-oxford/guidance-disabled-applicants [Accessed 2020-09-24]

[120] Henderson, K. (2001). 2001 college freshmen with disabilities: A biennial statistical profile (pp. 42). Washington, DC: Heath Resource Center.

[121] Gerber, P. J., & Brown, D. (1997). *Learning disabilities and employment*. Pro-Ed.

[122] Cameron, H., & Nunkoosing, K. (2012). Lecturer perspectives on dyslexia and dyslexic students within one faculty at one university in England. *Teaching in Higher Education*, *17*(3), 341-352. https://doi.org/10.1080/13562517.2011.641002

[123] Greenbaum, B., Graham, S., & Scales, W. (1996). Adults with learning disabilities: Occupational and social status after college. Journal of Learning Disabilities, 29, 167-173. https://doi.org/10.1177/002221949602900206

[124] Callens, M., Tops, W., & Brysbaert, M. (2012). Cognitive profile of students who enter higher education with an indication of dyslexia. *Plos One*, 7(6e38081). https://doi.org/10.1371/journal.pone.0038081

[125] Deacon, S. H., Cook, K., & Parrila, R. (2012). Identifying high-functioning dyslexics: is self-report of early reading problems enough?. *Annals of Dyslexia*, *62*(2), 120-134. https://doi.org/ 10.1007/s11881-012-0068-2

[126] Kirby, J. R., Silvestri, R., Allingham, B. H., Parrila, R., & La Fave, C. B. (2008). Learning strategies and study approaches of postsecondary students with dyslexia. *Journal of Learning Disabilities*, 41(1), 85-96. https://doi.org/10.1177/0022219407311040

[127] Pino, M., & Mortari, L. (2014). The inclusion of students with dyslexia in higher education: A systematic review using narrative synthesis. Dyslexia. 20(4), 346-69. https://doi.org/10.1002/dys.1484

[128] Simmons, F., & Singleton, C. (2000). The reading comprehension abilities of dyslexic students in higher education. *Dyslexia*, 6, 178-192. https://doi.org/10.1002/1099-0909 (200007/09) 6:3<178::AID-DYS171>3.0.CO;2-9

[129] Erskine, J. M., & Seymour, P. H. K. (2005). Proximal analysis of developmental dyslexia in adulthood: The cognitive mosaic model. *Journal of Educational Psychology*, 97(3), 406-424. https://doi.org/10.1037/0022-0663.97.3.406

[130] Connelly, V., Campbell, S., MacLean, M., & Barnes, J. (2006). Contribution of lower-order letter and word fluency skills to written composition of college students with and without dyslexia. *Developmental Neuropsychology*, 29(1), 175-196. https://doi.org/10.1207/s15326942dn2901_9

[131] Galbraith, D., Baaijen, V., Smith-Spark, J., & Torrance, M. (2012). The effects of dyslexia on the writing processes of students in higher education. Chapter 2.02.06 In M. Torrance, D. Alamargot, M. Castello, F. Ganier, O. Kruse, A. Mangen, L. Tolchinsky, & L. Van Waes (Eds): *Learning to write effectively: Current trends in European research*. Emerald Group Publishing.

[132] Sterling, C. M., Farmer, M., Riddick, B., Morgan, S., & Matthews, C. (1997). Adult dyslexic writing. *Dyslexia*, 4, 1-15. https://doi.org/10.1002/(SICI)1099-0909(199803)4:1<1::AID-DYS87>3.0.CO;2-F

[133] British Dyslexia Association (n.d.) *Modern Foreign Languages*. Available from https:// www.bdadyslexia.org.uk/advice/educators/teaching-for-neurodiversity/modern-foreign-languages [Accessed 2020-09-15]

[134] Block, D., & Cameron, D. (Eds.). (2002). *Globalization and language teaching*. Routledge.

[135] Lawes, S. (2000). Why learn a foreign language?. In K. Field (Ed.) *Issues in modern foreign languages teaching*, 41-51. Routledge Farmer

[136] Merritt, A. (2013). Why learn a foreign language? Benefits of bilingualism. *The Telegraph*. https:// www.telegraph.co.uk/education/2018/03/27/learn-foreign-language-benefits-bilingualism/

[137] European Parliament (2019). Multilingualism: The language of the European Union. Available from: https://www.europarl.europa.eu/RegData/etudes/BRIE/2019/642207/EPRS_BRI (2019)642207_EN.pdf

[138] Fuller, M., Healey, M., Bradley, A., & Hall, T. (2004). Barriers to learning: A systematic study of the experience of disabled students in one university. *Studies in Higher Education*, 29(3), 303-318. https://doi.org/10.1080/03075070410001682592

[139] Collinson, C., & Penketh, C. (2010). 'Sit in the corner and don't eat the crayons': Postgraduates with dyslexia and the dominant 'lexic' discourse. *Disability & Society*, 25(1), 7-19. https://doi.org/10.1080/09687590903363274

[140] Hutcheon, E. J., & Wolbring, G. (2012). Voices of "disabled" post-secondary students: Examining higher

education "disability" policy using an ableism lens. *Journal of Diversity in Higher Education*, 5(1), 39-49. https// doi.org/10.1037/a0027002

[141] Gibson, S., & Kendall, L. (2010). Stories from school: Dyslexia and learners' voices on factors impacting on achievement. *Support for Learning*, 25(4), 187-193. https://doi.org/10.1111/j.1467-9604.2010.01465.x

[142] Goode, J. (2006). 'Managing' disability: Early experiences of university students with disabilities. *Disability & Society*, 22(1), 35-48. https://doi.org/10.1080/09687590601056204

[143] Olofsson, A., Ahl, A., & Taube, K. (2012). Learning and study strategies in university students with dyslexia: Implications for teaching. *Procedia Social and Behavioural Sciences*, 47, 1184-1193. https://doi.org/10.1016/j.sbspro.2012.06.798

[144] Sharma, V. (2018). Soft skills: An employability enabler. *IUP Journal of Soft Skills*, *12*(2), 25-32. https://www.econbiz.de/Record/soft-skills-an-employability-enabler-sharma-vandana/10011989354

[145] Majid, S., Eapen, C. M., Aung, E. M., & Oo, K. T. (2019). The Importance of Soft Skills for Employability and Career Development: Students and Employers' Perspectives. *IUP Journal of Soft Skills*, *13*(4), 7-39. https://search-proquest-com.ejournals.um.edu.mt/docview/ 2330760547? accountid=27934

[146] Succi, C., & Canovi, M. (2020). Soft skills to enhance graduate employability: comparing students and employers' perceptions. *Studies in Higher Education*, *45*(9), 1834-1847. https://doi.org/10.1080/03075079.2019.1585420

[147] Theodoropoulou, S. (2010). Skills and education for growth and well-being in Europe 2020: are we on the right path. *EPC Issue Paper*, *61*. https://www.researchgate.net/profile/Sotiria_ Theodoropoulou2/publication/ 267574715_Skills_and_education_for_growth_and_well-eing_in_Europe_2020_are_we_on_the_right_path

[148] Brownlie, F., Feniak, C., & Schnellert, L. (2006). *Student diversity: Classroom strategies to meet the learning needs of all students*. Pembroke Publishers Limited.https://doi.org/10.1177/07419325030240060501

[149] Florian, L. (2015). Inclusive Pedagogy: A transformative approach to individual differences but can it help reduce educational inequalities. *Scottish Educational Review*, *47*(1), 5-14. https://www.scotedreview.org.uk/ media/microsites/scottish-educational-review/other-docs/2015_47-1_ May_03_Florian.pdf

[150] Lloyd, C. (2008). Removing barriers to achievement: a strategy for inclusion or exclusion? *International Journal of Inclusive Education*, *12*(2), 221-236. https://doi.org/10.1080/13603110600871413

[151] Schnotz, W. (2002). Towards an integrated view of learning from text and visual displays. *Educational Psychology Review*, 14, 101-120. https://doi.org/10.1023/A:1013136727916

[152] Kerr, S., & Baker, M. (2013). Six practical principles for inclusive curriculum design. In B. Tynan, J. Willems, & R. James (Eds.), *Outlooks and opportunities in blended and distance learning* (pp. 74-88). IGI Global.

[153] Wankat, P. (2002). *The effective efficient professor: Teaching, scholarship and service*. Allyn and Bacon.

[154] Milman, N. B. (2012). The flipped classroom strategy: What is it and how can it best be used? *Distance Learning*,

9(3), 85-7. https://tojdel.net/journals/tojdel/articles/v03i01/v03i01-04.pdf

[155] Charlton, J. I. (2000). *Nothing about us without us: Disability oppression and empowerment*. University of California Press

[156] Nunan, T., George, R., & McCausland, H. (2000). Inclusive education in universities: Why is it important and how might it be achieved. *International Journal of Inclusive Education*, 4(1), 63-88. https://doi.org/10.1080/136031100284920

[157] McNulty, M. A. (2003) Dyslexia and the life course. *Journal of Learning Disabilities,* 36(4), 363-381. https://doi.org/10.1177/00222194030360040701

[158] Singer, E. (2005). The strategies adopted by Dutch children with dyslexia to maintain their self-esteem when teased at school. *Journal of Learning Disabilities,* 38, 411-423. https://doi.org/10.1177/00222194050380050401

[159] Khan, M. (1964). Ego distortion, cumulative trauma, and the role of reconstruction in the analytic situation. *International Journal of Psycho-Analysis*, *45*, 272-279. https://www.pep-web.org/document.php?id=IJP.045.0272A

[160] Snyder, L. A., Carmichael, J. S., Blackwell, L. V., Cleveland, J. N., & Thornton, G. C. III. (2010). Perceptions of discrimination and justice among employees with disabilities. Employee Responsibilities and Rights Journal, 22, 5-19. https://doi.org/10.1007/s10672-009-9107-5

[161] Barga, N. K. (1996). Students with learning disabilities in education: Managing a disability. *Journal of Learning Disabilities*, 29, 413-421. https://doi.org/10.1177/002221949602900409

[162] Rao, S. (2004). Faculty attitudes and students with disabilities in higher education: A literature review. *College Student Journal*, 38(2), 191-198. https://go.gale.com/ps/anonymous?id=GALE%7CA119741925

[163] Bohdanowicz, K. (2015). How to End the Shame of Dyslexia? Education. *The Times Educational Supplement*, *5133*, 46. https://www.tes.com/news/how-end-shame-dyslexia-education

[164] Nalavany, B. A., Carawan, L. W., & Sauber, S. (2015). Adults with dyslexia, an invisible disability: The mediational role of concealment on perceived family support and self-esteem. *The British Journal of Social Work*, *45*(2), 568-586. https://doi.org/10.1093/bjsw/bct152

[165] Mortimore, T., & Crozier, W. R. (2007). Dyslexia and difficulties with study skills in higher education. *Studies in Higher Education*, 31(2), 235-251. https://doi.org/10.1080/03075070600572173

[166] Falzon, R., & Camilleri, S. (2010). Dyslexia and the school counsellor: A Maltese case study. *Counselling and Psychotherapy Research*, *10*(4), 307-315. https://doi.org/10.1080/14733140903370228

[167] Gerber, P. J., & Reiff, H. B. (1991). *Speaking for themselves: Ethnographic interviews with adults with learning disabilities* (No. 9). Univ of Michigan Press. DOI: 10.3998/mpub.9690752

[168] Gerber, P. J., Reiff, H. B. & Ginsberg, R. (1996) Reframing the learning disabilities experience.*Journal of Learning Disabilities,* 29(1), 98. https://doi.org/10.1177/002221949602900112

[169] Frymier, A. B., Wanzer M. B. (2003). Examining Differences in Perceptions of Students' Communication with Professors: A Comparison of Students with and without Disabilities. *Communication Quarterly* 51 (2), 174-191. https://doi.org/10.1080/01463370309370149

[170] Reiff, H. B.; Gerber, P. & Ginsberg, R. (1997) Exceeding expectations: Successful adults with learning disabilities. Pro-Ed.

[171] Duchane, K., Leung, R., & Coulter-Kern, R. (2008, October). Pre-service Physical Educator Attitude Toward Teaching Students with Disabilities. Clinical Kinesiology (Online) 62(3), 16-20. https://go.gale.com/ps/anonymous?id=GALE%7CA192975563

[172] Upton, T. D., Harper, D. C., & Wadsworth, J. S. (2005). Postsecondary attitudes towards persons with disabilities: A comparison of college students with and without disabilities. Journal of Applied Rehabilitation Counselling, 36 (3), 24-31. https://doi.org/10.1891/0047-2220.36.3.24

[173] Field, S., Sarver, M. & Shaw, S. (2003). Self Determination: A key to success in postsecondary education for students with learning disabilities. Remedial and Special Education, 24, 339-349. https://doi.org/10.1177/07419325030240060501

[174] Mishna, F. (2003). Learning disabilities and bullying: Double jeopardy. Journal of Learning Disabilities, 36, 1-15. https://doi.org/10.1177/00222194030360040501

[175] Hornstra, L., Denessen, E., Voeten, M., van den Bergh, L., & Bakker, J. (2010). Teacher attitudes toward dyslexia: Effects on teacher expectations and the academic achievement of students with dyslexia. Journal of Learning Disabilities, 43(6), 515-529. https://doi.org/10.1177/0022219409355479

[176] Higgins, E. L., Raskind, M. H., Goldberg, R. J., & Herman, K. L. (2002). Stages of acceptance of a learning disability: The impact of labelling. Learning Disability Quarterly, 25, 3-18. https://doi.org/10.2307/1511187

[177] Powell, J. J. (2013). From ableism to accessibility in the universal design university. *Review of Disability Studies: An International Journal*, *8*(4), 33-45.

[178] Hehir, T. (2017). How Did You Get to Harvard?. *Educational Leadership*, *74*(7), 36-40. Available from https://eric.ed.gov/?id=EJ1138116

[179] Bianco, M. (2005). The effects of disability labels on special education and general education teachers' referrals for gifted programs. Learning Disability Quarterly, 28(4), 285-293. https://doi.org/10.2307/4126967

[180] Solvang, P. (2007). Developing an ambivalence perspective on medical labelling in education: case dyslexia. *International studies in sociology of education*, *17*(1-2), 79-94. https://doi.org/10.1080/09620210701433779

[181] Taylor, L., Hume, I., & Welsh, N. (2010). Labelling and Self-Esteem: The impact of using specific vs. generic labels. Educational Psychology, 30(2), 191-202. https://doi.org/10.1080/01443410903494478

[182] Riddick, B. (1996). Living with dyslexia: The social and emotional consequences of specific learning difficulties. Routledge

[183] Kendall, L. (2018). Supporting students with disabilities within a UK university: Lecturer perspectives. *Innovations in Education and Teaching International*, *55*(6), 694-703. https://doi/full/10.1080/14703297.2017.1299630

[184] Ryder, D., & Norwich, B. (2019). UK higher education lecturers' perspectives of dyslexia, dyslexic students and related disability provision. *Journal of Research in Special Educational Needs*, *19*(3), 161-172. https://doi/epdf/10.1111/1471-3802.12438

[185] Parrila, R., Georgiou, G., & Crokett, J. (2007). University students with a significant history of reading

difficulties: What is and is not compensated? Exceptionality Education Canada, 17, 195-220. https://ir.lib.uwo.ca/eei/vol17/iss2/4/

[186] Dale, M. & Taylor, B. (2001) How adult learners make sense of their dyslexia. *Disability &Society,* 16(7), 997-1008. https://doi.org/10.1080/09687590120097872

[187] Schmar-Dobler, E. (2003). Reading on the Internet: The link between literacy and technology. *Journal of adolescent & adult literacy*, *47*(1), 80-85. Available from https://www.jstor.org/stable/40026906

[188] Ertmer, P. A., Ottenbreit-Leftwich, A. T., & Tondeur, J. (2015). Teachers' beliefs and uses of technology to support 21st-century teaching and learning. *International handbook of research on teacher beliefs*, 403-418. Available from http://hdl.handle.net/1854/LU-5815883

[189] Lysenko, L. V., & Abrami, P. C. (2014). Promoting reading comprehension with the use of technology. *Computers & Education*, *75*, 162-172. https://doi.org/10.1016/j.compedu.2014.01.010

[190] Harnad, S. (1991). Post-Gutenberg galaxy: The fourth revolution in the means of production of knowledge. *Public-access computer systems review*, *2*(1), 39-53. http://cogprints.org/1580/1/harnad91.postgutenberg.html

[191] Ok, M. W., & Rao, K. (2019). Digital tools for the inclusive classroom: Google chrome as assistive and instructional technology. *Journal of Special Education Technology*, 34(3), 204-211. https://doi.org/10.1177/0162643419841546

[192] Warschauer, M., & Matuchniak, T. (2010). New technology and digital worlds: Analyzing evidence of equity in access, use, and outcomes. *Review of research in education*, *34*(1), 179-225. https://doi.org/10.3102/0091732x09349791

[193] Castell, M. (1998). The End of Millenium, Vol. 3 of the Information Age.

[194] Castells, M. 1998. *End of Millenium.* Vol. 3 of *Information age: Economy, society, and culture*, Blackwell. Available from http://citeseerx.ist.psu.edu/viewdoc/download?doi= 10.1.1.457.4928&rep=rep1&type=pdf

[195] The Economist (2020, August 8-14). Briefing: COVID-19 and College. Uncanny University *The Economist,* 14-16. Also retrievable from https://www.economist.com/briefing/2020/08/08/ covid-19-could-push-some-universities-over-the-brink

[196] The Economist (2020), August 8-14), The absent student. *The Economist,* 7. Also retrievable from https://www.economist.com/weeklyedition/2020-08-08

[197] Prensky, M. (2001). Digital natives, digital immigrants. *On the horizon*, *9*(5). https://doi.org/10.1108/10748120110424816.

[198] Kennedy, G. E., Judd, T. S., Churchward, A., Gray, K., & Krause, K.-L. (2008). First year students' experiences with technology: Are they really digital natives? *Australasian Journal of Educational Technology*, *24*(1). https://doi.org/10.14742/ajet.1233

[199] UNESCO (n.d.) *Literacy.* Available from https://en.unesco.org/themes/literacy. [Accessed 2020/10/16]

[200] Clinton (1994, August 24). Statement on the Observance of International Literacy Day August 24, 1994. Authenticate US Government Information. https://www.govinfo.gov/content/pkg/WCPD-1994-08-29/pdf/WCPD-1994-08-29-Pg1713.pdf

[201] Alexander-Passe N (2016). The School's Role in Creating Successful and Unsuccessful Dyslexics. J Psychol Psychother 6: 238. doi:10.4172/2161-0487.1000238

Chapter 2

Effects of a Phonological Intervention on EEG Connectivity Dynamics in Dyslexic Children

Nicolas Bedo, Dikla Ender-Fox, Janet Chow, Linda Siegel, Urs Ribary and Lawrence M. Ward

Abstract

We examined the brain networks and oscillatory dynamics, inferred from EEG recordings during a word-reading task, of a group of children in grades 4 and 5 (ages 9–11), some of whom were dyslexic. We did this in order to characterize the differences in these dynamics between typical and dyslexic readers, and to begin to characterize the effect of a phonological intervention on those differences. Dyslexic readers were recorded both before and after they participated in a FastForWord (FFW) reading training program for approximately six months and typical readers were recorded once during this period. Before FFW dyslexic readers showed (i) a bottleneck in letter recognition areas, (ii) expansion in activity and connectivity into the right hemisphere not seen in typical readers, and (iii) greater engagement of higher-level language areas, even for consonant string stimuli. After FFW, dyslexic readers evinced a significant reduction in the engagement of language processing areas, and more activity and connectivity expanding to frontal areas, more resembling typical readers. Reduction of connectivity was negatively correlated with gains in reading performance, suggesting an increase in communication efficiency. Training appeared to improve the efficiency of the alternative (bilateral) pathways already used by the dyslexic readers, rather than inducing them to create new pathways more similar to those employed by typical readers.

Keywords: dyslexia, EEG, interregional connectivity, oscillatory dynamics, phonological intervention

1. Introduction

Having a reading disability, as seen in dyslexic children, is a very serious issue and often causes secondary emotional and cognitive consequences for the individual, as well as their family and their society [1]. Therefore, understanding the detailed underlying neurophysiological mechanisms of reading and their oscillatory brain network dynamics is of most importance.

Given the prevalence of phonological deficits in people with dyslexia [2, 3], it follows that training in phonological processing (and the underlying auditory processing therein) should improve reading ability. Indeed, there is evidence supporting this idea although there is some disagreement in the literature. Training and remediation programs that emphasize phonics and phonemic awareness have been shown to improve fluency and comprehension [4–8]. Neuroimaging results reflect these findings, showing increases of cortical activity in reading-related areas including left fusiform, IFG, and temporo-parietal cortex, as well as right STG and IFG areas following training [8, 9].

Although the aforementioned neuroimaging results are useful, the exact underlying brain dynamics across local and large-scale networks are largely unknown. In particular, previous studies have not addressed the way information flows throughout reading networks during the process of reading words, and how this might be changed by an intervention designed to improve reading performance. The present study concerns the brain-regional connectivity dynamics of reading before and after an interventional reading training program. Of particular interest is the relationship between improvement in reading performance and changes in connectivity. Understanding this relationship may offer new insights into reading disabilities as well as ideas about how to further optimize reading training programs to elicit the highest performance gains. In what follows, we describe an experiment that compared the connectivity dynamics of a typical-reading group of children with that of a group of same-aged children who are significantly reading-impaired. The typical readers were measured once (given limitation of EEG measurements in school environment), and the challenged readers were measured twice: once before a reading training program in which the latter children had been enrolled, and once after those children had experienced the training program for a period of 6 months.

Despite a growing literature on the development of impaired reading-related brain regions in dyslexia [8, 10], it is much less understood just how the communication between these regions also changes as a function of time on a millisecond scale. In what ways does the reading network become more or less efficient throughout development, and which connections are being utilized more or less effectively? These emergent local and large-scale brain network dynamics are very critical at the age of these children, with known developmental stabilization but also plasticity and vulnerability [11]. To that end, this study sought to investigate the development of reading-related brain connectivity in dyslexic children by comparing functional and effective connectivity measures prior to intervention and after 6 months of schooling supplemented by a phonologically-based reading training program.

Despite the evidence as to how specific brain sites develop or alter in response to this training, it remains unclear how the overarching reading networks develop as a function of this training. Moreover, with regard to laterality of reading functions in the brain, it is unclear as to whether connectivity in dyslexic children shifts to include more traditional left-hemispheric engagement, or if their reading networks instead continue to emphasize right-hemisphere networks [9, 12].

Importantly, some researchers have argued that neural oscillations – particularly in theta- and gamma-bands – play a critical role in the processing of written language [13–15]. In particular, these neural network oscillations are said to be perturbed in atypical brains such as those of dyslexic readers [16]. Thus, in our study we focused on oscillatory activity and functional and effective connectivity in theta- and gamma-bands.

We first needed to establish a "baseline" of brain network behaviour prior to the reading intervention program. The readers in the present experiment were in grades 4 and 5. Although children typically learn to read in grade 1, we chose this older group to study, reasoning that an additional three to four years of brain development – and particularly years of reading training – can produce very different reading network patterns from those just learning to read. Moreover, if children are still struggling to read in grade four, it is clear that they have a severe deficit that requires remediation. Finally, we reasoned that the additional years of brain development (potentially without reading improvement or intervention) would produce brain network behaviours in older children that were both different from those of typical readers, and also perhaps somewhat more resistant to change.

1.1 What happens 220 milliseconds after word presentation?

The temporal resolution of EEG affords the examination of brain activity at millisecond precision. Using such techniques, researchers have found specific moments in processing that reflect critical steps in the cognitive processing of words. Perhaps the most-commonly reproduced finding in reading is the N170 ERP component above the left fusiform gyrus in adult readers, in which a prominent negative peak is observed in the averaged EEG approximately 170 ms after word presentation [17–19]. This moment represents the orthographic processing step in word reading, where visual inputs are classified as orthography (written language) to then be passed along to higher-level language areas for further evaluation (e.g. extracting phonological information; [20]). In young children, this same processes is delayed somewhat to ~220 ms, as they are still developing the skills necessary to decode orthographic information [21–23]. So, when studying the neural dynamics of reading in children, this moment becomes critical in enhancing our understanding.

In this paper we focus our connectivity analyses on a specific window of time, 200–250 ms after word presentation, to capture the 5-dimensional brain oscillatory connectivity dynamics (across 3D space, time and frequency) of orthographic processing and the propagation of the reading information thereafter in the reading networks of dyslexic and typically-developing children. The lateralization of the connectivity, as well as the engagement of language areas in this time window may offer critical insights as to the neural underpinnings of dyslexia.

We hypothesized that, prior to intervention, children with reading difficulties would show altered and greater functional and effective connectivity in the theta and gamma frequency bands among reading-related sites compared to grade appropriate readers of the same age. These differences would arise because of the greater difficulty the impaired readers would have in decoding the orthographic symbols into language. We expected that these differences would be reduced after the intervention, at least to the extent the intervention ameliorated the reading difficulties and resulted in more fluid and effortless orthographic processing.

2. Methods

2.1 Participants

Twenty-eight students attending elementary schools in the Burnaby school district (BC, Canada) participated. In partnership with the school district, students in grades 4 and 5 were targeted to be a part of this study, making up a total potential pool of approximately 135 students. Parents of these students received information about the study and our consent forms through the schools. All eventual participants received parental consent and also gave verbal assent to participate. The protocol of the experiment was approved by the Behavioural Research Ethics Boards at the University of British Columbia and Simon Fraser University as well as by the Burnaby School Board in accordance with the provisions of the World Medical Association Declaration of Helsinki. Prior to our study, a subset of all grade 4 and grade 5 students had already been assessed by the schools as having specific reading difficulties and were already selected to be placed in an intervention program using FastForWord software (FFW; Scientific Learning, USA; see also [6, 7]) to practice core language skills such as phonemic awareness, auditory discrimination, and spelling. Thus, our sample of this group was an opportunity sample, granting us an opportunity to study the neurodynamics of challenged readers as they experienced this targeted intervention. Selection into the intervention program was determined over time, using a multi-tiered approach developed by the teachers and administrators prior to the start of our study. Selection criteria for the FFW program by the schools included apparent auditory processing deficits, difficulty in associating letters with sound, and reading 1.5–2 years below grade level—observations often further assessed by Woodcock-Johnson standardized achievement tests (Word Attack, Letter-Word Identification, and Passage Comprehension sub-tests), the Wechsler Intelligence Scale for Children – Fourth Edition (WISC-IV; Digit Span and Symbol Search sub-tests), and the Test of Auditory Processing Skills – Third Edition (TAPS-III; Word Discrimination, Phonological Blending, and Phonological Segmentation sub-tests). Guided by the district's selection criteria, Language Support Services (LSS; e.g. speech and language pathologists) were also involved as part of the process and aided in the admission into the FFW program. The FFW program was never used as the initial point of intervention; rather, students were only admitted into the targeted reading training if no other intensive strategies had worked or if students were showing very small gains with other methods. These LSS professionals eventually conducted the training during school hours. Ultimately, through this vetting process, 15 FFW-eligible students were given consent forms.

A set of typically developing readers (TYP, control sample), not enrolled in the interventional reading training programs, were selected at random, from among those students whose parents gave consent and also who gave verbal assent, from the classrooms of the dyslexic pre/post-FFW students to control for effects of teacher and general curriculum received. All participants had English as their first and primary language, and had normal or corrected-to-normal visual acuity. FFW students had been in the program for less than one month at the time of the initial experimental session. This effort was made to record a baseline measure before any targeted reading intervention occurred. In total, 11 FFW readers and 17 TYP readers were recruited for this experiment.

2.2 Experimental procedures

The experiment was conducted on-site at elementary schools in the Burnaby school district (Vancouver, Canada). A quiet room at each school was set aside for each session. First, children were asked to simply sit in a relaxed position for five minutes while their brainwaves were recorded using EEG during resting state. Participants then performed a lexical decision task in which they were asked to decide whether a letter string was a real word or not (i.e., "Is this a real word?"). Stimuli were classified into three conditions: real words (e.g., 'bread'), pseudowords (e.g., 'croll'), and consonant strings (e.g., 'rplcg'). A fixation cross was presented for 500 ms followed by a jittered inter-stimulus interval lasting between 800 and 1200 ms (**Figure 1**). Then a letter string was presented for 1500 ms or until the participant pressed a response, whichever occurred first. After a 1000 ms inter-trial interval, the next trial began. For the Word condition, single-syllable words were aggregated from lists found at https://www.ontrackreading.com.These lists have been assembled to be accessible to children and to represent a wide range of vowel sounds. Pseudowords were derived from the pool of real word stimuli by taking a word and changing a single letter (e.g. *bread* to *bream*). All participants, both pre-FFW (n = 11) and TYP (n = 17) students, participated in Session 1, but only the post-FFW (n = 9) student group

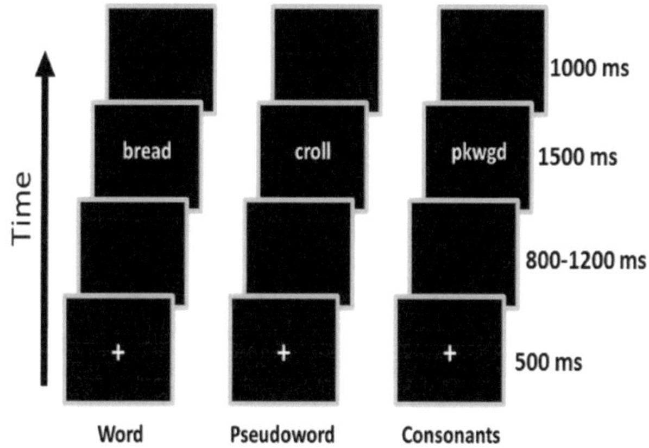

Figure 1.
Schematic of phonological lexical decision task. Participants were required to judge whether or not a letter string was a real word.

(also recorded in session 1) participated also in Session 2, which occurred about 6 months after Session 1. Unfortunately only the 9 post-FFW dyslexic students finished their training among the 11 who began it.

Stimuli from each condition consisted of 4- and 5-letter strings (60 trials each), each presented randomly for a total of 360 trials (120 trials per condition). Blocks of 40 trials were separated by self-timed rest breaks. Participants had the option to continue to the next block immediately upon reaching a break or they could rest as long as necessary before continuing. The task was performed on a laptop while sitting at a desk. A height-adjustable chin rest was used to reduce the possibility of head movements.

Presentation software (Neurobehavioral Systems, USA) was used to present stimuli in white font on a black background. All stimuli were centered on a 17-inch computer monitor placed 45 cm in front of the participants. All participants used their right hand to respond on the keyboard; however, the response buttons used for "Yes" and "No" were counterbalanced across subjects.

2.3 EEG acquisition

A portable BioSemi system, provided by the Behavioral and Cognitive Neuroscience Institute (BCNI), was used to record continuous EEG from 64 active electrodes at equidistant locations based on the International 10–10 system of electrode placement, referenced to the average of all scalp signals (except Iz). EEG signals were amplified and sampled at 512 Hz through an analog passband of 0.16–100 Hz. Eye muscle activity was recorded by electro-oculogram (EOG) from two periocular electrodes. All electrode impedances were below 20 kΩ.

All further offline processing and analysis was performed using MATLAB software (Mathworks, Natick, USA). All signals were re-referenced to an average reference, resampled to 256 Hz, and digitally filtered from 1 to 100 Hz using EEGLAB software [24], an open source MATLAB toolkit, and custom scripts. A digital notch filter from 55 Hz to 65 Hz was applied to reduce line noise. The continuous data were epoched into 3500 ms bins time-locked to the presentation of the letter strings, capturing 1500 ms before and 2000 ms after word presentation. In Session 1 each of the 28 participants contributed an average of 256.12 trials (SD = 73.41), for a total of 6659 trials for the experiment. In Session 2, each of the 9 participants from the FFW group contributed an average of about 250 trials for a total of 2250 trials. All further processing and analysis was performed using MATLAB software (Mathworks, Natick, USA).

2.4 Current source density

To reduce the impact of volume conduction on subsequent analyses, the EEG signals were first converted to current source density (CSD). CSD, the second spatial derivative of the scalp potential, acts as a spatial filter, emphasizing shallow sources close to each recording electrode thus reducing volume conduction and increasing confidence that the channels being analyzed did in fact represent predominantly activity of the brain regions over which the corresponding electrodes sat. Furthermore, CSD acts as a form of artifact rejection or attenuation, particularly of muscular artifacts that can heavily contaminate EEG signals [25]. CSD Toolbox for MATLAB with default parameter values for spline flexibility (spline interpolation constant $m = 4$) and smoothing (smoothing constant $lambda = 0.00001$) was used to compute the CSD values the continuous EEG data from each individual participant [26–28].

Cortical regions of interest (ROIs) for further analysis were selected based on reading-related brain areas as revealed in previous research (**Table 1**; [29]). The cortical Talairach coordinates of these sites were then cross-referenced to anatomical locations of electrodes based on the 10–10 system [30]. The nearest electrodes to these sites, as measured by Euclidean distance, were then selected for further analysis. The subset of electrodes selected in this manner were CP5, CP6, F5, F6, FT7, FT8, O1, O2, P7, P8, TP7, and TP8 (**Figure 2**). For ease of exposition the ROIs will be referred to by their closest cortical locations, but it must be remembered that in fact the data to be analysed are the CSD values computed for the electrode locations nearest those cortical locations and not the activation levels of cortical sources inferred through localization analysis.

	Talairach coordinates			
EEG channel	**x**	**y**	**z**	**Corresponding Brain Region**
F5	−51	27	25	L. IFG
F6	51	27	25	R. IFG
FT7	−59	3	−2	L. PreCG
FT8	59	3	−2	R. PreCG
CP5	−62	−46	23	L. AG/SMG
CP6	62	−46	23	R. AG/SMG
TP7	−64	−45	−4	L. MTG/STG
TP8	64	−45	−4	R. MTG/STG
P7	−56	−65	0	L. vOT
P8	56	−65	0	R. vOT
O1	−26	−93	8	L. Occip
O2	26	−93	8	R. Occip

Table 1.
EEG channels and their corresponding brain regions. EEG channels were selected for further analysis based on their proximity to previously established ROIs (Jobard et al., 2003) and their cross-hemispheric counterparts. Anatomic locations of EEG channels in Talairach space were derived from Koessler et al. (2009).

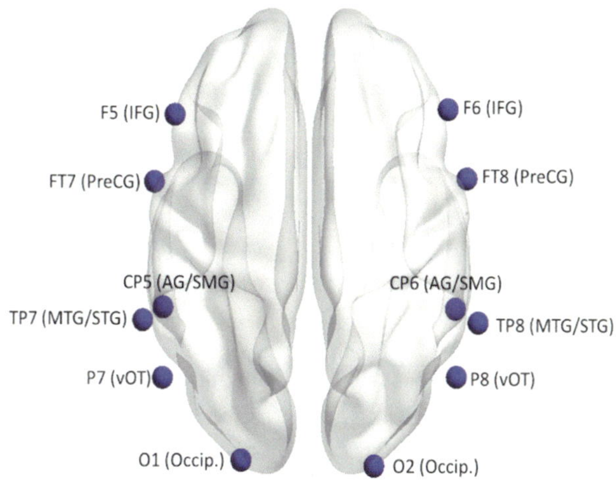

Figure 2.
Selected electrodes that overlap with reading-related brain areas. Visual representation of anatomical locations of channels as described in ***Table 1****.*

2.5 Event-related potentials (ERPs)

ERPs were computed by averaging each participant's epoched EEG activity in signal space and across trials. This was done separately for each condition. ERPs were baseline corrected relative to a 100 ms pre-stimulus window and low-pass filtered at 20 Hz. ERPs from each group were then compared using independent samples *t*-tests at each time point. Instances of significant differences between conditions sustained across multiple time points then informed the subsequent connectivity analyses as to which moments might provide insights into important network differences.

2.6 Event-related spectral perturbations (ERSPs)

ERSPs (10 log [power at time point *t*/average baseline power]; in dB units) allow us to observe the moment-to-moment fluctuations in oscillatory power at various oscillatory frequencies relative to a 100 ms pre-stimulus baseline. The powers at different frequencies were computed in 1.5 Hz increments from 3 Hz to 50 Hz using a sliding cosine wavelet (Hanning-windowed) with linearly increasing cycles from 1.8 cycles at 3 Hz to 30 cycles at 50 Hz. ERSPs were computed by EEGlab's *newtimef*() function across trials for each subject separately. This technique produced an output 400 time points in length, capturing ERSPs from −940 to 1440 ms of the original epoch.

Each ERSP output was then collapsed across each selected frequency band (i.e. theta and gamma) at each time point, such that the maximum absolute value of ERSP at any individual frequency in the band was used [31, 32]. This produced a time series for each channel that reflected its most prominent level of activation in a region at each time point. ERSPs from each condition were then compared using pairwise *t*-tests at each time point. Sustained instances of significant differences between groups then informed the eventual connectivity analyses as to which moments might provide insights into important network differences.

2.7 Phase synchrony

Phase synchrony analyses were conducted in order to assess inter-regional functional connectivity, or the degree to which two brain areas are sharing information, in theta- (3–8 Hz) and gamma- (30–50 Hz) bands. This was done by computing the phase-locking values (PLVs) between pairs of electrodes located over reading-related brain regions. PLVs were computed using the following formula [24]:

$$PLV_{1,2}(f,t) = \frac{1}{N}\sum_{k=1}^{N} \frac{W_{1,k}(f,t)W_{2,k}^{*}(f,t)}{\left|W_{1,k}(f,t)W_{2,k}(f,t)\right|} \quad (1)$$

where $Wi,k(f,t)$ are the wavelet coefficients for each time point, t, and frequency, f, for each EEG channel, i, and $k = 1$ to N is the index of epochs. The PLVs produced by these computations indicate the degree of constancy of the phase differences between signals at a specific oscillatory frequency across trials. PLVs range from 0 to 1, where 0 indicates the absence of any phase locking, and 1 indicates perfect phase locking, such that the phase difference between two channels at a given time point remains constant across all trials. Only stochastic phase locking, with $0 < \text{PLV} < 1$, is expected from any time series of brain activity because of neural noise [33].

PLVs were computed by EEGlab's *newcrossf*() function across subjects separately and for each time point for all channel pairs. This technique produced an output 400 time points in length, capturing ERSPs from −940 to 1440 ms of the original epoch. The phase lags of the significant PLVs were always significantly different from zero (as determined by circular t-tests, $p < 0.001$), indicating that volume conduction, which can cause spurious zero-phase-lag synchronization, could not have been responsible for any significant PLVs.

PLVs were baseline corrected by subtracting the mean of PLVs in the 100 ms window immediately preceding stimulus presentation from the dataset. Each output was then collapsed across each frequency band at that time point (theta and gamma bands), such that the maximum absolute value of PLV at any individual frequency in the band was used, identical to the process used for ERSPs. This consolidated the time series for each channel pair so that it reflected their degree of functional connectivity in this pair of regions at each time point. In order to differentiate PLV connectivity patterns between groups, two-tailed independent t-tests ($\alpha = 0.01$) were used.

In order to assess the connectivity patterns with each group, two-tailed one-sample t-tests ($\alpha = 0.001$) were employed to determine the statistical significance of these PLVs relative to zero at each time point. As a means to differentiate PLV connectivity patterns between groups, two-tailed independent t-tests ($\alpha = 0.01$) were used, comparing FFW and TYP groups at each time point.

To assess the statistical reliability of these t-tests, time points from 0 to 900 ms following the stimulus onset were divided into non-overlapping 50 ms time bins (i.e., 18 such bins). To control for multiple comparisons, and to exclude meaningless interactions, we adopted a conservative criterion and considered a 50 ms bin to contain meaningful evidence of greater functional connectivity for one group than for the other if at least half (5 or more of 9) of the time points in that bin reached the statistical threshold described earlier for either TYP > pre/post-FFW, or vice versa, and none did for the opposite comparison. To assess the experiment-wise error of this procedure, we used $p = 0.01$ ($q = 1 - p = 0.99$) as the probability of a success in a single binomial trial to compute the binomial probability of getting 5 or more significant time points by chance out of the total of 9 time points in each 50-ms bin [36]. This probability is 1.21×10^{-8} if all of the time points in a bin represented independent tests. This assumption of independence is probably not precisely correct as using consecutive time points will lack complete independence, although it is not too unreasonable because the tests were made across subjects, who were independent of each other. Since we made 66 (inter-regional) comparisons (each possible pairing of 12 different brain ROIs) for 18 time bins, there were 1188 such tests. At most (p = 0.01, with the minimum 5 of 9 significant data points per bin), the experiment-wise error probability for each set of t-tests, assuming independence, was 1188 x 1.21 x 10^{-8} = .0000144.

2.8 Transfer entropy

Whereas measures of functional connectivity show which brain areas are engaged and sharing information (i.e. functionally connected), these measures do not indicate the directional flow of the information. That is, a measure such as phase synchrony does not indicate which site is *sending* the information, and which site is *receiving* the information, or if a bi-directional relationship exists. In order to understand such relationships, effective connectivity analyses must be employed. To address this, we employed transfer entropy, a recently developed technique for revealing directed information flow without needing to specify or fit a model [34]. Transfer entropy from time series J to time series I is defined [34] as the (asymmetric) Kullback-Liebler entropy between two time series at a specified, non-zero, lag (k-l):

$$T_{J\to I} = \sum p\left(i_{n+1}, i_n^{(k)}, j_n^{(l)}\right) \log \frac{p\left(i_{n+1} \middle| i_n^{(k)}, j_n^{(l)}\right)}{p\left(i_{n+1} \middle| i_n^{(k)}\right)}. \quad (2)$$

Transfer entropy measures the extent to which the transition probabilities (dynamics) between states within one time series (say J) are *not* independent of the past states of another time series (say I). It is larger the greater the influence of the state of I on the transition probabilities of J. Both the influence of J on I and that of I on J can be computed in this way. With regard to information transfer between neural sources, transfer entropy computes the additional information predicted by one region that is not already predicted by another region's prior activity. Narrow-band transfer entropy (NBTE) is a variant of this, whereby transfer entropy is computed *within a specific frequency band* rather than over the broadband signal [35]. The TIM toolbox, developed by German Gomez-Herrero and Kalle Rutanen, for MATLAB (http://www.cs.tut.fi/~timhome/tim/tim.htm) was employed to compute theta- and gamma-band NBTE.

Theta-band (3–8 Hz) and gamma-band (30–50 Hz) oscillatory time series were obtained by filtering the CSD activations in the epochs using EEGlab's digital FIR filter. NBTE was then computed across trials for each subject at 30 ms and 50 ms lags. The lags used here span the range of lags found to contain significant NBTE in previous similar investigations [13, 35].

In order to assess the connectivity patterns within each group, two-tailed one-sample t-tests (α = 0.05) were employed to determine the statistical significance of these NBTE values relative to zero at each time point. As a means to differentiate NBTE connectivity patterns between groups, two-tailed independent t-tests (α = 0.01) were used, comparing FFW and TYP groups at each time point.

To assess the experiment-wise error of this procedure, we used p = 0.05 (q = 1 – p = 0.95) as the probability of a success in a single binomial trial to compute the binomial probability of getting 7 or more significant time points by chance out of the total of 13 time points in each 50-ms bin [36]. This probability is 9.85 x 10^{-7} if all of the time points in a bin represented independent tests. This assumption of independence is probably not precisely correct as using consecutive time points will lack complete independence, although it is not too unreasonable because the tests were made across subjects, who were independent of each other. Since we made

132 (inter-regional) comparisons (each possible pairing of 12 different brain ROIs in both directions) for 18 time bins, there were 2376 such tests. At most ($p = 0.05$, with the minimum 7 of 13 significant data points per bin), the experiment-wise error probability for each set of t-tests, assuming independence, was 2376 x 9.85 x $10^{-7} = 0.00234$.

2.9 Connectivity correlations

Measuring the brain activity from FFW participants at two distinct time points (pre-FFW and post-FFW) gave us the opportunity to examine the relationship between gains in reading performance and changes in network connectivity. Correlations were computed, both before and after the FastForWord intervention, between FFW participant assessment scores (WJ-WA and WJ-LW tests) and connectivity measures (PLVs and NBTE) for the nine post-FFW participants who participated at both times (session 1 and session 2). This process followed the exact set of methods in the synchrony and transfer entropy analyses, but used the difference in assessment scores (POST – PRE) and the differences in connectivity values (POST – PRE).

Correlations were employed to determine the statistical significance of these associations between brain connectivity and assessment scores at each time point ($\alpha = 0.01$ for PLVs, 0.05 for NBTE). To assess the experiment-wise error of this procedure, we used $p = 0.01$ ($q = 1 - p = 0.99$) as the probability of a success in a single binomial trial to compute the binomial probability of getting 5 or more significant time points by chance out of the total of 9 time points in each 50-ms bin for correlations with PLVs. This probability is 1.21 x 10^{-8} if all of the time points in a bin represented independent tests. This assumption of independence is probably not precisely correct as using consecutive time points will lack complete independence. Since we made 66 (inter-regional) comparisons (each possible pairing of 12 different brain ROIs) for 18 time bins, there were 1188 such tests. At most ($p = 0.01$, with the minimum 5 of 9 significant data points per bin), the experiment-wise error probability for each set of t-tests, assuming independence, was 1188 x 1.21 x $10^{-8} = .0000144$.

The experiment-wise error for the NBTE correlations required 7 or more significant time points out of 13 time points ($p = 0.05$) to consider a 50 ms to be significant. This probability is 9.85 x 10^{-7} if all of the time points in a bin represented independent tests. Since we made 132 (inter-regional) comparisons (each possible pairing of 12 different brain ROIs in both directions) for 18 time bins, there were 2376 such tests. At most ($p = 0.05$, with the minimum 7 of 13 significant data points per bin), the experiment-wise error probability for each set of t-tests, assuming independence, was 2376 x 9.85 x $10^{-7} = .000234$.

3. Results

3.1 Comparison of TYP and pre-FFW groups

3.1.1 Behavioural performance

Woodcock-Johnson tests (Word Attack and Letter-Word Identification) were conducted on a subset of all participants (9 pre-FFW (those who were tested twice), 11 TYP) by the experimenters to validate the differentiation of groups with regard to reading difficulties initially appraised by the schools (**Figure 3A**). The pre-FFW group showed significantly lower scores compared to the TYP group

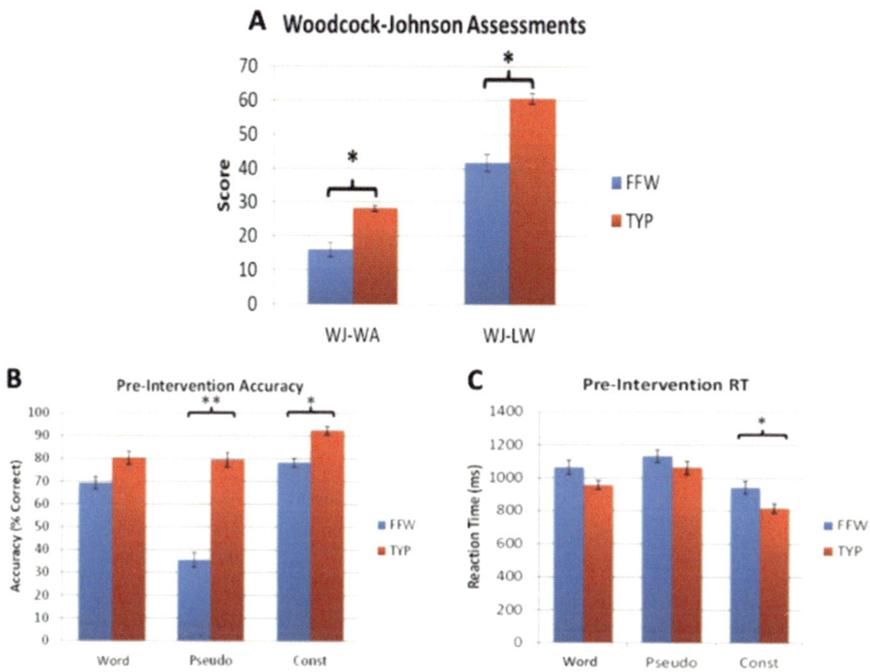

Figure 3.
*(A) Reading assessments of typical readers (TYP) and atypical (FFW) readers before starting the Fast Forword training program in both the Word Attack (WJ-WA) and Letter-Word Identification (WJ-LW) tests. *p < 0.0001. (B) Pre-FFW lexical decision task accuracy before starting training. Word = Word, Pseudo = Pseudoword, Const = Consonant Strings. *p < 0.05, **p < 0.0001. (C) Pre-FFW lexical decision task reactions times before starting training. Word = Word, Pseudo = Pseudoword, Const = Consonant Strings. *p < 0.05.*

in both the Word Attack subtest, $t(18) = 6.64$, $p < 0.0001$, and the Letter-Word Identification subtest, $t(18) = 5.14$, $p < 0.0001$.

Accuracy in each experimental task condition was measured as percentage of correct trials. The pre-FFW group was significantly less accurate than the TYP group in the Consonant condition, $t(23) = 2.15$, $p = 0.04$ (**Figure 3B**). The FFW was also significantly less accurate than in the TYP group in the Pseudoword condition, $t(23) = 5.37$, $p < 0.0001$. The accuracy difference between groups in the Word condition was not statistically significant ($t(23) = 1.83$, $p = 0.08$), although the 11% difference was in the direction of TYP > pre-FFW as for the other conditions.

With respect to reaction time, the pre-FFW group was significantly slower than the TYP group in the Consonant condition, $t(23) = 2.54$, $p = 0.02$ (**Figure 3C**). There was no significant difference in reaction time between groups in the Pseudoword condition, $t(23) = 1.11$, $p = 0.28$, or the Word condition, $t(23) = 1.49$, $p = 0.15$, although the TYP group was faster than the pre-FFW group in all conditions.

3.1.2 ERPs

ERPs from TYP and pre-FFW groups were compared at each time point for each condition using two-sample *t*-tests (**Figure 4A**). The pre-FFW group showed a more pronounced N170/220 component (early negative peak) at R.vOT and R.AG sites in all three conditions 200–250 ms following stimulus presentation ($p < 0.05$, uncorrected) as well as from L.AG in the Pseudoword condition. In the Pseudoword and Word conditions, the pre-FFW group also generated a larger P1 component at R.vOT 100–150 ms after stimulus presentation, as well as greater activation in

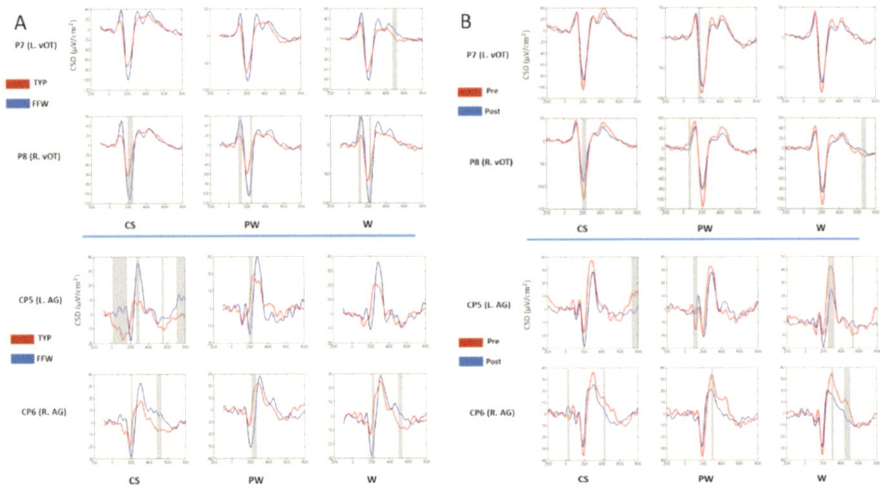

Figure 4.
(A) Event-related potentials (ERPs) during word reading for selected electrodes before Fast Forword training for typical readers (TYP) and atypical readers (FFW). Sections highlighted in grey indicate significant differences between groups (p < 0.05, uncorrected). CS = Consonant String; PW = Pseudoword; W = Word; vOT = ventral Occipito-Temporal cortex; AG = Angular Gyrus. (B) ERPs comparing engaged reading-related brain regions between sessions (pre-FFW vs. post-FFW). Sections highlighted in grey indicate significant differences between groups (p < 0.05, uncorrected). CS = Consonant String; PW = Pseudoword; W = Word; vOT = ventral Occipito-Temporal cortex; AG = Angular Gyrus.

L.vOT at 475–540 ms. At area L.AG, the pre-FFW group produced a significantly larger ERP immediately following stimulus presentation, as well as a more pronounced peak from 260 to 310 ms. The pre-FFW group produced late ERP components (>500 ms) in both L.AG and R.AG sites in the Consonants condition, while R.AG showed this effect in the Word condition, as well.

3.1.3 ERSPs

Spectral power dynamics were investigated at reading-related sites at theta (3–8 Hz) (**Figure 5A**) and gamma (30–50 Hz) (**Figure 5B**) frequency bands. Between-subjects *t*-tests revealed greater theta power for the pre-FFW group in the Consonants condition at L.AG from 210 to 280 ms, R.AG from 650 to 800 ms, and R.AG from 100 to 260 ms and 360–410 ms ($p < 0.05$, uncorrected). The pre-FFW group showed greater theta power at R.vOT in the Pseudoword condition from 180 to 240 ms. In the Word condition, the pre-FFW group showed greater theta power at R.AG from 195 to 300 ms and at R.vOT from 175 to 290 ms. These results highlight not only the greater amount of resources engaged by the pre-FFW group for written language, but also the bilateral nature of this processing, such that they utilize regions of the right hemisphere to an extent that TYP readers do not.

Between-subjects *t*-tests revealed greater gamma power for the pre-FFW group in the Consonants condition at R.vOT from 110 to 385 ms and 595–780 ms ($p < 0.05$, uncorrected). The pre-FFW group showed greater gamma power in the Pseudoword condition at R.AG from 270 to 305 ms, and at R.vOT from 300 to 405 ms. The TYP group showed greater gamma power in the Consonant condition at R.AG from 585 to 630 ms, in the Pseudoword condition at L.AG from 440 to 510 ms, and in the Word condition at R.vOT from 475 to 580 ms. Overall, The TYP group showed more gamma power later in the trial (>400 ms) in the right-hemispheric regions during Consonant and Word trials, as well as in L.AG during Pseudoword trials.

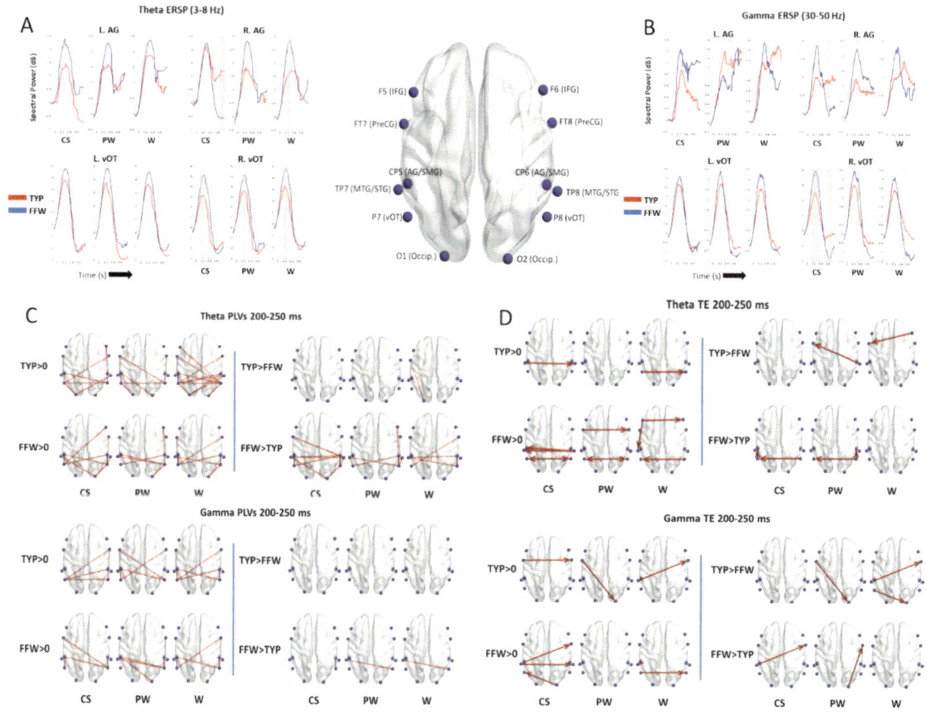

Figure 5.
(A) Theta-band ERSPs for both groups before training. Sections highlighted in grey indicate significant differences between groups (p < 0.05, uncorrected). (B). Gamma-band ERSPs for both groups before training. Sections highlighted in grey indicate significant differences between groups (p < 0.05, uncorrected). (C) (Top) Theta-band phase synchrony from 200 to 250 ms. (Left) Red lines between areas indicate significant changes in PLV compared to zero (p < 0.001); (Right) Red lines between areas indicate significant differences between groups (p < 0.01). (Bottom) Gamma-band phase synchrony from 200 to 250 ms. (Left) Red lines between areas indicate significant changes in PLV compared to zero (p < 0.001); (Right) Red lines between areas indicate significant differences between groups (p < 0.01). (D) (Top) Theta-band (3–8 Hz) NBTE from 200 to 250 ms. (Left) Red arrows between areas indicate significant changes in TE compared to zero; (Right) Red arrows between areas indicate significant differences between groups. (Bottom) Gamma-band (30–50 Hz) NBTE from 200 to 250 ms. (Left) Red arrows between areas indicate significant changes in TE compared to zero; (Right) Red arrows between areas indicate significant differences between groups. CS = Consonant String; PW = Pseudoword; W = Word; vOT = ventral Occipito-Temporal cortex; AG = Angular Gyrus.

3.1.4 Phase synchrony

As mentioned earlier, we focused our connectivity analyses on the time window 200–250 msec after word onset, as this window is critical for orthographic processing and transmitting the resulting information to areas downstream of the vOT cortex. Both groups showed distributed theta-band network functional connectivity relative to baseline across all conditions ($p < 0.001$; **Figure 5C**). Comparing groups, the TYP group show no instances of greater theta-band phase synchrony ($p < 0.01$) in any condition. The pre-FFW group showed greater theta-band PLVs between R.AG and L.PreCG, L.STG, L.vOT, and R.vOT in the Consonant condition, and between R.IFG and R.vOT in the Pseudoword condition. The pre-FFW group showed greater theta-band PLVs between L.STG and R.vOT, L.vOT and R.PreCG, and R.vOT and R.AG in the Word condition. Especially notable is the significant engagement of the vOT and AG regions in the right hemisphere across all conditions in the pre-FFW group.

Both groups showed distributed gamma-band network functional connectivity relative to baseline across all conditions ($p < 0.001$). Comparing groups, the TYP group did not yield any instances of greater gamma-band synchrony in any condition ($p < 0.01$). The pre-FFW group showed greater gamma PLVs between R.vOT and R.AG in the Consonant condition, and between R.vOT and L.STG in the Pseudoword and Word conditions. Again, especially notable is the engagement of the vOT region in the right hemisphere across all conditions.

3.1.5 Transfer entropy

The TYP group showed significant theta-band NBTE from L.STG to R.STG in the Consonant condition, as well as from L.vOT to R.vOT in the Word condition ($p < 0.05$; **Figure 5D**). The pre-FFW group showed significant NBTE from R.STG to L.STG and L.AG sites, in addition to a bi-directional relationship between L.vOT and R.vOT in the Consonant condition. The bi-directional relationship was present in the Pseudoword condition, accompanied by theta-band NBTE from L.PreCG to R.PreCG. In the Word condition, the pre-FFW group showed NBTE from L.IFG to L.STG and R.IFG, as well as from R.vOT to L.vOT. Comparing groups, the TYP group showed no instances of greater theta NBTE ($p < 0.01$) in the Consonant condition, although this group showed greater connectivity from R.STG to L.PreCG in the Pseudoword condition, and from R.IFG to L.PreCG in the Word condition. The pre-FFW group showed no instances of greater theta NBTE in the Word condition, but showed greater connectivity from R.vOT to L.vOT and from L.vOT to L.AG in the Consonant condition, and from R.vOT to L.vOT and from R.vOT to R.AG in the Pseudoword condition.

The TYP group showed significant gamma-band NBTE (relative to baseline) from L.PreCG to R.PreCG in the Consonant condition, from L.PreCG to R.Occipital cortex in the Pseudoword condition, and from L.STG to R.PreCG in the Word condition ($p < 0.05$, **Figure 5D**). The pre-FFW group showed significant gamma-band NBTE from L.AG to R.PreCG, from L.STG to R.STG, and from R.Occipital cortex to L.vOT in the Consonant condition, from L.vOT to R.vOT in the Word condition, and no gamma-band NBTE in the Pseudoword condition. Comparing groups, the TYP group showed greater gamma-band NBTE from L.PreCG to R.Occipital cortex in the Pseudoword condition ($p < 0.01$), from L.STG to R.PreCG and from L.vOT to R.Occiptial cortex in the Word condition. The pre-FFW group showed greater gamma-band NBTE from L.AG to R.PreCG in the Consonant condition and from R.Occipital cortex to R.PreCG in the Pseudoword condition.

3.2 Pre-post FFW intervention comparison

3.2.1 Behavioural performance

Whereas both WJ-WA and WJ-LW reading assessments revealed slight improvements after training in the post-FFW group, these improvements were overall not statistically significant. Participants showed increased scores for WJ-WA in the second session ($M = 18.73$, $SD = 4.34$) compared to session one ($M = 16$, $SD = 6.54$), though these gains were not statistically significant, $t(8) = 0.14$, $p > 0.05$. In the WJ-LW assessment, participants showed increased scores in the second session ($M = 44.64$, $SD = 6.86$) compared to session one ($M = 41.67$, $SD = 7.75$), although again not reaching statistical significance, $t(8) = 0.15$, $p > 0.05$. No significant difference in accuracy or reaction time on the experimental task was observed between sessions for the post-FFW group (**Tables 2** and **3**).

3.2.2 ERPs

In L.vOT, the POST session (post-FFW) yielded a less pronounced N170/220 negative peak from 170 to 190 ms in the Pseudoword condition ($p < 0.05$, **Figure 4B**).

Condition	Pre		Post			
	M	*SD*	*M*	*SD*	*t(8)*	*p*
Consonant	78.36	23.69	73.16	29.49	0.59	0.57
Pseudoword	35.47	27.67	44.60	26.09	1.02	0.34
Real Word	69.24	18.77	53.90	27.77	1.98	0.08

Table 2.
Dependent sample t-tests revealed no significant differences in accuracy (percent correct) between sessions. M = Mean; SD = Standard Deviation.

Condition	Pre		Post			
	M	*SD*	*M*	*SD*	*t(8)*	*p*
Consonant	943	132	871	123	1.69	0.13
Pseudoword	1134	130	1045	136	1.99	0.08
Real Word	1064	146	1012	128	1.14	0.29

Table 3.
Dependent sample t-tests revealed no significant differences in reaction times (in milliseconds) between sessions. M = Mean; SD = Standard Deviation.

In R.vOT, the POST session yielded a less pronounced negative peak from 195 to 240 ms in the Consonant condition, as well as a smaller ERP from 70 to 110 ms in the Pseudoword condition, and greater activation in the Word condition from 640 to 715 ms. In L.AG, the PRE session (pre-FFW) showed greater activations from 730 to 800 ms in the Consonant condition, while the POST session (post-FFW) showed greater activations from 95 to 140 ms in the Pseudoword condition. The PRE session showed greater activity from 290 to 315 ms in the Word condition, with the POST session showing greater activity from 525 to 550 ms. In R.AG, the POST session showed greater activity from 10 to 40 ms in the Consonant condition, while the PRE session showed greater activity from 415 to 435 ms. The PRE session yielded a greater response from 280 to 310 ms in the Pseudoword condition. In the Word condition, the PRE session showed greater activity from 290 to 315 and 425–505 ms. Although not always significant, there is a general trend of post-intervention ERP peaks being less pronounced compared to the same peaks in the first session, especially around ~210 ms at vOT sites. As well, the left and right AG regions tend to show more prominent positive peaks after ~300 ms in the first session.

3.2.3 Phase synchrony

Both sessions showed distributed theta-band network functional connectivity relative to baseline across all conditions ($p < 0.001$; **Figure 6A**). Comparing sessions, the POST session (post-FFW) showed greater theta-band phase synchrony between L.STG and R.IFG in the Pseudoword condition, and between left and right PreCG regions and left and right STG sites in the Word condition ($p < 0.01$). The PRE session (pre-FFW) showed greater theta-band PLVs between R.vOT and R.AG sites, as well as between R.vOT and R.PreCG in the Consonant condition. The PRE session displayed greater PLVs between R.AG and R.IFG for Pseudowords. In the Word condition, the PRE session showed greater PLVs between L.vOT and R.PreCG, between R.vOT and R.AG, and between L.PreCG and right occipital cortex.

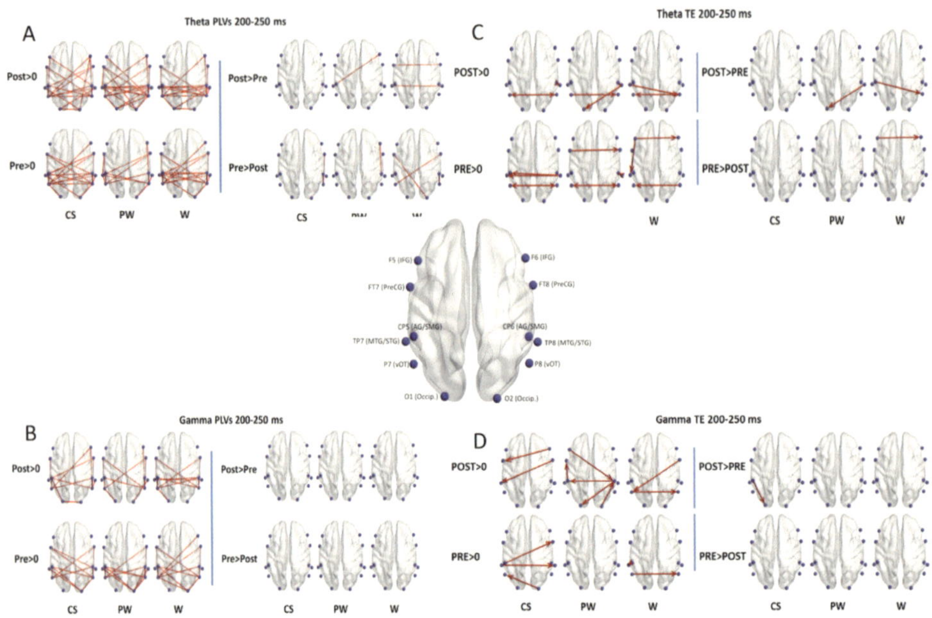

Figure 6.
(A) Theta-band phase synchrony from 200 to 250 ms before and after training for the FFW group. (Left) Red lines between areas indicate significant PLV compared to zero (p < 0.001); (Right) Red lines indicate significant differences comparing PRE- versus POST-training (p < 0.01) (greater connectivity in the PRE session suggests a significant decrease in the POST session). (B) PRE- and POST-training gamma-band phase synchrony from 200 to 250 ms. (Left) Red lines between areas indicate significant PLV compared to zero (p < 0.001); (Right) Red lines indicate significant differences comparing PRE- versus POST-training (p < 0.01). (C) Theta-band NBTE from 200 to 250 ms. (Left) Red arrows between areas indicate significant TE compared to zero (p < 0.001); (Right) Red arrows indicate significant differences in TE comparing PRE- versus POST-training (p < 0.01). (D) Gamma-band NBTE from 200 to 250 ms. (Left) Red arrows between areas indicate significant TE compared to zero (p < 0.001); (Right) Red arrows indicate significant differences in TE comparing PRE-versus POST-training (p < 0.01). CS = Consonant String; PW = Pseudoword; W = Word.

Both sessions (pre-FFW and post-FFW) showed distributed gamma-band network functional connectivity relative to baseline across all conditions ($p < 0.001$; **Figure 6B**). When comparing across sessions, however, neither showed any instances of greater gamma-band network functional connectivity.

3.2.4 Transfer entropy

The POST session (post-FFW) showed significant theta-band NBTE from R.AG to R.STG, as well as bi-directional connectivity between left and right vOT sites in the Consonant condition ($p < 0.05$; **Figure 6C**). In the Pseudoword condition, the POST session further showed significant connectivity from R.AG to R.STG, from L.vOT to R.vOT, and from R.STG to right occipital cortex. In the Word condition, the POST session showed theta NBTE from L.STG to R.vOT, as well as bi-directional connectivity between left and right vOT regions. The PRE session (pre-FFW) showed significant connectivity from R.STG to L.AG and L.STG, and between left and right vOT sites in the Consonant condition. For Pseudowords, the PRE session showed theta-band NBTE from L.PreCG to R.PreCG, and between L.vOT and R.vOT. In the Word condition, connectivity was observed from R.vOT to L.vOT, and from L.IFG to R.IFG and L.STG. Comparing groups, the POST session (post-FFW) showed greater theta-band NBTE from R.STG to left occipital cortex in the Pseudoword condition, and from L.AG to R.vOT in the Word condition ($p < 0.01$). The PRE session (pre-FFW) showed greater connectivity from L.IFG to R.IFG in the Word condition.

The POST session (post-FFW) showed significant gamma-band NBTE from R.PreCG to L.STG, and from R.IFG to L.PreCG in the Consonant condition ($p < 0.05$; **Figure 6D**). In the Pseudoword condition, the POST session showed significant connectivity from L.AG to L.PreCG, from L.IFG to R.AG, from R.AG to L.AG and left occipital cortex, and from right occipital cortex to R.AG. In the Word condition, the POST session showed gamma NBTE from R.PrecCG to L.vOT and from L.vOT to R.vOT. The PRE session (pre-FFW) showed significant connectivity from L.AG to R.PreCG, from L.STG to R.STG, and from right occipital cortex to L.vOT in the Consonant condition. For Pseudowords, the PRE session showed gamma-band NBTE from L.PreCG to R.PreCG, and between L.vOT and R.vOT. In the Word condition, connectivity was observed from R.vOT to L.vOT, and from L.IFG to R.IFG and L.STG. Comparing sessions, the POST session (post-FFW) showed greater gamma-band NBTE only from R.AG to left occipital cortex in the Consonant condition ($p < 0.01$).

3.3 Correlations between connectivity and assessment scores

Gains in performance (POST-PRE scores) on two reading assessments – WJ-WA and WJ-LW – were correlated with changes in brain connectivity. Increases in theta-band phase synchrony between R.vOT and R.IFG in the Pseudoword condition were significantly correlated with WJ-WA performance gains ($p < 0.01$, **Figure 7A**). Significant correlations were also observed between R.vOT and L.IFG for Words. Negative correlations in the Consonant condition were observed between R.AG and L.AG, between R.AG and L.STG, and between R.vOT and right occipital cortex. In the Word condition, correlations were observed between R.STG and L.PreCG, and between R.vOT and R.STG. Increases in theta-band synchrony between R.vOT and R.PreCG in the Consonant condition were significantly correlated with WJ-LW performance gains ($p < 0.01$). In the Pseudoword condition, correlations were observed between R.vOT and L.IFG and between L.vOT and R.STG. Correlations were also observed between R.vOT and L.IFG, between R.vOT and R.AG, and between R.AG and R.PreCG for Words. Negative correlations in the Pseudoword condition were observed between L.AG and R.STG, between R.AG and L.STG, and in the Word condition between L.IFG and R.IFG, and between right occipital cortex and R.STG, L.STG, and left occipital cortex.

Increases in gamma synchrony between L.vOT and R.PreCG in the Consonant condition were significantly correlated to WJ-WA performance gains ($p < 0.01$, **Figure 7B**). Negative correlations in the Consonant condition were observed between L.IFG and left occipital cortex. In the Word condition, negative correlations were observed between L.AG and right occipital cortex. Increases in gamma synchrony between L.IFG and left occipital cortex in the Pseudoword condition were significantly correlated to WJ-LW performance gains ($p < 0.01$). In the Word condition, correlations were observed between R.IFG and left and right vOT regions, as well as with left occipital cortex. Negative correlations in the Consonant condition were observed between R.PreCG and L.IFG, and between R.PreCG and R.IFG. In the Pseudoword condition, negative correlations were observed between R.PreCG and right occipital cortex. In the Word condition, negative correlations were observed between R.PreCG and left and right occipital cortex sites.

Increases in theta-band NBTE from L.AG and R.PreCG to right occipital cortex in the Pseudoword condition were significantly correlated to WJ-WA performance gains ($p < 0.05$, **Figure 7C**). Significant correlations were also observed from L.IFG to L.PreCG for Words. Negative correlations in the Consonant condition were observed from L.AG to L.vOT, and from left occipital cortex to right occipital cortex. In the Pseudoword condition, correlations were observed from left occipital

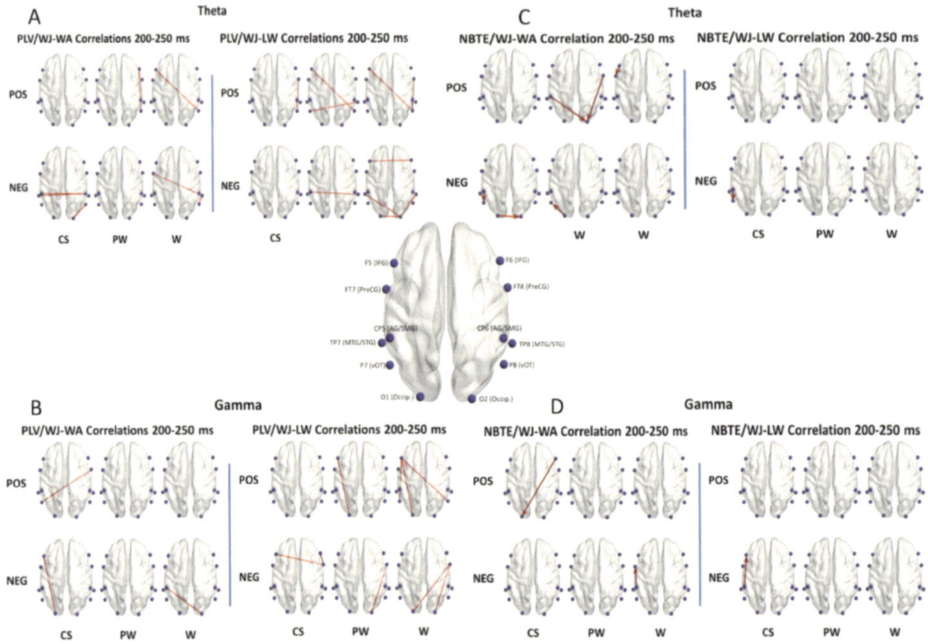

Figure 7.
(A) Significant correlations (red lines between areas) between changes in theta-band PLVs from 200 to 250 ms and gains in behavioural performance in WJ-WA (Left) and WJ-WA (Right) assessments after FFW intervention for the FFW group only. (B) Significant correlations between changes in gamma PLVs from 200 to 250 ms and gains in behavioral performance in WJ-WA (left) and WJ-WA (right) assessments post FFW intervention. (C) Significant correlations between changes in theta NBTE from 200 to 250 ms and gains in behavioral performance in WJ-WA (left) and WJ-WA (right) assessments following FFW intervention. (D) Significant correlations between changes in gamma-band NBTE from 200 to 250 ms and gains in behavioral performance in WJ-WA (left) and WJ-WA (right) assessments following FFW intervention. CS = Consonant String; PW = Pseudoword; W = Word.

cortex to L.vOT. Gains in theta NBTE from L.AG to R.IFG were significantly positive correlated to WJ-LW performance gains in the Pseudoword condition ($p < 0.05$), and from R.IFG to L.vOT in the Word condition. Negative correlations in the Consonant condition were observed from L.AG to L.vOT.

Increases in gamma-band NBTE from R.IFG to left occipital cortex in the Consonant condition were significantly correlated to WJ-WA performance gains ($p < 0.05$, **Figure 7D**). Significant negative correlations in the Word condition were observed from L.AG to L.PreCG. Changes in gamma-band NBTE did not show significant positive correlations with WJ-LW performance gains in any condition ($p < 0.05$). Negative correlations in the Consonant condition were observed from L.AG to L.IFG.

3.4 Comparing post-intervention dyslexic and typical reading networks

The FFW group's phase synchrony measures from both PRE and POST intervention sessions were compared to the networks of typical readers from Session 1 (TYP). Across all conditions in the PRE session, pre-FFW readers showed widespread occipito-temporal theta-band connectivity that was significantly greater than TYP readers (**Figure 8A**; $p < 0.05$). In the POST session, post-FFW readers showed occipito-temporal theta-band connectivity that was significantly greater than TYP readers in the pseudoword and word conditions, but show no differences in the consonant condition ($p < 0.05$). Following the interventional training program, the reading networks of dyslexic children more resemble those of

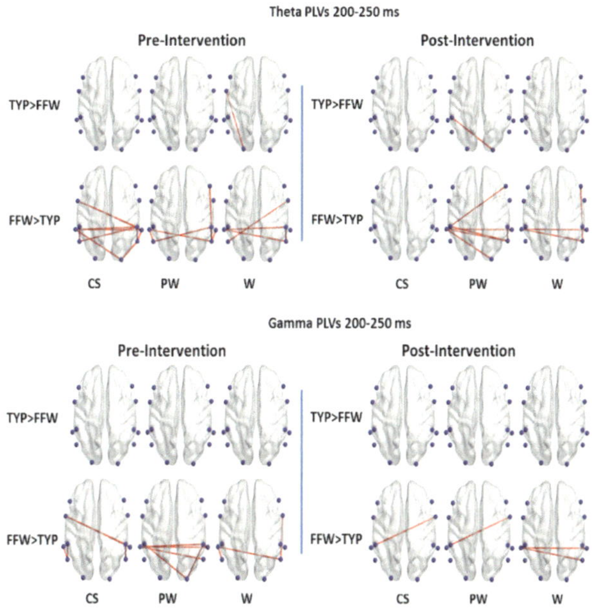

Figure 8.
(Top) Comparing dyslexic and typical theta-band network connectivity dynamics before and after intervention. (Left) Theta PLVs, comparing the dyslexic group (pre-FFW) to their typically-developing classmates prior to intervention. (Right) Comparing the dyslexic group after six months training (post-FFW) to the typical group (only session). (Bottom) Comparing dyslexic and typical gamma-band networks before and after intervention pre/post-FFW). (Left) Gamma PLVs, comparing the dyslexic group to their typically-developing classmates prior to intervention. (Right) Comparing the dyslexic group after six months to the typical group (only session). CS = Consonant String; PW = Pseudoword; W = Word.

typically-developing classmates when processing basic orthography (consonants). However, when processing pseudowords and words the post-FFW group continued to use pathways that were dissimilar to those used by typically-reading children when processing the same information.

Across all conditions in the PRE session, pre-FFW readers showed occipito-temporal gamma-band connectivity (**Figure 8B**), as well as occasional engagement of frontal sites, that was significantly greater than in TYP readers ($p < 0.05$). In the POST session, post-FFW readers showed single instances of greater gamma-band connectivity (than the TYP group) between L.AG and R.PreCG in the Consonant and Pseudoword conditions, as well as occipito-temporal connectivity in the Word condition. Comparing PRE and POST sessions, the gamma-band connectivity in the Pseudoword condition is much more sparse following intervention. Following the intervention program (post-FFW), however, the reading networks of dyslexic children, viewed from gamma-band connectivity, do more closely resemble those of typically-developing classmates, particularly in the Pseudoword condition.

4. Discussion

The present study examined the differences in neural processing dynamics between typically developing readers (TYP) and dyslexic readers who have been enrolled in a reading training program (FastForWord, FFW), prior to training (pre-FFW) and after the training (post-FFW). Our initial hypothesis of dyslexic readers generating more functional connectivity (phase synchrony) in response to words was supported. With regard to information flow connectivity (NBTE), results supported the hypothesis for theta-band NBTE, but were somewhat ambiguous for the gamma band.

Both groups in this experiment showed pronounced N170/220 components at reading-critical sites in response to orthographic stimuli. However, the pre-FFW group showed more pronounced negative peaks across all conditions in the R.vOT region – a right-hemispheric analog to the so-called visual word-form area (VWFA, or L.vOT), which is thought to be critical to the processing of sub-lexical orthographic information [37, 38]. These results may reflect a similar specialization for orthographic processing that is leveraged by dyslexic readers to compensate for under-developed regions in the left hemisphere. Or it could reflect a less efficient (more effortful) bilateral form-processing response to orthographic stimuli, as the original function of these areas is visual form processing [37].

Observing underlying oscillatory activity at specific frequency bands allows for more nuanced examinations of neural oscillations that help to further characterize patterns observed in ERPs. To that end, we investigated the fluctuations in theta- and gamma-band power following the presentation of written words. Similar to the ERP results, the pre-FFW group showed significantly larger bursts of theta-band power from R.vOT at the same time as the N170/220 component, a relationship that has been documented in prior studies of the oscillatory dynamics of reading in the brain [13].

The connectivity results further corroborated this assertion of a right-hemispheric network at play in dyslexic children during reading. Neuroimaging studies have repeatedly identified regions in the right hemisphere producing stronger activations in dyslexic individuals in response to reading tasks [9, 10, 12, 39, 40]. Here we showed that, at the moment that orthographic information is first being processed, each group leverages distinct neurocognitive networks to carry out this process – such that dyslexic children display more inter-hemispheric connectivity, as well as right-sided intra-hemispheric connectivity in response to written language, not seen in typical readers.

Pre-FFW readers showed robust posterior (occipito-temporal) connectivity across all three conditions. Notably, this includes the Consonants condition, in which the stimuli lacked any linguistic content to be evaluated by the central question "Is this a real word?" Presumably, if dyslexia only involves processing beyond simple orthographic decoding, then the two groups should be identical until such processing is required. Our interpretation of the overactive connectivity in the Consonant condition is that there is a "bottleneck" in processing in early dyslexic language networks. Note that regardless of the actual linguistic content in the stimuli, the string still must be evaluated as though it *may* have linguistic content, which is enough to engage various aspects of the reading network to evaluate the content [20]. This window 200–250 ms after stimulus onset captures the moment in which orthographic decoding occurs and information is relayed to other sites to be further evaluated for content. For pre-FFW readers, a set of alternative processes and pathways is engaged to handle the consonants. First, as we saw with ERPs and ERSPs, the right hemisphere plays a large role for dyslexic readers, particularly in posterior sites. In the decoding and transmission of orthographic information, the lack of expertise in dyslexic children means that they must spend more time processing the stimuli in order to make their judgement.

Theta-band NBTE results are consistent with this framing, with dyslexic readers showing greater effective connectivity from R.vOT to L.vOT, then from vOT sites to AG regions. Whereas pre-FFW network connectivity was constrained to occipito-temporal sites in posterior cortex, the TYP group showed greater engagement of frontal sites.

Across all behavioral scores – reading assessments (WJ-WA and WJ-LW), task accuracy, and reaction time – the pre-FFW vs. post-FFW comparison was not significant for either task accuracy or reaction time. Despite the overall FFW group lacking significant gains in aggregate, however, some readers did improve their performance after intervention. This fortuitous result in turn informed the correlation analysis between changes in reading performance and changes in oscillatory connectivity. Between sessions (post-FFW vs. pre-FFW), localized brain activity (ERPs) at reading-related sites showed a general reduction in intensity, such that positive and negative peaks of interest (e.g. N170 component) were less pronounced in the POST session (post-FFW) [17, 18, 22, 23, 41]. These findings are in line with neuroimaging studies of other dyslexia interventions, whereby improved reading ability was linked to decreases in general activation due to more efficient and specialized processing, as well as a shifting in regional activations [42, 43].

Functional connectivity findings, as measured by phase synchrony, displayed several differences in connectivity patterns between sessions (post-FFW vs. pre-FFW) and across conditions. Theta-band phase synchrony has been shown to reflect network connectivity patterns over time during reading [13, 31]. In the present study, a reduction of theta synchrony was observed in the Consonant condition of the POST session (post-FFW) at the time window most critical for pre-lexical orthographic processing in children (200–250 ms). Interestingly, the Consonant condition requires no additional reading training to identify its semantic or phonological properties, and yet orthographic expertise seems to have had an effect even here. Just as with ERPs, this result suggests a reduction in executive engagement during orthographic processing, thus requiring fewer resources to accomplish the same task [20, 44].

Further supporting this account, the correlations between behavioral performance and brain network connectivity also showed significant negative correlations between occipito-temporal posterior connectivity and reading assessment scores. In other words, children who showed the lowest performance gains also tended to exert more resources among posterior sites involved in the early stages of reading, whereas individuals who showed the largest performance gains in their reading assessments instead tended to show brain connectivity patterns engaging more frontal sites, suggesting the engagement of higher-level language areas.

Price and Devlin [20] have argued for a framework of occipito-temporal cortical dominance in word reading that emphasizes the role of connectivity and communication between these and other regions, such that orthographic information is resolved by comparing bottom-up inputs with top-down expectations. In this framework, unfamiliar or difficult content would require substantially more frequent evaluations to resolve the perceptual inputs before sending that information to higher-level language-processing regions, resulting in slower overall performance. The results presented here indeed suggest that readers who showed the greatest behavioral improvements required fewer resources at earlier stages, allowing for earlier engagement of frontal sites.

In general, the most improved readers showed greater theta-band connectivity within frontal brain areas whereas the least improved readers showed greater posterior occipito-temporal connectivity patterns instead. Following Price and Devlin's framework, whereas poor readers are still resolving the orthographic and initial linguistic content, more developed readers are evaluating (or at least engaging with) higher-level linguistic content in the frontal language processing centers. In this case, we suppose that the higher levels of occipito-temporal connectivity in the poor readers reflect a delay or disruption in sensory processing, in that more experienced readers are already accessing linguistic information beyond simple pre-lexical orthography [45].

Frontal lobe connectivity changes have been shown to be a predictor of reading performance gains. Hoeft and colleagues [10] have shown that structural connectivity linked to R.IFG is a predictor of performance gains in children with developmental dyslexia. In the present study, our functional and effective connectivity results did not clearly corroborate this account, since R.IFG showed distinct instances of increased connectivity both in PRE- and in POST-training sessions, as well as both positive and negative correlations to gains in assessment scores. Thus, it seems that structural connectivity alone is not enough – there must be functional and effective connectivity accompanying it for reading performance to be bettered.

Although we did not measure the TYP group's reading networks a second time, a meaningful comparison is still possible to address the question of whether the intervention (plus the intervening time period and other school activities) caused the post-FFW reading networks to more closely resemble the already substantially more skilled TYP reading networks. We found that indeed there was some closer resemblance in theta-band connectivity in the POST session, but only for the consonant strings. Even after six months of intervention, however, the FFW group's theta-band networks in the Pseudoword and Word conditions remained robustly distinct from the TYP group. These findings suggest that whereas some aspects of the reading network brain connectivity dynamics may have come to resemble more closely typical processing at early (i.e. pre-lexical) stages, the later and more complex stage processes still utilized alternative pathways. It remains unclear if this is because of a compensated efficiency in alternative pathways or because of poor coordination from typical regions (e.g. ectopias, that is, distorted cortical layering, disrupting processing in the left hemispheric language areas, [46]), or both.

In the gamma band, PRE- and POST-training session differences were somewhat less pronounced, but it is clear that the post-FFW network connectivity in the Pseudoword condition more closely resembles the TYP group after the training. The nature of the task is such that the Pseudoword condition is particularly taxing on phonological processing skills of the reader, forcing them to sound out the letter strings. In this regard, the improved performance of the post-FFW group in reading assessments may be related to their networks being more optimal (i.e. closer to the typical organization).

The underlying premise for this comparison between post-intervention FFW and TYP readers was to examine if a targeted reading intervention would shape the reading network connectivity dynamics in dyslexic children at the ms time scale to be more closely aligned to their typically-developing classmates, or if the training would instead optimize their existing "compensational" networks. These results suggest that for early orthographic processing, post-FFW readers' theta-band networks do seem to shift in such a way that orthographic processing follows pathways more similar to those of TYP readers. However, after this initial processing, as the orthographic information needs to be made available to the rest of the reading network (e.g. for phonological or semantic processing), post-FFW readers continue to use alternative bilateral pathways to achieve improved behavioral results.

This divergence in results between theta and gamma bands may be addressed by explanations proposing different functional properties of each frequency band [47], whereby theta-band PLVs represent long distance communication (e.g. occipito-frontal; [48]), whereas gamma-band oscillations work in conjunction with theta-band oscillations to aid in more localized computations. As for gamma-band connectivity, Lehongre and colleagues [14] showed a reduced ability for dyslexic individuals to synchronize their auditory processing at a gamma rate compared to controls. Goswami [15] went on to posit that this gamma synchrony deficit might account for phonological processing difficulties seen in dyslexic readers [16], as the average speed at which phonemes are read is at a gamma rate. This has the result that, when dyslexic readers attempt to string together speech sounds from text, they do so in an uncoordinated manner, resulting in poor reading performance.

What remains unclear is why phonological processing networks in the gamma band would shift toward a more typical organization, but the orthographic (consonant strings) or semantic processing (words) did not show so drastic a change. It is possible that more complex processing using higher language networks requires more time to remediate because plasticity across large-scale networks must be coordinated (see [16]).

Another perspective to consider is whether or not the presence of ectopias has altered the micro-structure of the reading-related brain regions to the point that pathways connected to these regions are under-utilized by the dyslexic reading networks in favor of alternative pathways (e.g. right hemisphere). An ectopia is a distortion of the cortex during development in which many neurons fail to migrate to their proper layer, ending up as clumps in layer I of cortex. Ectopias not only affect the operation of the cortical area in which they occur, but also they cause distorted processing in areas to which the affected area is connected [46]. In rats, ectopias cause difficulties in auditory processing specifically [46]. Ectopias are found in the brains of some dyslexic readers (post mortem) and are hypothesized to be at least one cause of the disorder [46]. If ectopias in the left hemisphere have disrupted the brain's ability to develop effective pathways and networks in the left hemisphere, then their coordination is also likely disrupted, and perhaps accounts for the challenges in phonological processing and compensation via expansion to the right hemisphere. These results suggest that, at least in the gamma band, enough coordination was shored up to the extent that the post-FFW networks statistically more closely resembled the TYP network, compared to the PRE training session. This and other conclusions would be strengthened by a similar experiment that would include a group of dyslexic students who did not receive training (perhaps because of unavailability; not done here due to ethical considerations), but who could then be compared to the trained dyslexic readers, thus characterizing in this population the effects of training plus classroom instruction and general development in contrast to the latter two alone.

5. Conclusion

EEG brain imaging indicated significant differences in local and largescale brain network connectivity dynamics between typical and dyslexic readers. Prior to FastForWord (FFW) training, a "bottleneck" in early orthographic decoding leads to greater posterior occipito-temporal connectivity with expansion into the right hemisphere in dyslexic readers compared to neurotypical readers.

After cognitive training, the "bottleneck" is relieved for consonant strings, while pseudowords and real words continue to utilize right- and cross-hemispheric networks rather than typical left-hemispheric networks, but involving more frontal areas overall. As dyslexic readers become more proficient, they are able to engage higher-level language areas faster and thus reduce posterior engagement. Brain-based cognitive training programs, such as FastForWord, further indicate significant potential for improving reading ability by accelerating reading network development in dyslexic children.

What are the implications of this study for treatment of dyslexia? It is clear that more research is needed to more precisely characterize both the brain network dynamics characterizing dyslexic reading, and also the effects of interventions such as FastForWord on these dynamics. We have mentioned several such possible studies earlier. In particular, however, a prospective study with more participants and an untreated control group is critical. More generally, however, it would be desirable to identify children at risk of dyslexia as early as possible in their reading training, and engage them in a reading training program, so as to take advantage of brain plasticity in guiding the reading networks in the most efficient trajectory. Equally important, however, is the implication that such programs will not help all children equally. Even in our small sample we found a range of outcomes from the FastForWord program, from no improvement to significant improvement. How much will be gained from enrollment in such a program will depend on many factors, among them are the precise nature of the brain impairment causing the difficulty, and the amount of effort and motivation a student can bring to the program. Moreover, if the cause of the dyslexia is a brain abnormality, for example an ectopia in the left temporal lobe, then specific training likely will not result in a "normal" reading network because the ectopia cannot be "cured." Nonetheless, improvement of the alternative, more right-hemisphere-oriented, network resulting from a training program can be expected in these cases.

Acknowledgements

We thank the school district of Burnaby, BC for their kind assistance in providing access to their students and also for providing a venue where the EEG and reading testing could take place.

This research was supported by grant A9958 from the Natural Sciences and Engineering Research Council of Canada to LMW, by the BC Leading Edge Endowment Fund to UR, and by an in-kind grant from the Behavioural and Cognitive Neuroscience Institute (BCNI) at Simon Fraser University (UR, Director).

Author details

Nicolas Bedo[1], Dikla Ender-Fox[2], Janet Chow[3], Linda Siegel[4], Urs Ribary[5,6,7]*
and Lawrence M. Ward[1,7]*

1 Department Psychology, University of British Columbia (UBC), Vancouver, Canada

2 Ramat Hasharon, Israel

3 School District, Burnaby, BC, Canada

4 Department Educational Counselling Psychology and Special Education UBC, Vancouver, Canada

5 Behavioral Cognitive Neuroscience Institute (BCNI), Simon Fraser University, Vancouver, Canada

6 Department of Pediatrics and Psychiatry UBC, Vancouver, Canada

7 Brain Research Centre UBC, Vancouver, Canada

*Address all correspondence to: urs_ribary@sfu.ca and lward@psych.ubc.ca

References

[1] Livingston-Hirst E, Siegel LS, Ribary U. Developmental dyslexia: emotional impact and consequences. Australian Journal of Learning Difficulties, 2018; 23: 107-135. DOI: 10.1080/19404158.2018.1479975

[2] Liberman IY. Segmentation of the spoken word and reading acquisition. Bulletin of the Orton Society, 1973; 23: 65-77.

[3] Tallal P. Improving language and literacy is a matter of time. Nature Reviews Neuroscience, 2004; 5: 721-728.

[4] Byrne B, Fielding-Barnsley R, Ashley L. Effects of preschool phoneme identity training after six years: Outcome level distinguished from rate of response. Journal of educational psychology, 2000; 92(4): 659.

[5] Hatcher PJ, Hulme C, Ellis AW. Ameliorating early reading failure by integrating the teaching of reading and phonological skills: The phonological linkage hypothesis. Child development, 1994; 65(1): 41-57.

[6] Merzenich MM, Jenkins WM, Johnston P, Schreiner C, Miller SL, Tallal P. Temporal processing deficits of language-learning impaired children ameliorated by training. Science, 1996; 271: 77-81.

[7] Tallal P, Miller SL, Bedi G, Byma G, Wang X, Nagarajan SS, Schreiner C, Jenkins WM, Merzenich MM. Language comprehension in language-learning impaired children improved with acoustically modified speech. Science, 1996; 271: 81-84.

[8] Temple E, Deutsch GK, Poldrack R. Miller SL, Tallal P, Merzenich MM, Gabrieli JDE. Neural deficits in children with dyslexia ameliorated by behavioral remediation: evidence from functional MRI. Proceedings of the National Academy of Sciences of the United States of America, 2003; 100(5): 2860-5.

[9] Eden G, Jones K, Cappell K, Gareau L. Neural changes following remediation in adult developmental dyslexia. Neuron, 2004; 44: 411-422.

[10] Hoeft F, McCandliss BD, Black JM, Gantman A, Zakerani N, Hulme C, Lyytinen H, Whitfield-Gabrieli S, Glover GH, Reiss AL, Gabrieli JDE. Neural systems predicting long-term outcome in dyslexia. Proceedings National Academy of Sciences of USA, 2011; 108: 361-366.

[11] Benasich AA, Ribary U. Emergent Brain Dynamics: Prebirth to Adolescence. MIT Press: Cambridge, MA, 2018.

[12] Hoeft F, Hernandez A, McMillon G, Taylor-Hill H, Martindale JL, Meyler A., Whitfield-Gabrieli S. Neural basis of dyslexia: a comparison between dyslexic and nondyslexic children equated for reading ability. The Journal of Neuroscience, 2006; 26(42): 10700-10708.

[13] Bedo N, Ribary U, Ward LM. Fast dynamics of cortical functional and effective connectivity during word reading. PloS ONE, 2014; 9(2): e88940.

[14] Lehongre K, Ramus F, Villiermet N, Schwartz D, Giraud AL. Altered low-γ sampling in auditory cortex accounts for the three main facets of dyslexia. Neuron, 2011; 72(6): 1080-1090.

[15] Goswami U. A temporal sampling framework for developmental dyslexia. Trends in Cognitive Sciences, 2011; 15(1): 3-10.

[16] Ribary U, Doesburg SM, Ward LM. Unified principles of thalamocortical network dynamics: A framework for typical/atypical functional connectivity.

In Magnetoencephalography, Supek S Aine CJ, eds, Springer, Cham, 2019, p. 1-28. DOI: 10.1007/978-3-319-62657-4_19-1

[17] Dujardin T, Etienne Y, Contentin C, Bernard C, Largy P, Mellier D, Rebaï M. Behavioral performances in participants with phonological dyslexia and different patterns on the N170 component. Brain and Cognition, 2011; 75(2): 91-100.

[18] Mahé G, Bonnefond A, Gavens N, Dufour A, Doignon-Camus N. Impaired visual expertise for print in French adults with dyslexia as shown by N170 tuning. Neuropsychologia, 2012; 50(14): 3200-3206.

[19] McCandliss BD, Cohen L, Dehaene S. The visual word form area: expertise for reading in the fusiform gyrus. Trends in Cognitive Sciences, 2003; 7(7): 293-299.

[20] Price CJ, Devlin JT. The interactive account of ventral occipitotemporal contributions to reading. Trends in Cognitive Sciences, 2011; 15(6): 246-253.

[21] Brem S, Bach S, Kucian K, Guttorm TK, Martin E, Lyytinen H, Brandeis D, Richardson U. Brain sensitivity to print emerges when children learn letter-speech sound correspondences. Proc. Natl. Acad. Sci. USA, 2010; 107: 7939-7944.

[22] Hasko S, Groth K, Bruder J, Bartling J, Schulte-Körne G. The time course of reading processes in children with and without dyslexia: an ERP study. Frontiers in Human Neuroscience, 2013; 7: 570.

[23] Hasko S, Groth K, Bruder J, Bartling J, Schulte-Körne G. What does the brain of children with developmental dyslexia tell us about reading improvement? ERP evidence from an intervention study. Frontiers in Human Neuroscience, 2014; 8: 441.

[24] Delorme A, Makeig S. EEGLAB: an open source toolbox for analysis of single-trial EEG dynamics including independent component analysis. Journal of Neuroscience Methods, 2004; 134(1): 9-21.

[25] Fitzgibbon SP, DeLosAngeles D, Lewis TW, Powers DMW, Whitham EM, Willoughby JO, Pope KJ. Surface Laplacian of scalp electrical signals and independent component analysis resolve EMG contamination of electroencephalogram. International Journal of Psychophysiol, 2015; 97(3): 277-284.

[26] Kayser J. Current Source Density (CSD) Interpolation Using Spherical Splines–CSD Toolbox (Version 1.1). New York State Psychiatric Institute: Division of Cognitive Neuroscience. 2009.

[27] Kayser J, Tenke CE. Principal components analysis of Laplacian waveforms as a generic method for identifying ERP generator patterns: I. Evaluation with auditory oddball tasks. Clinical Neurophysiology, 2006; 117(2): 348-368.

[28] Kayser J, Tenke CE. Principal components analysis of Laplacian waveforms as a generic method for identifying ERP generator patterns: II. Adequacy of low-density estimates. Clinical Neurophysiology, 2006; 117(2): 369-380.

[29] Jobard G, Crivello F, Tzourio-Mazoyer N. Evaluation of the dual route theory of reading: a metanalysis of 35 neuroimaging studies. NeuroImage, 2003; 20(2): 693-712.

[30] Koessler L, Maillard L, Benhadid A, Vignal JP, Felblinger J, Vespignani H, Braun M. Automated cortical projection of EEG sensors: anatomical correlation via the international 10-10 system. Neuroimage, 2009; 46(1): 64-72.

[31] Bedo N, Ward LM (submitted). Fast brain network dynamics of reading words compared to those of "reading" consonant strings.

[32] Doesburg SM, Bedo N, Ward LM. Top-down alpha oscillatory network interactions during visuospatial attention orienting. NeuroImage, 2016; 132: 512-519.

[33] McDonnell MD, Ward LM. The benefits of noise in neural systems: bridging theory and experiment. Nature Reviews Neuroscience, 2011; 12(7): 415-426.

[34] Schreiber T. Measuring information transfer. Physical Review Letters, 2000; 85: 461.

[35] Wibral M, Rahm B, Rieder M, Lindner M, Vicente R, Kaiser J. Transfer entropy in magnetoencephalographic data: quantifying information flow in cortical and cerebellar networks. Progress in Biophysics and Molecular Biology, 2011; 105(1-2): 80-97. http://doi.org/10.1016/j.pbiomolbio.2010.11.006

[36] Onton J, Delorme A, Makeig S. Frontal midline EEG dynamics during working memory. Neuroimage, 2005; 27(2): 341-356.

[37] Dehaene S. Reading in the Brain. The science and evolution of a human invention. 2009; 2008:4, Viking.

[38] Cohen L, Dehaene S, Naccache L, Lehéricy S, Dehaene-Lambertz G, Hénaff M, Michel F. The visual word form area: spatial and temporal characterization of an initial stage of reading in normal subjects and posterior split-brain patients. Brain : A Journal of Neurology, 2000; 123: 291-307.

[39] Temple E, Poldrack R. Salidis J, Deutsch GK, Tallal P, Merzenich MM, Gabrieli JD. Disrupted neural responses to phonological and orthographic processing in dyslexic children: an fMRI study. Neuroreport, 2001; 12(2): 299-307.

[40] Temple E. Brain mechanisms in normal and dyslexic readers. Current Opinion in Neurobiology, 2002; 12(2): 178-183.

[41] Jucla M, Nenert R, Chaix Y, Demonet JF. Remediation effects on N170 and P300 in children with developmental dyslexia. Behavioural Neurology, 2010; 22(3-4): 121-129.

[42] Schlaggar BL, Church JA. Functional neuroimaging insights into the development of skilled reading. Current Directions in Psychological Science, 2009; 18(1): 21-26.

[43] Shaywitz BA, Shaywitz SE, Pugh KR., Mencl WE, Fulbright RK, Skudlarski P., Gore JC. Disruption of posterior brain systems for reading in children with developmental dyslexia. Biological Psychiatry, 2002; 52(2): 101-110.

[44] Johnson MH. Interactive specialization: a domain-general framework for human functional brain development. Developmental Cognitive Neuroscience, 2011; 1(1): 7-21.

[45] Wolf M. Proust and the squid: The story and science of the reading brain. Cambridge: Icon. 2008.

[46] Galaburda AM. Dyslexia—A molecular disorder of neuronal migration. Annals of Dyslexia, 2005; 55(2): 151-165.

[47] Ribary U, Doesburg SM, Ward LM. Unified principles of thalamo-cortical processing: The neuronal switch. Biomedical Engineering Letters, 2017; 7: 229-235. DOI: 10.1007/s13534-017-0033-4

[48] Ward LM. Synchronous neural oscillations and cognitive processes. Trends in Cognitive Sciences, 2003; 7: 553-559.

Chapter 3

Dyslexia and the Speech Pathologist

Jane Roitsch

Abstract

Dyslexia is a complex condition. Timely identification of this disorder is imperative to its optimal management. Students benefit most when the skill sets of specialists trained to recognize markers and characteristics of dyslexia are effectively utilized. This chapter provides a real-life case study describing the process by which a student with a language literacy disorder such as dyslexia was assessed by a speech-language pathologist (SLP). Supporting literature is embedded throughout the case study to enhance learning and support the decisions made by the SLP. The role that the SLP can take in working with students with language literacy disorders such as dyslexia is also discussed. Therefore, the aims of this chapter are threefold: to (a) provide guidance for SLPs who may work with students with language literacy disorders such as dyslexia; (b) educate parents of children, with language literacy disorders such as dyslexia, about SLPs; and (c) support teachers and educational professionals by providing information about professionals who can serve as a resource for students.

Keywords: speech pathologist, speech therapist, assessment

1. Introduction

Dyslexia is a neurological learning disability that impairs a person's ability to read. Estimates suggest that dyslexia is a condition that affects nearly 13% of school-aged children in the United States [1] and more than 10% of populations worldwide [1, 2]. Although not a comprehensive list, the following characteristics are commonly associated with dyslexia [1]:

- Difficulty with the development of phonological awareness and phonological processing skills.
- Difficulty in accurately decoding nonsense or unfamiliar words.
- Difficulty in reading single words in isolation.
- Inaccurate and labored oral reading.
- Lack of reading fluency.
- Various degrees of learning the names of letters and their associated sounds.

IntechOpen

- Difficulty with learning to spell.
- Difficulty in word finding and rapid naming.
- Variable difficulty with aspects of written composition.
- Variable degrees of difficulty with reading comprehension.

Vocabulary limitations, poor phonological awareness, and comprehension problems often associated with reading challenges such as dyslexia can become more pronounced in elementary school when the students begin to read to learn [3, 4]. Often, when higher cognitive-level reading processes are required, (i.e., not only reading words but retaining and applying information from what they have read), reading difficulties such as dyslexia often become more apparent as students progress in school. During these developmental years, the effects that reading challenges have on students with dyslexia can be quite apparent. The long-reaching effects of weak reading skills can be devastating. The impact of dyslexia on an individual can lead to poor self-esteem and limited awareness of social, emotional, and academic deficits [5]. Effective identification of dyslexia helps students, parents, and educators to manage the disorder, establish support, and reduce the impact of the condition.

Most students are diagnosed with dyslexia by an educational psychologist following referral from a teacher or other educational professional. It has been well-recognized that reading specialists and special educators provide critical support to students with dyslexia. Often lesser known is that differential assessment and management of language literacy disorders such as dyslexia can be supported by multiple disciplines, such as speech-language pathology or speech therapy [6]. The following section provides insight into the utility of the speech-language pathologist (SLP) in the identification and management of such students.

2. Speech-language pathology and dyslexia

The position statement of the American Speech-Language-Hearing Association (ASHA) states that SLPs "play a critical and direct role in the development of literacy for children and adolescents with communication disorders" and "make a contribution to the literacy efforts of a school district or community on behalf of other children and adolescents" [7]. In order to effectively and appropriately perform these roles, ASHA emphasizes the need for collaboration with written language development experts and those with expertise in each student's specific situation(s) [7]. ASHA states that SLPs are uniquely trained in "normal and disordered language acquisition, and their clinical experience in developing individualized programs for children and adolescents, prepare them to assume a variety of roles related to the development of reading and writing. Appropriate roles and responsibilities for SLPs include, but are not limited to (a) preventing written language problems by fostering language acquisition and emergent literacy; (b) identifying children at risk for reading and writing problems; (c) assessing reading and writing; (d) providing intervention and documenting outcomes for reading and writing; and (e) assuming other roles, such as providing assistance to general education teachers, parents, and students; advocating for effective literacy practices; and advancing the knowledge base" [7].

As students with dyslexia are often characterized as having appropriate language comprehension skills but poor reading abilities, it stands to reason identification of dyslexia in children and adolescents can be aided by literacy and language assessments from SLPs (i.e., professionals uniquely trained in the assessment and management of expressive and receptive language and speech skills). As will be seen, the role that the SLP can play in assessment and treatment planning for students with language literacy disorders such as dyslexia can be a crucial and pivotal one.

3. Case study

3.1 Methodology

For this chapter, a single-participant case report style was employed. This research methodology is often selected when a work seeks to answer a descriptive or explanatory research question. The question this chapter aims to answer is, "What can a trained SLP do to provide assessment and intervention for students with language literacy disorders such as dyslexia?"

Selection of a case study method is not without limitations. Certainly, generalization of John's outcomes cannot be made to all students with dyslexia and reporting of a single study lacks the rigor of a blinded, systematic, multiple-subject research project. Further, the student selected, the instruments used, and the outcomes reported are at the discretion of the SLP and this author.

However, because a case study report allows for in-depth explanations that are not provided by other methods (e.g., qualitative research designs with multiple participants), John's story is able to be told. A case study design also allows for a real-world context, such as John's to be provided. Thus, the benefits of a case study research design lie in its ability to study real-world situations and address important research questions [8].

3.1.1 Ethical considerations

John's mother consented for his participation in the initial assessment at the SLP's clinic on a university campus in the United States. She also consented for the use of his assessment, outcomes, and history to be included in this work. The author is a professor at the clinic where the SLP works and was granted access to his case study by his mother who consented and the SLP who provided the reporting results. The Human Subject and Institutional Review Board at the university agreed that the author did not need to submit materials for approval, since this case study chapter is one case study in a book chapter and thus does not meet the federal definition of "generalizable." Had this chapter involved a large-scale case study project involving multiple cases, research approval may have been required. All identifying markers were removed and his name was changed to preserve anonymity. His age was also changed by a month.

3.2 Participant

John[1] is a 8-year-, 9-month-old English-speaking male brought for a speech and language assessment by his parents who expressed concerns with his language and literacy abilities. He attends third grade at a local elementary school. John works hard in school, but struggles academically, especially with reading. Specifically, John often writes with letter reversals, omits or substitutes basic sight words when reading aloud, and skips punctuation. **Legible handwriting, appropriate use of**

[1] Name changed.

punctuation, omitting words and reversals of letters in writing can be characteristics of dyslexia [9].

John's birth history and hearing screening history are unremarkable. The first indications of John's language challenges were noted at the age of 3. He reportedly was able to combine up to three words yet had a lexicon of only about 45 words. He scored below average in expressive language (SS = 80) on The Preschool Language Scale-5 (PLS-5) [10] and his total communication index score fell in the low average range (SS = 85). **Dyslexia has been linked to deficits in expressive and receptive language skills** [11].

When John was in second grade, his academic performance warranted psychoeducational testing by the school's educational psychologist. Overall, John's cognitive functioning was noted higher than average on the Wechsler Intelligence Scale for Children—Fifth Edition (WISC-V; [12]). **Students with dyslexia do not typically test below average on intelligence tests** [13].

On the Wechsler Individual Achievement Test—Third Edition (WIAT-III) [14], John demonstrated strong mathematic abilities. However, his comprehension, sight word reading, phonetic decoding, and written expression were below average. **The presence of early speech sound disorders has been shown to be related to poor phonemic skills and spelling at the age of 5½ and difficulty with reading words at the age of 8** [15].

Although John's listening comprehension was above average range in receptive vocabulary, his oral discourse comprehension score was in the lower average range, indicating possible processing problems. **Weaknesses in semantics, syntax, and oral expression have been shown to contribute to reading difficulties in children with dyslexia** [16].

Presently, John receives speech-language pathology and reading specialist services at his school. The school SLP is targeting articulation of /r/ and /r/ blends in all positions of words in all contexts. **Articulation errors have been identified among students with dyslexia** [17].

In his most recent report card, John received passing grades in all areas except reading. His classroom teachers stated that he is not a fluent reader and his comprehension of written text seems inconsistent based upon the given task and its requirements. He also has reported difficulty with word recall and story event sequencing and challenges with spelling and decoding. **Persons with dyslexia often demonstrate inaccurate word recognition and comprehension, poor spelling and difficulty with decoding** [18]. John receives classroom accommodations and is allowed to read aloud in a quiet area during reading tasks.

His teacher and parents state that John is aware of his reading difficulties, and this increases his anxiety and impedes his academic performance. **Children with dyslexia may demonstrate low self-esteem and anxiety, among other feelings because they must work harder in school to keep up with their classmates,** [17]. The SLP determined they needed to assess his language skills in-depth.

4. Assessment

4.1 John's speech-language pathology assessment

The tests that the SLP selected for use with John were (1) tests within the discipline's scope of practice and that (2) utilized both formal and informal measures. Specifically, the SLP selected the Comprehensive Test of Phonological Processing—Second Edition (CTOPP-2) [19], Test of Word Reading Efficiency—Second Edition (TOWRE-2) [20], the Test of Integrated Language and Literacy Skills (TILLS; [21]), the TILLS Student Language Scale (SLS Questionnaire; [21]), the AIMSweb Spelling and Reading Maze Curriculum Based Measures [22], the Gray Oral Reading Test—Fifth Edition (GORT-5) [23], a morphological awareness probe, and a writing sample.

The International Dyslexia Association (IDA) suggests the following areas be examined to ensure a comprehensive educational dyslexia assessment: Phonological awareness, phonological/language-based memory, rapid automatic naming, receptive vocabulary, phonics and de-coding abilities, decoding of both reading and nonsense words, oral reading fluency, spelling and writing of single words, sentences, paragraphs [1].

4.1.1 Comprehensive Test of Phonological Processing Second Edition (CTOPP-2)

The CTOPP-2 assesses phonological processing skills [19]. As noted previously, phonological processing skills underlie word reading efficiency and deficits in these skills are a key characteristic of language literacy disorders such as dyslexia [3]. Often identified as a fundamental building block of reading, phonological awareness is the ability to attend, reflect on, or manipulate speech sounds in words. Phonological memory is the ability to encode and store phonological information (i.e., speech sounds) [24]. Rapid symbolic naming refers to the ability to quickly name a series of letters, numbers, familiar objects, or colors [25]. Therefore, the SLP opted to employ three subtests to determine John's phonological awareness, phonological memory, and rapid symbolic naming abilities. **Results revealed John scored two standard deviations or more below the mean on all three subtests, scoring lowest on the phonological memory subtest.**

4.1.2 Test of Word Reading Efficiency: Second Edition (TOWRE-2)

The TOWRE-2 includes the subtests of sight word efficiency and phonemic decoding efficiency to determine the ability to pronounce printed words [20]. It has been suggested that persons with reading difficulties have more challenges retaining sight words in memory than readers without difficulties [26]. Additionally, phonemic decoding has been shown to be challenging for students with language literacy disorders such as dyslexia [27]. Thus, the TOWRE-2 subtests lend information about a reading efficiency at the word-level. Word reading efficiency leads to effective reading comprehension and reading ability.

For each subtest, John was instructed to read as many words as he could from the list, as quickly and accurately as possible in 45 seconds. He was permitted to skip words he did not know by saying "pass." He correctly read 42 sight words and 11 pseudowords. He made errors on eight other pseudowords. For the sight word efficiency subtest, John received a scaled score of 77, placing him at the 6th percentile. For the phonemic decoding efficiency subtest, he received a scaled score of 74, placing him at the 4th percentile. His total word reading efficiency index (i.e., a combination of both the sight word and phonemic decoding efficiency tests) was a scaled score of 74, placing him at the 4th percentile. **In sum, his performance on these subtests was significantly below average.**

4.1.3 The Test of Integrated Language and Literacy Skills (TILLS)

The TILLS is an assessment of oral and written language and literacy abilities from the single-sound level to discourse level and is used to (1) identify a language/literacy disorder, (2) describe patterns of strengths and weaknesses, and (3) track changes over time [21]. To minimize fatigue and optimize time (as John was going to have numerous assessments to complete during his comprehensive evaluation), the SLP selected subtests that would provide the core, sound/word composite, and written language composite scores.

John's identification core composite raw score of 17 was less than 34, which is the cut score for 8- to 11-year-olds. His score was consistent with having a language/literacy disorder. The sound/word composite evaluated John's intact morphological and phonological awareness abilities across writing, reading, and oral language tasks. John's sound/word raw composite score of 35 was considered low, and translates to a standard score of 69, which is three standard deviations below the mean, and **indicates a significant deficit at the sound/word level.** John scored within the average range on the nonword repetition and reading fluency subtests, but below average on the phonemic awareness, nonword reading, nonword spelling, and written expression-word subtests. **Deficits at the sound/word level are a defining characteristic of dyslexia.**

Two sentence/discourse subtests, the Listening Comprehension and Vocabulary Awareness subtests were administered. John achieved a standard score of 7 and a percentile rank of 14 in Listening Comprehension, indicating borderline average ability. On the Vocabulary Awareness subtest, John achieved a standard score of 6 and percentile rank of 8 (i.e., one standard deviation below the mean). On the written composite score, John achieved a standard score of 69 (i.e., three standard deviations below the mean), **indicating a significant written language deficit.**

4.1.4 The TILLS Student Language Scale (SLS Questionnaire)

The Student Language Scale (SLS) from the TILLS is used to screen for language/literacy disorders by asking parents and teachers to rate their perceptions of student ability. When teachers or parents rate more than two areas on items 1–8 as less than 5, SLS results indicate the student may have a language and/or literacy disorder [21].

Overall, parent and teacher ratings of John's language and literacy abilities were very similar, **indicating John is at risk for language and literacy deficits.** The homeroom teachers rated John below 5 in 7 out of 8 areas, the reading and writing teacher rated John below 5 in 6 out of 8 areas, and John's mother rated him below 5 in 8 out of 8 areas.

4.1.5 AIMSweb Spelling and Reading Maze Curriculum-Based Measures

4.1.5.1 The AIMSweb Spelling Benchmark

The AIMSweb Spelling Benchmark uses two cut scores to identify at-risk students and those in need of intervention. Students who score below the Tier 1 cut score (which is the 45th percentile) are considered at moderate risk; those who score below the Tier 2 cut score (which is the 15th percentile) are considered at severe risk. For John's third grade level, the Tier 1 cut score is 83 and the Tier 2 cut score is 55. John received a score of 56, placing him just above the Tier 2 cut score of 55, **indicating risk for spelling difficulties and the need for intervention.** John spelled two words correctly out of a total of 17 words, and he scored 56 out of 112 for correct letter sequences, determined by pairs of letters that are correctly sequenced within a word [22].

4.1.5.2 AIMSweb Reading Maze Benchmark

The AIMSweb Reading Maze Benchmark uses two cut scores to identify risk for reading comprehension deficits. Students who score below the Tier 1 cut score (which again corresponds to the 45th percentile) are considered at moderate risk, and those who score below the Tier 2 cut score (which again corresponds to the 15th percentile) are considered at severe risk. For John's third grade level, the Tier 1 cut score is 11 and the Tier 2 cut score is 6. John received a score of 3.5, placing him below the Tier 2 cut score and **indicating significant risk for reading comprehension difficulties and the need for intervention.** John did not finish reading the passage within the time limit, leaving 31 mazes unanswered. **It is possible that the cognitive challenge of decoding at the word level inhibited John's reading rate and adversely affected his overall fluency and comprehension.**

4.1.6 GrayOral Reading Test: Fifth Edition (GORT-50)

The Gray Oral Reading Test (GORT-5) assesses rate, accuracy, fluency, and comprehension. Fluency and comprehension are combined to provide an oral reading index score. For this assessment, John's scaled scores of reading fluency (i.e., rate and accuracy) and comprehension were assessed. First, he was timed while reading short texts aloud, then each section of text was read out loud for John to answer questions [23].

He received a scaled score of 6 for fluency and 7 for comprehension. The mean for each scaled score is 10, with a standard deviation of 3. **This indicates that John's reading fluency is below average.** John's comprehension score fell at the borderline/low average range. His oral reading index was 81, placing him in the 10th percentile, indicative of a below average performance. More specifically, John did not attempt to sound out words (i.e., he did not attempt to decode) but instead skipped over words as the difficulty of the story increased.

4.1.7 Probe of morphological awareness

Morphological awareness refers to the ability to identify morphemes (i.e., the base and any prefixes and suffixes) in words. Research shows that morphological awareness is related to word reading and spelling, vocabulary, and reading comprehension. Probes of morphological awareness often assess morphology and word order by asking for adding or removing word endings [28].

The SLP assessed John's awareness of morphemes in words, relations between words that have common morphemes, and his ability to apply this knowledge when spelling words. Specifically, the examiner said a word and then a sentence with a missing word at the end. John was asked to complete the sentence by making a new word from the word provided at the beginning. For example, the examiner said, "Skip. As he crossed the street, Paul ____." In this instance, the correct answer is "skipped." John answered 90% of the items correctly.

Next, he was asked to spell the complex word (base + suffix). When shown the spelling of the base word, he spelled 40% of the complex words correctly. However, when he was *not* shown the base word, he did not spell *any* of the complex words correctly. **The difference in spelling accuracy levels with and without the base indicates he can use the base to help him spell the complex words, but is unable to accurately generate the spelling of the base on his own.**

Given his performance, morphological awareness would appear to be a strength of John's oral language despite his difficulty in spelling when the base word was removed. John's dichotomy in ability is not an uncommon finding. **Researchers have found phonological challenges can limit the segmenting of affixes (i.e., word-endings) in students with dyslexia** [29].

4.1.8 Writing sample

The examiners prompted John to write an expository text about his favorite sport. The length of the text John submitted was short. Given 10 minutes, he wrote a three-sentence, 29-word paragraph, with an average of 9.8 words per sentence. John's sentence complexity was limited, including 1.3 clauses per sentence and only one compound sentence (using the conjunction "but"). John's writing sample provided basic organization and content as well as some key writing mechanic skills for his grade level. He effectively communicated the basics of the topic he selected, but his explanation lacked supporting details. No errors occurred in subject-verb agreement, capitalization, or punctuation. **Writing samples have been used to identify the specific strengths and weaknesses in persons with dyslexia and language impairment** [30].

Frequent spelling errors were more common with complex words (base + affix) than simple words (base word only). For instance, he spelled "baskle" for basically. This demonstrates that this word may be in his lexicon, but he is not able to spell it correctly likely due to phonological processing and morphological awareness deficits. Additionally, he substituted "b" for "p" as in "bast" for pass.

Overall, John's performance on the independent writing sample illustrated difficulties with syntax and spelling that are consistent with his performance on other tests. These difficulties at the sound, word, and sentence level may have contributed to briefness of the exposition, requiring increased cognitive load and appearing effortful.

4.1.9 Test results and recommendations

Results of testing indicate that John presented with a language/literacy disorder. John's profile is consistent with characteristics of dyslexia in that he tested significantly below average at the sound/word level, including on tests of phonological processing, word reading, and spelling.

The SLP recommended intensive and direct services for both oral and written language (literacy). Further, it was suggested that oral language services to be provided by an SLP, and written language services provided by an SLP and/or teacher or educator trained in evidence-based literacy intervention, with a focus on phonological and morphological, and orthographic abilities.

5. Future considerations and practice implications

To date, our understanding of dyslexia hypothesizes that it is a literacy disorder involving deficits in use and understanding of phonological systems such as decoding and encoding [18]. The interconnection between speech sounds, language production skills, and dyslexia has been suggested in research and practical situations. Indeed, deficits in the phonological systems of students provide an explanation for many students with dyslexia, such as John. Challenges in phonological awareness and their representations also appear to manifest long after language develops, creating ongoing disruptions for students with dyslexia [31].

As previously noted, the sooner a student is identified with a language literacy disorder such as dyslexia, the better their long-term educational, mental, and emotional outcomes become. After dyslexia is suspected, a student is often referred by a teacher or learning specialist to an educational psychologist who can confirm a diagnosis of dyslexia. Because of the volume of students in the school systems, the chance for a student's language literacy disorder to be missed or at very least, not be identified until later in their schooling, is a legitimate concern. The importance, then, of other skilled professionals such as SLPs to take an active role in assessing students at risk for language literacy disorders cannot be understated. With a background in language and literacy development, the SLP can serve as a valuable resource for students, parents, and educators alike. Such was the case for John, whose language literacy disorder was identified by an SLP well trained in assessment and treatment of students with language literacy disorders.

Based on phonological training and knowledge of all the subsystems of language, the SLP can serve as a valuable resource for identification and management of dyslexia in students. The use of formal assessments and information means (i.e., written and oral language samples), parent and teacher reports, and collaboration with reading specialists give insight into the unique needs of each student with dyslexia as well. Future research into the influence of other language subsystems such as semantics, syntax, and morphology may provide further insight into identification and treatment of dyslexia.

Author details

Jane Roitsch
Old Dominion University, Norfolk, VA, USA

*Address all correspondence to: jroitsch1@gmail.com

References

[1] International Dyslexia Association. Dyslexia assessment: What is it and how can it help? 2020. Available from: https://dyslexiaida.org/dyslexia-assessment-what-is-it-and-how-can-it-help-2/ [Accessed: 12 August 2020]

[2] Sprenger-Charolles L, Siegel LS, Jimenez JE, Ziegler JC. Prevalence and reliability of phonological, surface, and mixed profiles in dyslexia: A review of studies conducted in languages varying in orthographic depth. Scientific Studies of Reading. 2011;**15**(6):498-521. DOI: 10.1080/10888438.2010.524463

[3] Pennington BF, Bishop DVM. Relations among speech, language, and reading disorders. Annual Review of Psychology. 2009;**60**:283-306. DOI: 10.1146/annurev.psych.60.110707.163548

[4] Chall JS. Literacy: Trends and explanations. Educational Research. 1983;**12**(9):3-8. DOI: 10.2307/1174721

[5] Polychroni F, Koukoura K, Anagnostou I. Academic self-concept, reading attitudes and approaches to learning of children with dyslexia: Do they differ from their peers? European Journal of Special Needs Education. 2006;**21**(4):415-430

[6] Viscomi C. The speech-language pathologist's role in diagnosing dyslexia. The ASHA Leader Live. 2018. Available from: https://leader.pubs.asha.org/do/10.1044/the-speech-language-pathologists-role-in-diagnosing-dyslexia/full/ [Accessed: 12 August 2020]

[7] American Speech-Language-Hearing Association. [Internet]. Roles and responsibilities of speech-language pathologists with respect to reading and writing in children and adolescents [Position Statement]. Available from: www.asha.org/policy [Accessed: 14 August 2020]

[8] Yin RK. A (very) brief refresher on the case study method. Applications of Case Study Research. 2012;**3**:3-20

[9] Rief S, Stern J. The Dyslexia Checklist a Practical Reference for Parents and Teachers. 1st ed. San Francisco, Calif: Jossey-Bass; 2010

[10] Zimmerman IL, Steiner VG, Pond RE. The Preschool Language Scale-5. San Antonio, TX: Pearson; 2011

[11] Nash HM, Hulme C, Gooch D, Snowling MJ. Preschool language profiles of children at family risk of dyslexia: Continuities with specific language impairment. Journal of Child Psychology and Psychiatry. 2013;**54**:958-968. DOI: 10.1111/jcpp.12091

[12] Wechsler D. Wechsler Intelligence Scale for Children. 5th ed. Bloomington: Pearson; 2014

[13] Das JP, Mishra RK, Kirby JR. Cognitive patterns of children with dyslexia: A comparison between groups with high and average nonverbal intelligence. Journal of Learning Disabilities. 1994;**27**(4):235-242. DOI: 10.1177/002221949402700405

[14] Wechsler D. Wechsler Individual Achievement Test. 3rd ed. San Antonio, TX: Pearson; 2009

[15] Hayiou-Thomas ME, Carroll JM, Leavett R, Hulme C, Snowling MJ. When does speech sound disorder matter for literacy? The role of disordered speech errors, co-occurring language impairment and family risk of dyslexia. Journal of Child Psychology and Psychiatry. 2017;**58**:197-205. DOI: 10.1111/jcpp.12648

[16] Xiao X-Y, Ho CS-H. Weaknesses in semantic, syntactic and oral language expression contribute to reading difficulties in Chinese dyslexic children.

Dyslexia. 2014;**20**:74-98. DOI: 10.1002/dys.1460

[17] Al-Zoubi S, Al-Zoubi S. Prevalence of articulation errors among Jordanian gifted students with dyslexia. Journal for the Education of Gifted Young Scientists. 2020;**8**(1):533-547. DOI: 10.17478/jegys.682635

[18] Lyon GR, Shaywitz SE, Shaywitz BA. A definition of dyslexia. Annals of Dyslexia. 2003;**53**:1-14. DOI: 10.1007/s11881-003-0001-9

[19] Wagner RK, Torgesen JK, Rashotte CA, Pearson NA. Comprehensive Test of Phonological Processing-Second Edition (CTOPP-2); Austin, Tex: Pro-Ed; 2012. Available from http://www4.parinc.com/Products/Product.aspx?ProductID=CTOPP-2

[20] Torgesen JK, Rashotte CA, Wagner RK. TOWRE 2: Test of Word Reading Efficiency. Austin, Tex: Pro-Ed; 2012

[21] Nelson NW, Plante E, Helm-Estabrooks N, Hotz G. Test of Integrated Language and Literacy Skills. Baltimore, MD: Paul H. Brookes; 2016

[22] Shinn MR, Shinn MM. AIMSweb Training Workbook. Eden Prairie, MN: EdInformation, Inc; 2002

[23] Wiederholt JL, Bryant BR. Gray Oral Reading Tests—Fifth Edition (GORT-5). Austin, TX: Pro-Ed; 2012

[24] Perrachione TK, Ghosh SS, Ostrovskaya I, Gabrieli J, Kovelman I. Phonological working memory for words and nonwords in cerebral cortex. Journal of Speech, Language, and Hearing Research. 2017;**60**(7):1959-1979. DOI: 10.1044/2017_JSLHR-L-15-0446

[25] Vander Stappen C, Reybroeck MV. Phonological awareness and rapid automatized naming are independent phonological competencies with specific impacts on word reading and spelling: An intervention study. Frontiers in Psychology. 2018;**9**:320. DOI: 10.3389/fpsyg.2018.00320

[26] Casalis S, Colé P, Sopo D. Morphological awareness in developmental dyslexia. Annals of Dyslexia. 2004;**12**(9):114-138. DOI: 10.1007/s11881-004-0006-z

[27] Puranik CS, Lombardino LJ, Altmann LJ. Writing through retellings: An exploratory study of language-impaired and dyslexic populations. Reading and Writing. 2007;**20**:251-272. DOI: 10.1007/s11145-006-9030-1

[28] Ehri LC. Sight word learning in normal readers and dyslexics. In: Blackman BA, editor. Foundations of Reading Acquisition Dyslexia: Implications for Early Intervention. New York: Routledge; 2013

[29] Snowling MJ. Phonemic deficits in developmental dyslexia. Psychological Research Psychologische Forschung. 1981;**43**:219-234. DOI: 10.1007/BF00309831

[30] Bernstein SE, Flipse JL, Jin Y, Odegard TN. Word and sentence level tests of morphological awareness in reading. Reading and Writing. 2020;**33**:1591-1616. DOI: 10.1007/s11145-020-10024-6

[31] Alt M, Hogan T, Green S, Gray S, Cabbage K, Cowan N. Word learning deficits in children with dyslexia. Journal of Speech, Language, and Hearing Research. 2017;**60**(4):1012-1028. DOI: 10.1044/2016_JSLHR-L-16-0036

Chapter 4

"It's a Battle!": Parenting and Supporting a Child with Dyslexia

Helen Ross

Abstract

Parents and carers supporting their children with dyslexia liken their experiences to battle, when trying to secure appropriate educational provision for their children. This chapter expands our understanding of parents'/carers' experiences through exploration of both academic studies, reviews and gray literature since the Assent of the Children and Families Act 2014 in England. Using a Bourdieusian framework underpinned by Jenkins' 'levels of interaction', this chapter studies parental/carers' experiences of dyslexia and procurement of appropriate educational provision for their children with dyslexia. Parents'/carers' internal sense-making of dyslexia is explored. Connections are made between this sense-making and the nature of parents'/carers' interactions with their children and education professionals. These interactions, as underpinned by individuals' understandings of dyslexia are then explored in the context of the social positions occupied by parents/carers relative to others within the field of education. Parents'/carers' capacity to engage with professionals, and contribute meaningfully to decision-making processes through embodiment of necessary habitus is exposed through analysis of individual sense-making, interactional exchanges and institutional relationships. Practical and theoretical implications of parents'/carers/sense-making of dyslexia, their interactional experiences, and embodiment of habitus are then described in a 'Who, What, When and How' overview of parents/carers supporting a child with dyslexia.

Keywords: dyslexia, SEND, parent voice, Bourdieu, inclusion

1. Introduction

In this chapter, 'levels of interaction' [1] are combined with Bourdieusian concepts of habitus, field and practice to explore parents' experiences of their children's dyslexia within an English policy context. Dyslexia is a contested phenomenon [2–4] within literature, practice and media [5–7]. This is despite the British Dyslexia Association [8] providing a robust definition, which incorporates 'testable' characteristics to allow for diagnostic assessment of difficulties.

However, some institutions refute the existence of dyslexia as a discrete phenomenon [2], leading to rejection of or refusal to diagnose [9, 10]. For parents this leads to challenges in supporting their children. If dyslexia does not exist, then literacy difficulties are the 'fault' of the child, the parents are overreacting and schools are not obliged to make concessions to support children or their parents. This chapter explores how parents at the 'individual level' make sense of their children's dyslexia and reframe it as an 'inclusive' and positive phenomenon. As interaction between professionals and parents can be problematic [10–12], we explore at the 'interactional level' how parents' sense-making and reframing of dyslexia underpins their interactions with their children and empower them to engage with schools [13]. Where communication is problematic, barriers to positive interaction are delineated and contextualized within wider structures. Political constructs within education in England place the onus for inclusion on professionals, settings and Local Authorities [14]. However, studies have found that parental participation is not always productive or meaningful, despite policy expectations [10, 15, 16]. As such, exploration of institutional roles and policy within this chapter is important to understand structures which impede parents' active participation in their children's education. Habitus and transformations within parents, professionals and wider structures are discussed, so that practical recommendations can be drawn from literature and exploration of each level of interaction.

2. Dyslexia: what is it?

Dyslexia is a condition whose definition and existence are contested. Some research disputes its existence as a scientifically 'testable' condition [2]. Other work explicitly states that those with dyslexia and 'poor readers' should not be conflated [3]. Rather, Frith [3] and the British Dyslexia Association [8] argue that dyslexia is an underlying neurological difference that is the root cause of some reading difficulties. Formal definition of the neuro-biological impairment that leads to dyslexic-difficulties is outside of the scope of this chapter (significant work has been undertaken on this elsewhere [3, 17, 18]). However, a functional working definition of dyslexia and an understanding of its characteristics is necessary. It is also important to understand the connection between medicalized and social models of dyslexia. This underpins exploration of parents' personal conceptualizations of dyslexia at the 'individual level', during their interactions with other individuals and through their interactions with institutions.

Medicalized views of dyslexia locate its root causes within the individual with little-to-no reference to structural factors affecting it [19]. Solvang [20], Ross [15] and Calfee [19] found that language surrounding 'diagnosis' of dyslexia frame it as an internal 'impairment' within the individual. This serves to explain why children experienced difficulties and removes parents' 'fault' for their children's dyslexic difficulties. Others argue that external, structural factors should be considered in the conceptualization of dyslexia. Riddick [4] suggested that locating cause purely within the individual is an oppressive model, which disempowers individuals to argue for changes within their environment.

Other work locates causes of dyslexia outside of the individual to define dyslexia through cultural and social norms [21]. However, this view of dyslexia does not consider neurological differences between individuals, which predispose them to dyslexic difficulties. This is also problematic, as there is potential for individuals to understand reasons for their difficulties as being outside of their control, leading to disempowerment and oppression when they experience dyslexic-type difficulties. As such this paper draws on a bio-social model of dyslexia congruent with earlier work by MacDonald [22] and Ross [11, 15]. This model allows for consideration of underlying impairments within the individual, and external, social factors which act to emphasize or minimize effects of that underlying impairment.

Although various definitions of dyslexia exist [23, 24], which draw on both internal difficulties and consider effects of social factors on individuals, for the purposes of this chapter, the British Dyslexia Association definition of dyslexia [8] will be used:

DOI: http://dx.doi.org/10.5772/intechopen.93948

> *"...[dyslexia is] a learning difficulty that primarily affects the skills involved in accurate and fluent word reading and spelling. Characteristic features of dyslexia are difficulties in phonological awareness, verbal memory and verbal processing speed. Dyslexia occurs across the range of intellectual abilities. It is best thought of as a continuum, not a distinct category, and there are no clear cut-off points. Co-occurring difficulties may be seen in aspects of language, motor co-ordination, mental calculation, concentration and personal organization, but these are not, by themselves, markers of dyslexia. A good indication of the severity and persistence of dyslexic difficulties can be gained by examining how the individual responds or has responded to well-founded intervention.*
>
> *In addition to these characteristics: The British Dyslexia Association (BDA) acknowledges the visual and auditory processing difficulties that some individuals with dyslexia can experience, and points out that dyslexic readers can show a combination of abilities and difficulties that affect the learning process. Some also have strengths in other areas, such as design, problem solving, creative skills, interactive skills and oral skills."*

It describes both behavioral manifestations and also outlines diagnostic criteria, namely poor phonological awareness, memory and processing. This is useful when considering the experiences of non-professionals, and how they understand dyslexia and its effects.

3. Dyslexia, Bourdieu and Jenkins: theorizing dyslexia and identity within education

Dyslexia, Bourdieu and Jenkins may be an unlikely grouping in the development of theoretical frameworks. While dyslexia and identity have been considered sociologically [4, 22], a unified theory to facilitate exploration and analysis of its effects on individuals, their identities and interactions, and ability to engage with social structures is lacking. Ross' [11, 15] work pragmatically knitted together 'levels of interaction' [1] to explore stakeholders' experiences in the development of support interventions for young people in school. Key concepts are defined in this section. They are then related to the field of education, and the specific area of interest for this chapter: dyslexia-support for young people and the experiences of their parents/carers.

3.1 Bourdieu's 'field', 'habitus' and 'practice'

The ground-breaking concepts of 'field', 'habitus' and 'practice' described in Bourdieu's seminal work 'Outline of a Theory of Practice' [25], are central to understanding how dyslexia influences an individual's experiences of education and related interactions in that field. Bourdieu [26] argued that the social world around us is produced through social interactions, actions and thoughts of social actors.

Of the three central tenants of his sociological project, the 'field' is perhaps the easiest to define. Bourdieu [27] viewed the field as "a simple idea: it designates a system of objective relationships between positions, implies a relative autonomy etc. but it is difficult to put into practice". Largely, when operationalizing the concept of field in line with Bourdieu's sociological project, it is best understood as the space within which social actors' relationships are defined by their relative positions in that space. The field of education is where parent-professional interactions relating to dyslexia support for young people take place. Within the field relative positions of parents/carers and parents are defined and (re-)produced through those interactions.

The set of social norms and expectations associated with different roles/social positions within a field is viewed by Bourdieu as both an internal process and an externally perceptible object. He named this set of norms and processes 'habitus', a concept that he continually revisited and developed for the duration of his sociological project. Defined as, "both a system of schemes of production of practices and a system of perception and appreciation of practices ... habitus produced practices and representations which are available for classification which are objectively differentiated," Bourdieu's [26] concept of 'habitus' encapsulates these sets of expectations, as something that is 'done' within a social setting. When these expectations are then embodied, produced and reproduced by others within a field, propagating social positions they become the 'done thing'. The embedded set of 'done thing' habitus can then be described as a set of 'practices'.

Through the lens of these cornerstone concepts within Bourdieu's sociological project, we can explore the experiences of parents and carers within the field of education as they navigate systems for supporting young people with dyslexia. As parents/carers make sense of dyslexia, the habitus necessary for positive, constructive engagement with other individuals implicated in supporting their children and the wider institutions of the field is delineated. The capacity of parents/carers to embody that habitus and engage with social structures at institutional level can then be investigated.

3.2 Roles and values in education

Prior to discussion of different roles in education, it is important to address underlying philosophical assumptions associated with it. Bourdieu [25] argued that practices and values associated with education are largely white and middle class. He viewed the field of education as a site of production and reproduction (propagation) of social positions, relationships and power differentials. The power differentials encapsulated in the social relationships between individuals in a social field thus act to maintain a status quo. With this in mind, he reasoned that teachers, and other 'state functionaries,' are inculcated by the habitus of their social position and role to exclude actors whose habitus does not align with that of positions of power within education. Where values do mis-align, individuals experience a 'clash' in values, known as a 'dialectical confrontation' [28], which may result in modification of that individuals' embodied habitus. However, where personal values do not align with the values of the education system, and the actor's embodied habitus remains unchanged, their difficulties in meaningfully accessing systems related to education will remain [28].

Bourdieu [25, 26, 29] considered the 'State' as controlling some social categories, defined by him as 'official identities.' These identities, and the roles occupied by social actors are objective social structures according to him [25, 29]. Within education, the 'State', via universities and training providers, acts as gatekeeper to the status of 'Qualified teacher' in England. The status is granted following successful completion of academic and work-based elements of government-approved teacher-training programs and an in-school 'induction year' [30]. Other professionals, such as educational psychologists, occupational therapists, and physiotherapists must also acquire professional qualifications. These qualifications allow those professionals access to formal positions in the field of education, based on those credentials. These professionals then are afforded, by their professional status, the capacity to affect the type of support available to young people. In many cases they act as gatekeeper to that support. In so doing, congruent with Bourdieu's findings, these professionals' actions act to propagate their dominant positions within the field, affording them power over other social actors.

Within a school, the 'Special Educational Needs Coordinator' (SENCo) and other teachers are responsible for provision of support for young people with Special Educational Needs and/or Disability (SEND) [14]. They act as stewards for resources and support for those who have identified need. However, in some cases identification of need can only be undertaken by certain professionals, such that needs are not always formally and fully identified. Mainstream teachers and SENCos cannot formally identify need without further training. The lack of formal diagnosis or identification of need may then impact on young people's ability to access appropriate resources and provision. Teachers may be aware of need but not know how to support young people appropriately.

Within education, the propagated, middle-class values which call for children and young people to conform to 'normative' values [31] act to exclude young people with special educational needs and disability (SEND). They rarely conform to normative expectations and often require specialized support. Thus, within the field of education, a young person with SEND may be unable to embody the necessary habitus to successfully navigate the practices of the field. Despite being expected to actively engage in decision-making processes relating to their own educational provision [14], in reality, young people are often subordinate and unable to meaningfully access these processes [11, 16]. Their views are more likely to be represented by their parents/carers in formal settings, reinforcing their subordinate, oppressed position within that field.

In policy the role of parents/carers in supporting their children with SEND appears to be relatively straightforward: they are expected to be fully "involved in discussions and decisions about their individual support" [14]. This expectation reflects legislative directives [32]. Other stakeholders should make adjustments where necessary to facilitate parental/carer involvement in decision-making relating to support for young people. However, the detail as to how this should be undertaken has not been given. In fact, research has shown that the enactment of this legislation and guidelines has been unsuccessful in ensuring the active and meaningful participation of parents/carers in discussions about provision for their children [16, 33, 34]. This is indicative of a system that is not fulfilling its brief. Where parents'/carers' roles are unclear, their capacity to positively, meaningfully and productively engage in decision-making processes for their children's education is hindered, and their capacity to enact agency and effect change is severely limited. This can leave them feeling powerless and impact negatively on future interactions with actors in the 'field' of education due to the negative effects of oppression and powerlessness on their internal sense-making of their situation.

3.3 Identity construction

A significant volume of psychological and sociological research has explored the processes which underpin the formation of identity. In this chapter, we focus on work that considers identity as a social process. That is, that identity is constructed both through internal sense-making of self in relation to one's social position within a network and also through interactions with others in that network. Social position is a key factor in identity construction within the sociologies of Bourdieu [25] and Jenkins [1], as well as in social-psychological studies.

Within Bourdieu's sociology, institutions and 'roles' may act as social agents, acting to oppress and promote others within their field depending on their relative positions and roles. As such, a broader framework is necessary so that different types of interaction between different types of social actor may be considered intersectionally. The sociological work of Richard Jenkins [1] around identity and its formation suits this purpose ideally. He believes that the social world and its interactions influence how identity is constructed and reconstructed constantly through social relationships. Thus, his theoretical concepts may be interweaved with Bourdieu's sociological project to produce a powerful theoretical framework to explore roles, relationships and power-differentials within social fields.

3.4 Bourdieu and Jenkins

At first glance, Jenkins and Bourdieu may not appear an obvious 'pairing'. Jenkins [35] viewed elements of Bourdieu's sociological project as unsuccessful in their attempts to bridge the subjectivist-objectivist gap. It is argued that Bourdieu's frameworks inadequately consider people's own individual agency [35]. Jenkins viewed 'structuralism' as imposing itself on actors, and minimizing their individual capacity to enact agency [35]. However, a central tenet of both Bourdieu's and Jenkins' work is that external structures exist within the social world and influence the identity, interactions and actions of social agents within a field. 'Levels of interaction' [1] model the social world through exploration of interactions at three levels and Bourdieu's 'habitus', 'practice' and field also explore social actor's interactions within their social context. Both Jenkins [1, 35] and Bourdieu [25–27] viewed the social actors and their context as inseparable. It is this unifying feature which allows for combining of their sociological frameworks through which to explore the social world.

3.5 Levels of interaction and dyslexia

As has been shown elsewhere, Bourdieu's concepts of 'habitus', 'field' and 'practice' [25–27] and Jenkins' 'levels of interaction' [1] have been successfully knitted together to develop a strong theoretical framework to analyze social interactions [11, 15]. Through this framework, barriers to parents' meaningful participation in discussions about provision for their children have been uncovered [15], and teachers' roles in provision for young people have been explored. This was done through the analysis of habitus, practice and field at different 'levels of interaction' [1].

The 'levels of interaction' are defined thus [1]:

- "the individual order is the human world as made up of embodied individuals and what-goes-on-in-their-heads;
- the interaction order is the human world as constituted in relationships between individuals, in what-goes-on-between-people;
- the institutional order is the human world of pattern and organization, of established-ways-of-doing-things."

Young people's views are traditionally represented by their parents in policy forums, as parents (or carers) are legally responsible for them [36]. This is despite expectation that young people's own views are considered independently [14, 16]. Therefore, it is vital to understand how parents conceptualize dyslexia and subsequently their children's identity as a 'dyslexic,' as this will affect how their children's views are represented. As noted in [1], identity and social interactions are inseparable and mutually constructing. The 'concepts of self', informed by dyslexia thus influence parents' interactions with teachers at the 'interactional' level. Objective structures such as age, gender and social class influence interactions significantly. At the institutional level, these structures act to impede or facilitate social exchanges due to the requisite habitus and its (lack of) embodiment. Parents' capacity to embody a habitus affects their ability to successfully navigate structures around SEND provision for their children [15]. Insights relating to this suggest that barriers are complex and habitus 'clashes' occur [28].

Using this theoretical framework, this chapter will explore formal academic literature and 'gray literature' [37] to further develop our understanding of parents' participation in processes related to supporting their children with dyslexia. Individual understandings of dyslexia will be discussed, and then interactions between stakeholders in decision-making processes will be outlined. Finally, systemic relationships will be uncovered, and their implications described.

4. Making sense of it all: parents' understandings of dyslexia

In this section, how parents make sense of their children's dyslexia is discussed. The varied understandings and sources of parental information are highlighted. The internal conceptualization of a 'dyslexia' which bolsters them in supporting their dyslexic children, as discussed in [15], is expanded upon. We then reflect on the sense making that takes place and how it underpins parent's interactions with others in relation to their child's dyslexia. In so-doing we draw on Ingram's [28] understanding of 'dialectical confrontation', and Bourdieu's [25, 26] concepts of habitus and field.

4.1 Dyslexia: a parental understanding

Parental conceptualization of dyslexia is not a static phenomenon. It is a dynamic and ongoing process, altering as parents progress along their journey as 'parents of dyslexic children'. Prior to their child's diagnosis, Ross [15] found that parents located difficulties within their child. Young people's struggles were their own fault, rather than due to something outside of their control. Although writing in the early 1980s, Hartwig [6] had already ascertained what much research now reinforces: there was (and still is) much debate about the nature of dyslexia, its causes and its effects [2]. Parents did not, and do not always have a full understanding of dyslexia and its implications. A diagnosis or mention of SEND may strike significant fear into parents. They may be aware of potential battles ahead [7] or fear that their children are not 'normal'. This is particularly the case for parents who have dyslexia-type difficulties themselves and experienced education adversely [38]. Dyslexia is often not understood by parents [5] who may view their children as weak academically, and not realize the effects of the underlying impairment. That said, parents were largely aware of the external manifestations of their children's dyslexia; their children were poor spellers, reluctant writers and unenthusiastic readers.

However, upon 'diagnosis', parents' reframing process began. Solvang [20] notes that parents drew upon medicalized discourses which placed blame for young people's literacy difficulties squarely at the feet of their dyslexia. There was a reason for their difficulties: an internal force that young people could not control or overcome without support. Medicalization of dyslexia to relocate blame is a common theme in literature. The label of dyslexia became a source of relief and strength for parents; they could definitively say why their children had difficulties [12]. There was something 'wrong' with their children, but it wasn't theirs, or their children's fault [15, 20]. Dyslexia was something tangible, making learning difficult for their children.

4.2 My child has dyslexia: what next?

Once parents begin to make sense of their children's dyslexia as the root of their difficulties, then a sense of 'what next' arose. Ross [15] found that a significant aspect of parents' individual sense making and conceptualization of dyslexia linked to positive reframing of it. However, Woodcock [7] found that dyslexia can be a distressing and demanding experience for families. This chimes with other reports of anxiety and stress connected to schooling [39]. However, assessment and subsequent diagnosis of dyslexia has been found to be a source of empowerment for parents and children alike in much work [4, 20, 40].

The guilt, for blaming children for their dyslexic-difficulties, experienced by many parents [10, 15] acted as impetus for them to find out more. As noted in [41], "Acquiring knowledge is the basis of increased confidence". Information about dyslexia and its implications is a key factor highlighted in much literature. For some parents, a diagnosis of dyslexia may be a means to support their child and build up their self-esteem [9]. Parents seek the positives around dyslexia. They search for affirmations that there are benefits in the label, looking to their peers, media sources and celebrity role models for a sense of their child's potential [41]. Spaces in which parents could make sense of dyslexia and its impact are a key theme noted [15, 42]. Through the reframing of dyslexia positively and inclusively, "to include more affirmative, strength-based perspectives" [13], parents' can embrace their child's dyslexia, and see benefits as well as its drawbacks.

While sense-making and reframing of dyslexia positively take place at the individual level, internally within each individual [1], foundations are laid at this level for inter-personal interactions and the presentation of 'self' in these interactions. The 'sense-made' of dyslexia, encapsulated at the individual level underpins, parents' interactions with other individuals as they support their child within the field of education [11, 15].

4.3 Moving forwards and outwards

To conceptualize how parents move forwards as 'parents of young people with dyslexia,' we need to understand their internal sense-making and its subsequent role underpinning interactions with individuals around them. Ingram [28] discusses the habitus of working-class boys, rooted in their home-setting and how, when they are exposed to the conflicting 'habitus' of their school setting, a 'dialectical confrontation' takes place. She argues that habitus, in the Bourdieusian sense can be formed across mismatched fields. In the case of dyslexia and schooling, the central 'field' is education (their children's school) and their parenting habitus. We can draw on this concept when considering parental reactions to their children's dyslexia diagnosis.

Within literature there are commonalities documented in parental experience before their children receive a diagnosis of dyslexia. High stress is commonly documented and frustration that their children find engaging with education difficult. As noted above, parents frequently blame their children for the difficulties they have in school. They believe that lack of effort or attention are the root cause of their children's educational difficulties. Their habitus as parents is formed around their role of parent of a 'lazy' child, who is academically underachieving without 'good' reason. However, receipt of a 'diagnosis' of dyslexia exposes parents to a new habitus. A new 'field' becomes accessible to them in that moment: parenting a child with an educational need. Their position has shifted. They become a parent whose child has a need, which is making learning difficult for them. This new position initiates a 'dialectic confrontation' where their familiar habitus is disrupted and space created for adaptation. In processing this 'dialectic confrontation,' parents seek knowledge, and reflect on dyslexia and its meaning. This reflection underpins attempts to reframe dyslexia positively as a means for them to present a positive view of dyslexia to themselves. This allows them to construct a sense of self and parenting habitus, based around 'positive dyslexia'. When parents conceptualize dyslexia positively at the 'individual level', this positivity permeates their interactions at the 'interactional level' [11, 15].

5. Working with other people: parents' interactions with other individuals

Parents' interactions with others are underpinned by their conceptualization of dyslexia and their relationships with those connected to supporting their children. Here we explore parents' interactions with professionals. The effects of dyslexia on parents and their interactions with their children are also explored, with reference to sibling and parent-child relationships.

5.1 Parents and young people

Dyslexia has a profound impact on parents and other members of the family alike. As noted in [42], views shared with young people about dyslexia may be negative. Young people's self-esteem can be adversely affected by negative discourse, such that they are in need of positive messages about dyslexia. Hartwig [6] in a personal capacity notes the effect of *not* knowing about his son's dyslexia, stating that his parenting would have improved markedly if he had known earlier. He states tension and friction within his household, and subsequent anxiety were rooted in difficulties that he and his wife had in supporting both their son and their other children. Ross [15] uncovered similar experiences, with parents describing problematic interactions with all of their children, as a result of one of their children having dyslexia. Relationships suffer and non-dyslexic children may resent their dyslexic siblings. Dyslexic children often need a larger proportion of their parents' time for homework, extra money is spent on tuition and emotional labour is given to supporting their self-esteem [6, 15].

Positive reframing of dyslexia is a common strategy used by parents to support their children when discussing dyslexia with them [9, 15]. Where young people view dyslexia negatively and they are subject to poor academic expectations, positive reframing by parents aims to highlight young people's strengths and potential. To do this, parents draw on their internal conceptualization of a 'positive dyslexia' so that they can present this to their children. Parents provide context, safe spaces and advice [42, 43] for their children, to support them in positively reframing their own dyslexia, to construct a positive sense of self and their potential. Thus, parents' internal sense-making at the 'institutional level' serves to empower them in supporting their children via their exchanges at the 'interactional level'.

5.2 Parents and professionals

Positive relationships best underpin meaningful interactions between parents and professionals [12, 15, 40]. Where parents can frame dyslexia positively, and are confident in their knowledge of its characteristics, schools take their views seriously, which resulted in improved provision for young people [15]. Norwich et al. [12] found that appropriate provision for children was secured, not based on knowledge or formal diagnosis, but based on interactions and interpersonal relationships. Their study found that personal input from an independent professional, who advocated with teachers on behalf of parents, at times positively influenced provision for young people. This is particularly the case where parents felt unequipped to engage with teachers in relation to provision for their children. In such instances, parents may procure support to facilitate engagement with their child's school.

Lichtenstein [44] writes that in the United States, many parents feel unheard when raising concerns about their children's dyslexic-tendencies. He found that parents regularly had to commission private diagnostic assessments for their children. This echoes [12, 40]. Parents' understandings of their children's needs served to empower them to bypass the state school system and seek a private assessment of need. In obtaining a private diagnosis for their children, parents' hope is that they will be able to secure appropriate provision for their children. However, this may not be the case.

A common struggle experienced by parents is getting their children's needs identified and recognized [15, 45]. Schools may be reluctant to formally label young people as 'dyslexic' [4] or unwilling/unable to commission a formal diagnostic needs assessment for them [12]. The underlying reasons for schools' lack of capacity to identify need are varied and diverse. It may be that schools lack professional knowledge of dyslexia or that they view parents as overreacting to their children's perceived difficulties [12, 40]. Where schools have not adequately identified need, Ferguson [5] suggests that parents should advocate for their children, requesting regular updates, feedback, and progress reports from schools. She recommends working with schools to ensure that they quantify progress and provide cross-curricular feedback. However, in practicality this may be difficulty.

Parent-partnership is a problematic framework for both parents and teachers to engage in. Within policy they are responsible for provision for young people and are framed as experts. However, within the same policy framework, parents are also experts whose views must be considered [14]. In engaging with professionals, parents have reported that their own professional background had provided useful tools. Ross [15] found that parents, who had worked within the field of education could better engage with teachers supporting their children. They felt that their views were taken seriously as they were familiar with the habitus of education, and could access the language and practice of the field. Key in engaging with the school was an understanding of the required habitus. This chimes with other work [40], which agrees that mutual understanding and compassion is necessary. However, they 'flip' the view that parents must undergo battle [7, 10] to secure support for their children. Instead they argue that the onus for 'work' should be on professionals, as 'gatekeepers' to resources [12, 40]. They argue that professionals should adapt their communication strategies so that parents feel able to approach them personally to engage in discussion around provision for their children. However, such adjustment is not always readily achievable during interactions between parents and professionals.

5.3 Interacting on a level

As noted above, there is often a disjoint between teachers and parents when discussing provision for young people with dyslexia. Parents may have significant knowledge of dyslexia and how to support their children, whereas teachers have less knowledge but are in the position of gatekeepers to resources for young people [10]. There is a tension between teachers and parents where visions for support and expectations around provision differ; teachers grant access and parents may feel powerless. Research asserts that teachers, schools, and other professionals should make allowances when working with parents to facilitate their participation in decision-making processes about provision for young people [12, 40]. While in theory this is an excellent and inclusive strategy, on the ground some parents do not find that professionals make concessions or are approachable [12, 15]. There are social, cultural, and power-based barriers which impede parents' meaningful participation in decision-making processes at school.

Where parents had professional experiences working with teachers or as teachers themselves, it was often easier for them to discuss their children's support with professionals [15]. This is echoed elsewhere [12, 13, 42]. Knowledge and experience build parents' confidence, which can form part of an embodied habitus that aligns well with teacher's professional habitus. Such an alignment of habitus facilitates positive interaction and reduces social distance between parents and professionals.

Where social distances are minimal and habitus is shared, power differentials are minimized. Bourdieu's social project focusses on social relationships with a field, noting that those in an advantageous position will act to maintain their power. Those who are disadvantaged usually do not challenge power structures. However, within the field of education, parents with knowledge of dyslexia and policy frameworks have increased confidence and feel able to engage with teachers (in advantageous, gatekeeper positions). They feel better able to challenge decisions relating to their children, whether through their own actions, or with the support of legal counsel. Such engagement and challenge demonstrate parents' newly embodied habitus, initiated by their own internal sense-making of dyslexia at the 'individual level' [15]. This capacity to challenge individuals through social exchanges lays foundations for parents to act to challenge systemic barriers to participation and the roles embodied by individuals and institutions.

6. Engaging with the system

As parental confidence to engage with professionals increases, their capacity to challenge systemic barriers to participation in decision-making processes around support for their children improves. However not all parents are able to engage meaningfully. Within a Bourdieusian framework this is largely due to external structures which act to constrain them, impede their own free-agency and inculcating them to act in certain ways. Here, systemic structures are discussed and parents' positions within these are highlighted, with reference to power differentials between them and professionals. These differentials act to facilitate or impede meaningful, collaboration between parents and professional to support young people with dyslexia.

6.1 Parental roles in policy

Traditionally, parents have represented their children's views within policy frameworks [36]. Although within [32], and the 0–25 SEND Code of Practice [14], young people's views are sought, it is expected that parents/carers actively engage with educational settings in decision-making processes relating to provision and support for their children. Early 21st-century, policy reviews [12, 41] found that policy frameworks were inadequately supporting parental engagement, with resources inequitably allocated and young peoples' needs not met. Current policy frameworks were piloted under the Coalition Government, beginning in 2011 [46]. The aim of the revised policy frameworks was to facilitate parental engagement, remove unnecessary bureaucracy and streamline provision for young people with SEND. However, governmental evaluations of this framework found that parental engagement was not substantially improved [16]. Power imbalances, lack of transparency and inaccessible processes which impede parental participation remained within renewed policy structures.

Bourdieu [25] argues within his sociological project that dominant groups within a social field act to propagate their own advantageous position. The practices of a field and their associated habitus are constructed by dominant groups and then re-constructed through their continued (re-)embodiment by social agents within the field. Thus, within the field of education, while nominally, the role of parents within decision-making processes has been bolstered by new legislation, in practice parents feel that there is little difference. Parents felt disempowered [12], as do parents under current policy [15, 16]. They are still constrained by oppressive structures unless they experience a 'dialectical confrontation' [28], where their habitus is modified, facilitating their capacity to engage with professionals.

What parental engagement looks like and how their habitus modifies varies from individual to individual. Some parents commission external support and representation to facilitate their engagement with schools; they 'hire' knowledge and those who embody the habitus needed to access resources for their children [9, 15]. Other parents can engage in the role of 'active participants' without external support. They can embody knowledge of dyslexia, habitus and practice needed to secure resources within the field of education at institutional level. This is often connected to their professional or educational background [15]. Where parents embody the role of 'active participant' in their children's education, their habitus is such that they can enact agency, engage meaningfully with policy processes and potentially challenge dominant power structures. Where this is the case, the role of teachers and other professionals is questioned. This causes tension within the 'self-propagating structures' [27] constructed by and within institutions, risking loss of their advantageous position.

6.2 Other roles in policy

Bourdieusian sociology argues that teachers occupy a privileged position within policy and legal frameworks. Their position is that of state appointed 'gatekeeper' to resources and support, acting as intermediary between the school institution and parents [26, 29]. Where young people have dyslexia and other SEND, the SENCo in a school is the holder of resources, budget and staffing to provide support for them [14]. Others [10, 41] have also located teachers as keyholders to resources, whose positions make them inaccessible to some parents. This is particularly important to note, given that [12] found schools and professionals' accessibility and inclusivity lacking. Rose [24] highlighted similar issues, as did the 2010 Coalition Government [47]. Then, under a revised policy framework, further studies found that parents continued to be systemically impeded from meaningfully engaging in decision-making processes about their children's provision [10, 15].

The lack of 'movement' and adaptation within the field of education demonstrates the accuracy of Bourdieu's [25, 27] view that education is a site where a status quo is maintained, and self-propagating power-structures are in place. 'Levels of interaction' [1] support analysis of parental experiences within current frameworks and comparison with studies undertaken in previous policy-contexts. Through this, we can see that despite internal sense-making at the individual level, positive engagement with professionals at the 'interactional level'. The role of parent is nominally bolstered within the Children and Families Act [32] and the most recent SEND Code of Practice [14]. However, the reality, for many parents whose social position precludes them from being able to embody the necessary habitus at the interactional level, is that their children's needs are inadequately met. Institutionally, structures exist such that parents cannot embody their institutionally 'expected' role and challenge the provision for their children, or the systems that implement it.

7. The habitus of education: parenting-dyslexia embodied

Jenkins' [1] 'orders of interaction' allow us to delineate parents' individual sense-making of their children's dyslexia. Making sense of dyslexia, then reframing it positively through exposure to new knowledge and practice relating to dyslexia exposes parents to a new habitus of parenting. This new way of parenting incorporates dyslexia, and its associated challenges and strengths. A new habitus, may develop through the 'dialectical confrontation' [28] which occurs when families discover that a child has dyslexia. This creates space for parents to focus on dyslexia as the reason for their children's difficulties in learning at school. The 'space' created for dyslexia as root-cause of difficulties modifies parents' previous understandings for their children's difficulties, such as poor focus, laziness or poor academic potential. Where parents can make the shift to positively reframe their understanding of their children's dyslexia and educational difficulties, their capacity to present a 'positive dyslexia' to their children and others is supported at the 'interactional level.'

Interactionally, parents often found it challenging to interact with professionals, despite both professionals and parents (and policy) believing that positive interactions and partnership were key elements of effective intervention and support for young people. Where interaction was positive, parents' professional and educational backgrounds underpin it. They may have common experiences and understanding of the field of education; parents embody the habitus of the field and social distance between parents and teachers is reduced. Where parents do not operate within the field of education, but interactions are productive and meaningful their professional or personal experiences are such that social distance between them and professionals is minimal. Minimal social distance leads to compatible habitus, facilitating engagement between agents.

Where parental habitus does not align with that of education, but interactions are positive, professionals' personal attributes and concessions act to bridge social distances between individuals. This facilitates engagement and leads to better, more meaningful interactions. However, this was not always the case and some parents found that interpersonal interactions were not productive. Through their modified habitus, they knew their rights, but could not enact their agency without external support. Instead the modified individual, internal habitus of these parents empowered them to seek representation or advocacy to facilitate their involvement in decision-making processes relating to their children's educational provision. However not all parents can commission such support; structural barriers exist which make it impossible for them to do so.

Institutional barriers acted to maintain the social position of parents, despite nominal legislative changes which sought parents' views relating to their children's educational provision. The role of parents within policy is to play an active role in decision making, but roles of teachers and other professionals as 'gatekeepers' to labels and resources can limit parents' capacity to participate. Where parents could not engage meaningfully with schools, professionals and other institutions, their role of 'parenting dyslexic child' at times became overwhelming and they, "just wanted to be a parent but found themselves performing additional roles" [9]. Parents often required support to access language, practice and other habitus linked to institutions within fields, despite the onus for facilitating inclusion lying with schools in policy [14]. This suggests that fundamental change of the system is required so that roles within policy do not create barriers which agents cannot overcome interactionally, despite experiencing significant habitus modification through dialectical confrontation individually.

While there is relatively little work documenting parental experiences of supporting their children with dyslexia through education, the extant work shares common themes. Parents feel constrained and often frustrated by processes. There is relatively little work currently published using 'orders of interaction' [1] to support Bourdieusian analysis of lived experiences. However, the framework shows great promise at highlighting where barriers to participation and engagement exist for parents whose children have dyslexia. Knowing at what level barriers exist means support to overcome barriers can be implemented, and to ultimately ensure that dyslexic young people can access appropriate support.

8. Conclusions: supporting a child with dyslexia: who, what, when and how

In this chapter, we have seen how'orders of interaction' [1] effectively underpin a Bourdieusian analysis of how parents experience support systems for their children with dyslexia. The theoretical framework developed in this chapter allows for a clear delineation at each level of who, what, when and how different interactions support or impede parental involvement and effective support for young people. Concluding remarks here give a brief overview of practical implications uncovered by this theoretical framework in exploration of parental experiences off dyslexia support. These recommendations are relevant for parents, but also for practitioners and policy makers.

8.1 Who and what

Individually, parents need access to robust knowledge of strengths associated with dyslexia. This knowledge empowers them to empower their children through positive, inclusive understandings of dyslexia. Practitioners and other professionals, interactionally must ensure that they act to facilitate parental participation in decision-making about provision for young people. Where they do, and parents are actively included, power differentials and associated structures shift. This then leads to changes in habitus, and systemic practice. Changes in systemic practice lead to institutional transformations, which develop real capacity for parents' empowerment and meaningful participation in their children's education.

8.2 When

Individually, parents' need for robust knowledge of dyslexia and support interventions tends to accompany their child's 'diagnosis' of dyslexia. However, prior to this, many parents also seek information around their children's difficulties with learning. Prior to diagnosis, professionals may dismiss parental concerns and following diagnosis, visions for support interventions may differ. At all times, the onus of 'inclusivity' is on professionals within the current policy-framework in England. They "must ensure that children, young people and parents are provided with the information, advice and support necessary to enable them to participate in discussions and decisions about their support" [14]. This should be an on-going process, so that parents are continually supported to actively participate in decisions around their children's provision.

8.3 How

In research, various methods have been suggested to facilitate parental participation in decision-making and securing of appropriate support for their children:

- Peer support groups for parents to share experiences [42]
- Therapeutic groups for parents [48]
- Independent support and advice for parents [12]
- Advocacy and representation to liaise between parents and settings [12, 49]
- Policy-makers and legislators must be amenable to interactions with parents, acting to ensure they are inclusive in their practice, and that institutional structures do not create barriers to participation [12, 49].
- Access to resources should not be contingent on parental means; assessment for and diagnosis of dyslexia should be undertaken in a timely fashion within the state-education system [12].

While this chapter largely focuses on provision withing the English system, there are transferable principles that apply elsewhere. Material within this piece is taken from various legislative and policy settings, which demonstrates the strength of the theoretical framework in delineating parents' experiences and highlighting barriers to their participation in their children's education. However, further work using this framework is necessary to gain deeper insight into how parents can support young people with dyslexia.

Acknowledgements

No funding has been granted to support this project.

Conflict of interest

The author declares no conflict of interest.

Notes/Thanks/Other declarations

I would like to thank Dr. Tina Skinner at the University of Bath, UK, for her encouragement in pursuing further study of dyslexia and neurodiversity.

I would like to thank Dr. David Skidmore at the University of Bath for his guidance and support during and following my PhD.

I would like to thank John Hicks, Parenting and Neurodiversity Coach at Parenting Dyslexia for supporting me as we worked on together to gather, process and analysis responses from parents, about their experiences supporting their dyslexic children.

Author details

Helen Ross
Helen's Place Education Consultancy, Trowbridge, England

*Address all correspondence to: helen@helensplace.co.uk

References

[1] Jenkins R. Social Identity. London: Routledge; 2008. DOI: 10.4324/9780203463352

[2] Elliott J, Grigorenko E. The Dyslexia Debate. New York: Cambridge University press; 2014. 271. DOI:10.1017/CBO9781139017824

[3] Frith U. Paradoxes in the definition of dyslexia. Dyslexia: An International Journal of Research and Practice. 1999; 5:4:192-214. DOI: 10.1002/(SICI)1099-0909(199912)5:4%3C192::AID-DYS144%3E3.0.CO;2-N

[4] Riddick B. Dyslexia and inclusion: time for a social model of disability perspective. International Studies on Sociology of Education. 2001;11(3):223-236. DOI: 10.1080/09620210100200078

[5] Ferguson JL. Beyond dyslexia fonts: What parents can do to help kids who struggle with reading. The Washington Post [Internet]. 2016 October 21 [Cited 2020 July 25]. Available from: https://www.washingtonpost.com/news/parenting/wp/2016/10/21/beyond-dyslexia-fonts-what-parents-can-do-to-help-kids-who-struggle-with-reading/

[6] Hartwig LJ. Living with Dyslexia: one parent's experience. Annals of Dyslexia 1984; 34: 313-318. DOI: 10.1007/BF02663628

[7] Woodcock C. Mothers of Children with Dyslexia Share the Protection, "In-Betweenness," and the Battle of Living with a Reading Disability: A Feminist Autoethnography. The Qualitative Report 2020; 25 (6) pp 1637-1657

[8] British Dyslexia Association (BDA) About dyslexia What is dyslexia? 2010. Available from: https://www.bdadyslexia.org.uk/dyslexia/about-dyslexia/what-is-dyslexia [Accessed 2020-06-30]

[9] Leitão S. Dzidic P. Claessen M. Gordon J. Howard K. Nayton M. Boyles ME. Exploring the impact of living with dyslexia: The perspectives of children and their parents. International Journal of Speech-Language Pathology, 2019; 19: 322-334. DOI: 10.1080/17549507.2017.1309068

[10] Earey A., Parental experiences of support for pupils with dyslexia: ignoring the effect on pupils. Support for Learning, 2013; 28 (1): 35-40

[11] Ross H. An exploration of teachers' agency and social relationships within dyslexia-support provision in an English secondary school. British Journal of Special Education. 2017;44 (2):189-202. DOI: 10.1111/1467-8578.12174

[12] Norwich B. Griffiths C. Burden B. Dyslexia-friendly schools and parent partnership: inclusion and home–school relationships. European Journal of Special Needs Education, 2005; 20 (2): 147-165. DOI: 10.1080/08856250500055628

[13] Watt J. Splashes of light: Parents of children with dyslexia explore experiences through visual arts. International Journal of Education Through Art, 2020; 16 (1): 115-128. DOI: 10.1386/eta_00020_1

[14] Department for Education (DfE); Department for Health (DfH). Special Educational Needs Code of Practice. London: DfE and DfH. 2015.

[15] Ross H. Supporting a child with dyslexia: how parents/carers engage with school-based support for their children. British Journal of Special Education. 2019; 46 (2):136-157. DOI: 10.1111/1467-8578.12254; 0952-3383

[16] Craston M. Thom G. Johnson R. Spivack R. Purdon S. Bryson C. Lambert C. James N. Knibbs S. *Oliver D.*

Smith L. Vanson T. Department for Education, Evaluation of the SEND Pathfinder Programme: Process and Implementation Research Report. London: The Stationary Office. 2013

[17] Snowling M. Language Skills and Learning to Read: The Dyslexia Spectrum. In: Snowling M, Stackhouse J, editors. Speech and Language A Practitioner's Handbook. London: Whurr Publishers; 2006. p. 1-14.

[18] Stein JF. The magnocellular theory of developmental dyslexia. Dyslexia, 2001; 7: 12-36

[19] Calfee R. The Mind of the Dyslexic. Annals of Dyslexia. 1983;33(1):7-28. DOI: 10.1007/BF02647993

[20] Solvang P. Developing and Ambivalence Perspective on Medical Labelling in Education: Case Dyslexia. International Studies in Sociology of Education. 2007;17 (1-2):79-84. DOI: 10.1080/09620210701433779

[21] McKay J. Neal J. Diagnosis and disengagement: exploring the disjuncture between SEN policy and practice. Journal of Research in Special Educational Needs. 2009; 9 (2):164-172.

[22] MacDonald SJ. Towards a Sociology of Dyslexia: Exploring Links Between Dyslexia, Disability and Social Class. Saarbrücken: VDM Verlag Dr Müller Aktiengesellschaft & Co. KG; 2009. 284 p.

[23] British Psychological Society (BPS) Division of Educational and Child Psychology (DECP) (1999) A framework for psychological assessment and intervention. Division of Educational and Child Psychology Newsletter, 1999;89: 6-12.

[24] Rose J. Independent Review of the Primary Curriculum. London: DCSF. 1999. Available from: https://webarchive.nationalarchives.gov.uk/20100202112739/http://publications.teachernet.gov.uk//DownloadHandler.aspx?ProductId=DCSF-00499-2009&VariantID=Independent+Review+of+the+Primary+Curriculum%3a+Final+Report+PDF& [Accessed 2020-07-04]

[25] Bourdieu P. Outline of a Theory of Practice. Cambridge: Cambridge University Press. 1977. 248 p. DOI: 10.1017/CBO9780511812507

[26] Bourdieu P. Social Space and Symbolic Power. Sociological Theory. 1989;7(1):14-25. DOI: 10.2307/202060

[27] Bourdieu P. Séminaires sue le concept de champ. Actes de la rercherche en sciences sociales, 1972-1975; 200: 4-37.

[28] Ingram N. Within School and Beyond the Gate: The Complexities of Being Educationally Successful and Working Class. Sociology, 2011;45 (2): 287-302. DOI: 10.1177/0038038510394017

[29] Bourdieu P. Scattered Remarks. European Journal of Social Theory. 1999;2 (3):334-340. DOI: 10.1177/13684319922224563

[30] National College for Teaching and Leadership (NCTL). Teaching Regulation Agency (TRA). Qualified teacher status (QTS): qualify to teach in England [Internet]. 2020. Available from: https://www.gov.uk/guidance/qualified-teacher-status-qts [Accessed 2020-07-04]

[31] Glazzard J. A Critical Interrogation of the Contemporary Discourses Associated with Inclusive Education in England. Journal of Research in Special Educational Needs. 2010:13 (3);182-188. DOI: 10.1111/1471-3802.12018

[32] Children and Families Act 2014. London: The Stationary Office.

[33] Knight C. What is dyslexia? An exploration of the relationship between teachers' understandings of dyslexia and their training experiences. Dyslexia. 2018;24 (3):207-219. DOI: 10.1002/dys.1593

[34] Harper K. Kurtzworth-Keen K. Marable M. Assistive technology for students with learning disabilities: A glimpse of the livescribe pen and its impact on homework completion. Education & Information Technologies. 2017;22 (5):2471-2483. DOI: 10.1007/s10639-016-9555-0

[35] Jenkins R. Pierre Bourdieu, 2nd ed. London: Routledge; 2002. 206 p.

[36] Wyness M. Childhood and Society. Basingstoke: Palgrave MacMillan; 2012. 330 p.

[37] Sulouff P, Bell S, Briden J, Frontz S, Marshall A, Learning about grey literature by interviewing subject librarians,. College and Research Libraries News. 2005; 66 (7):510-515. DOI: 10.5860/crln.66.7.7475

[38] Bonifacci, P. Massi L. Pignataro V. Zocco S. Chiodo S. Parenting Stress and Broader Phenotype in Parents of Children with Attention Deficit Hyperactivity Disorder, Dyslexia or Typical Development. International Journal of Environmental Research and Public Health, 2019; 16: 1878-1892. DOI: 10.3390/ijerph16111878

[39] Winn DM. Raising a Child with Dyslexia: What every parent needs to know. US: Cardboard Box Adventures; 2019. 262p

[40] Long L. McPolin P. Psychological assessment and dyslexia: parents' perspectives. Irish Educational Studies, 2009; 28 (1): 115-126. DOI: 10.1080/03323310802597424

[41] Buswell Griffiths C. Norwich B. Burden B. Parental agency, identity and knowledge: mothers of children with dyslexia. Oxford Review of Education, 2004; 30 (3): 417-433. DOI: 10.1080/0305498042000260511

[42] Antonelli L. Bilocca S. Borg D. Borg S. Boxall M. Briffa L. Debono C. Falzon R. Farrugia V. Gatt L. *Formosa M.* Mifsud D. Mizzi K. Scurfield L. Scurfield M. *vella* GL. Drama, Performance Ethnography, and Self-Esteem: Listening to Youngsters With Dyslexia and Their Parents. SAGE Open, 2014; 4(2). DOI: 10.1177/2158244014534696

[43] Rimkute L. Torppa M. Eklund K. Jari-Erik N. Lyytinen H. The impact of adolescents' dyslexia on parents' and their own educational expectations. Reading and Writing 2014; 27: 1231-1253. DOI: 10.1007/s11145-013-9484-x

[44] Lichtenstein R. Parent Advocates Champion Evidence-Based Practice Under the Banner of Dyslexia- Part 3. Communiqué 2019; 47 (5): 16-18.

[45] Samuels CA. Parent-Driven Group Wields Influence in Dyslexia Issues. Education Week, 2015; 35 (14): 8.

[46] Education Act 2011. London: The Stationary Office

[47] Department for Education (DfE). Support and Aspiration: a new approach to special educational needs and disability: a consultation. London: DfE; 2010.

[48] Multhauf, B. Buschmann A. Soellner R. Effectiveness of a group-based program for parents of children with dyslexia. Reading and Writing 2016; 29: 1203-1223. DOI: 10.1007/s11145-016-9632-1

[49] Lichtenstein R. Parent Advocates Champion Evidence-Based Practice Under the Banner of Dyslexia- Part 2. Communiqué 2019; 47 (4): 14-16.

Chapter 5

The Three Educational Faces of Dyslexia: Identification and Remediation in the Orthographic Phase

Diane Montgomery

Abstract

Frith defined a her 3-phase and 6-step psychological model of dyslexia. The three phases were named Logographic, Alphabetic and Orthographic in which sometimes the steps in reading and at other times spelling were in the lead. Using this model, it was possible to consider what teachers would experience when meeting dyslexic pupils in the different phases and resulted in being able to identify three different educational faces. In the process of this research the dyslexic characteristics were more clearly illustrated and identified in the written work of dyslexics rather than in their reading. What they wrote displayed in concrete terms their knowledge of the alphabetic system and the structure of words. Many able readers were identified who found it almost impossible to write a legible, coherent and correctly spelled script at any age but the poorest spellers were able to read much more than they could write. It was found that nearly 20% of pupils in a range of schools had dyslexic-type spelling problems but these were generally ignored if they could read adequately. In this publication the subject is the Orthographic face and what teachers may do to help.

Keywords: dyslexia, orthographic stage, spelling, remediation, cognitive process strategies, word pattern

1. Introduction

Dyslexia is an unexpected difficulty in learning to read and spell in relation to age and ability by the methods normally used in classrooms. However the reading difficulties became the predominant concern in education and psychological research. For example in England the Department for Education stated, "dyslexia or reading difficulties" [1] in its guidance on special needs. This reflected the widespread opinion in both education and psychological research that reading was the essential component and the main target for investigation and remediation. The major focus of the National Literacy Strategy [2] for example was also reading.

Spelling teaching had become a neglected area in England since the 1950s when the Look and Say reading teaching method was introduced and replaced phonics teaching systems. Thereafter spelling was "caught" rather than taught [3, 4] and the only spelling "teaching" method left over from the earlier era was in copywriting.

The British Dyslexia Association (BDA) [5] was established in the 1970s by Marion Welchman with help of like-minded colleagues. The purpose of the BDA was to promote understanding and research into dyslexia. Welchman had seen a method developed by Gillingham and Stillman [6] in the US work with her dyslexic son. It was adapted from the original phonics methods imported from England in the earlier part of the 20th century. The G and S system introduced multisensory phonogram training and explicit strategies for teaching reading and spelling linking them through synthetic phonics and cursive handwriting, the particular expertise of the remedial teacher Bessie Stillman. The method only progressed at the learning rate of the individual dyslexic. The programme was imported into the UK by Kathleen Hickey [7, 8] who developed an anglicised version. But it was not widely adopted because it was the antithesis of the prevalent reading teaching orthodoxy and use of print script copywriting. It remained largely unknown except in specialist dyslexia centres in a band across the south of England whose leaders had attended the original training events promoted by the Bath Dyslexia Association and the Invalid Children's Aid Association [9].

In the multisensory Alphabetic-Phonic-Syllabic-Linguistic (APSL) programme of Hickey there was a balance between reading and spelling using reading and spelling pack phonogram cards linked with cursive handwriting training. All of which was in contrast to the "Look and Say" practices when phonics and spelling teaching was introduced later once reading was established and in some classrooms not at all. This was despite the researches by Chall [10, 11]; Clark [12] and Ferreiro, et al. [13] that showed that more dyslexia resulted in Look and Say regimes rather than Phonics in a ratio of 4 to 1–1.5. **Table 1** below shows results from APSL programmes balancing spelling and reading teaching methods and teacher-designed programmes emphasising reading.

Data on 50 teachers [14] using the Hickey Multisensory Language Course but leaving out the spelling pack work and dictations has been excluded from the table. Her results were Reading Age = 1.21 and Spelling Age = 0.96 showing how essential the spelling component is in a dyslexia remedial programme.

The 2-year effectiveness criterion was established by Vellutino [15] and this was that an effective remediation programme at 10 years for example must give at least 2 years uplift in each year of intervention. One year's progress is equivalent to one Standard Deviation in statistical terms but to make progress and catch up with peers the rate must be 2 years, or 1 year in 6 months. Any intervention that does not achieve this should be discontinued and another system implemented. After no progress for a year or two it is not enough for success to be claimed for an improvement of 3 or 4 months as is often the case.

Despite effective remediation offered by the specialist dyslexia programmes some problems remain. Adult recovered dyslexics have residual spelling difficulties that arise when they meet new and technical vocabulary and they are generally slower at reading. In addition the remedial programmes are most effective when they are begun early [16, 17] preferably well before the dyslexic is the age of 7 years. Recent research has shown that it can be most effective when given in the Reception Year [18]. It is therefore problematic that most specialist dyslexia provision in the

Reading age uplift	2.83 (APSL)	0.76 (non APSL)
Spelling age uplift	2.24 (APSL)	0.38 (non APSL)
	N = 179	172

Table 1.
Meta-analysis showing dyslexics' progress in 1 year in APSL and non-APSL programmes.

UK is not considered until a child is at least 7 years old and this "rule" has been in operation since before the Bullock Report [19] endorsed the practice. Later it was endorsed in the government Code of Practice [20] insisting on School Action and School Action plus before referral for specialist intervention.

This orthographic research began in the 1980s with the development of a Bachelor of Education honours programme on Learning Difficulties for teacher education students. This made links with the local education authority dyslexia teaching Reading Centre where the teachers had been trained by Hickey. The four teachers there were helped to write their variant of Hickey's Multisensory Language Course (HMLC) [7, 8] as their in-service updating project and it was called Teaching Reading Through Spelling (TRTS) [21–23] and it was this that was introduced to the B.Ed students.

During the teaching of this course it emerged that some of the student teachers had either been diagnosed as dyslexic at school or now realised that they had been dyslexic and it had not been identified. They all did have residual spelling problems to varying degrees and some had slow reading problems. However a number of them reported that they had never had reading problems and a few had even learned to read self-taught. This did not fit with the general perspective on dyslexia then prevalent.

However whatever the origins of their difficulties there was a clear need to offer them some remedial support but what this should be was not clear since they were beyond the remit of the APSL programmes. The investigation began by setting up individual lunchtime clinics to which students could refer themselves. Here it was found that their spelling correcting strategies were limited to rote learning of the correct versions, visualisation, look-cover-write-check, "does it look right" and asking a friend to proof read what they had written before they handed in any work. It was in examinations that they became most vulnerable to detection for their own proof reading too often missed the errors.

Why they had residual spelling problems seems to arise because reading is easier to learn because it is a recognition skill and all the details are already present on the page. Spelling is a recall skill and the words have to be constructed from letters by the learner and put down correctly on the page in handwriting. Some more able learners have such good visual recall that in the early years they can remember words "photographically" and only begin to falter at the age of about 8 as the vocabulary in their books broadens. They appear suddenly to "become dyslexic" especially in spelling.

For others it only becomes a problem at degree level. They do not receive remedial help because they read well but they lose marks and reach lower standards because of their spelling problems. It was this group that was termed "dysorthographics." The ratio of dyslexic males to females was thought to be 4 to 1 [5] but it is from referral data. Out in the community in 10,000 international cases it was found to be 1.5 to 1 males to females [24] and in England 1.2 to 1. [25]. Girls' needs were being overlooked.

Amongst both dyslexics and dysorthographics were a subset that in addition had handwriting coordination problems – dysgraphia and this caused them even more difficulties in associating sounds with symbols in the early years and in producing a legible speedy script later on [26–28]. It seemed from these studies that spelling was a more fundamental problem in literacy learning than had previously been supposed and a better balance in general teaching schemes needed to be established to include spelling and handwriting. In addition something needed to be done to help those with residual spelling difficulties already in the system to raise their achievements whatever their level of ability.

Frith in 1985 [29] had provided a psychological model of dyslexia in which there were three phases and 6 steps in which sometimes reading was the pacemaker and at other times it was spelling. The three phases were the **Logographic phase** in which dyslexics were thought to have difficulties moving from an early phase of acquisition in which reading was visually based (logographic), to the **Alphabetic phase** when children were able to use letter-sound associations for both reading and spelling. Later some dyslexics failed to move on into the **Orthographic phase** where reading and spelling were automatic and considered to be independent of sound.

Using this model it was possible to identify in the data collections three different educational aspects or "faces" connected with the psychological phases that teachers would meet and need to deal with. Over time it was also possible to devise identification and intervention procedures related to each "face" that proved to be effective. The identification procedures involved collecting the free writing scripts of all subjects referred and undertaking a spelling analysis. A range of researchers, Gentry [30], Read [31], Rosencrans [32], Bourassa et al., [33] and Ehri [34] have all shown that the errors that students make when they write are not casual or unintentional but reveal very clearly their level of literacy knowledge and level of development.

The successful intervention methods were found to be Multisensory Articulatory Phonogram Training (MAPT) in the Logographic phase [18], Alphabetic-Phonic-Syllabic-Linguistic (APSL) training in the Alphabetic phase [35] and Cognitive Process Spelling Strategies (CPSS) in the orthographic phase under consideration here. It means that dyslexics will already have learned sound-symbol correspondence during the alphabetic phase and can spell most common words. Government guidelines now insist all pupils should be taught using systematic synthetic phonics (SSP) and when this does not work in severe dyslexia cases the pupil may receive individual intervention by trained dyslexia tutors. Even then a few do not benefit from the methods especially if not of the APSL kind for them SSP is necessary but not sufficient. However most dyslexics do move on to the orthographic phase with just a few phonic errors to clear up. These are usually problems with consonant digraphs in particular the "wh" digraph in question words; the "ou" and "ow" diphthongs, homophones and inflectional suffixes.

2. The development of the cognitive process strategies for spelling

The research began with a real problem to solve and this was how to help intending teachers correct their misspellings and in the process learn how to help their pupils do the same. At the time there were few techniques and no programmes available to do this. The students had a history of being told to "use a dictionary" but not how to use it and "learn the rules" but which ones and why? Others said they must not be lazy or careless and just memorise the correct spelling.

Although there were no available programmes there was spelling teaching advice for example in *Logical Spelling* [36]; *Dyslexia The Problems of Spelling* [37], Cowdery et al. *The Spelling Notebook* 1983–7 [21–23], and Moseley's research [38]. He used a range of techniques to help improve the spelling of 13–15-year old poor spellers. His experimental group gained 3.7 months per month over a 5-month period. Controls using Look-Cover-Write-Check (LCWC) made no such progress.

The strategies were as follows:

- Say the word to suit the spelling
- Trace and say
- Sky-write

- Visualise the word and count the letters
- Use a mnemonic
- Use spelling patterns and some rules
- Focus on the tricky parts
- Say the alphabet names
- Make a rhyming word

Focusing on the tricky parts, patterns and rules might be most appropriate for adult learners but if we do not know how to spell a particular word how do we try to construct it? In this reflective frame of mind a list of strategies was invented that might assist in correcting misspellings. These worked out to a maximum of 12 and became the "cognitive process" or "brain engage" strategies that could serve as alternatives to the major rote learning procedures. The most widely used of these were mnemonics, visualisation, singing and rhyming and Look-Cover-Write-Check. It was hoped that the 12 strategies would prove to be more effective and be generalizable to more than one word at a time.

The original categorisations of spelling and reading errors were developed in a survey of studies by Spache [39] and have remained largely unchanged since then. The Neale Reading Analysis [40, 41] for example used Omissions, Inversions, Substitutions, Reversals, Additions, Transpositions (e.g., librety) and these have remained unchanged in test updates and revisions.

It was in analysis of these reading error types that it became clear that the most important information for the teacher was to know exactly what the learner had substituted, reversed, omitted or transposed rather these labels. They might just reflect the spelling knowledge to date and be similar to errors made by younger children. When this was tested and the same spelling test was given to dyslexics and controls who were 3 years younger it was found the spelling errors made were not significantly different [42]. This meant that the popular description of dyslexic errors as "bizarre" needed to be challenged for it was likely that the error merely reflected a much lower level of spelling development that was unexpected in a student of that age.

In order to find out if there were any more strategies in use a set of 12 difficult to spell words was selected and these words were deliberately misspelled to mislead. The subjects were to be asked to spell the words correctly and explain the strategies they found themselves using.

Spelling test: Ass-ee-9, Brag-ar-doh-chio, Virr-mill-aeon, Rare-ee-figh, Im-pahst-err, Row-cocoa, Lick-we-fye, Sack-ree-lidge-ious, Pav-ill-aeon, Ack-come-oh-dait, Se-pehr-ate, Dessy-kate.

Cohorts of students and experienced teachers on in-service training courses were each presented visually and orally with the misspelling test and were asked to write the words correctly, reflect on their mental processes in doing this and later share what strategies they were using.

The limited range of most people's strategies soon became apparent. They syllabified, used phonics and analogies with known words, wrote it then tried to assess if it "looked right." Some used meaning and the knowledge of another language. Many suggested how useful mnemonics (a verse or device for aiding the memory) could be. It was explained that finding a mnemonic was often a lengthy process and then only corrected the one misspelling making it not so useful as they might believe. Strategies were needed that would generalise to a range of words and misspellings.

In the developmental period 1700 subjects had been tested. Over time several thousand responses were recorded and no participant ever scored 12. Only a handful of subjects from this large group had scored more than 8 correct. Many had scored only 1 or 2 points to their great surprise and indignation. The best spellers appeared to have the largest range of strategies.

Twelve CPS strategies had been devised and in all the feedback from the subjects no more than these 12 were ever recorded. To convert them into a programme for intervention each needed an explanation to show how it could be used. Teachers would then have a general toolkit to use to help their pupils and their own spelling development and correct misspellings. The main problem that remained was that once a spelling had been corrected it must remain so and not reappear in subsequent days. This was a second problem that needed to be dealt with.

3. Testing the 12 CPSS for effectiveness

The students were invited to come individually for spelling help to lunchtime clinics and asked to bring a list of their misspellings from a recent essay plus the essay itself so that other errors they might have missed could be found and included. Together with the tutor they worked on correcting two errors per session using the list of 12 strategies below to give them ideas. The plan was for them to decide on two strategies to help them remember the correct spelling. First they must look up the correct spelling in a "good" dictionary. The "good" dictionary must contain 5 forms of information (1) correct spelling, (2) meaning, (3) pronunciation, (4) origins, (5) related words and uses.

The second strategy was for backup such as a "Funny."

3.1 The 12 cognitive process strategies for spelling

Lower order strategies

- **Articulation** - The misspelled word is clearly and precisely articulated for spelling - citation mode

- **Over articulation** - The word is enunciated with an emphasis on each of the syllables or unstressed sound. e.g., parli (a) ment, gover (n) ment, w(h)ere

- **Cue articulation** - The word is pronounced almost incorrectly, e.g. Wed - nes - day, Feb - ru - ary.

- **Syllabification** - The word is broken down into syllables, misdemeanour - mis/de/mean/our.

- **Phonics** - A comprehensible articulatory skeleton or phonetic word scaffold is made to build upon – km, cm then cum, may appear before come.

- **Rule** - A few rules can help unravel a range of spelling problems e.g. the l - f - s rule, these letters are doubled in one-syllabled words after a short vowel sound - ball, puff, dress. The exceptions are made into several sentences e.g.; "YES," the BUS runs on GAS PAL, IF you pay NILyou get turned off.

I before E except after C rule – receive, perceive to keep the "c" soft.

3.2 Higher order strategies

- **Origin** - The root in another language may give clues - op/**port**/unity; an opening, a **port** or a haven

- **Linguistics** - Syllable types - open, closed, accented and unaccented need to be taught as well as the 4 suffixing rules which govern most words e.g. Add, Double, Drop, Change

- **Family/base word** - Family helps reveal silent letters and correct representation for the "schwa" unstressed vowel e.g. Canada, Canadian; bomb, bombing, bombardier, bombardment; sign, signature signal, resign, resignation. Basewords can make families of words e.g. form, reform, forming, deformed, formation

- **Meaning** - Separate is often misspelled as sep/e/rate. The dictionary meaning shows it means to divide or part or even to pare. The pupil then just needs to remember "cut or part" and "pare" to separate.

- **Analogy** - comparison of the word or the key part of it with a word the pupil does know how to spell. "it is like boot - hoot, root; 'hazard' one 'z'" as in haze, maze

- **Funnies** - Sometimes it is not possible to find another strategy and so a "funny" can help out e.g. "cess pit" helped me remember how to spell "necessary."

Over time and use the 12 strategies were divided into lower and higher order strategies as in the above. This was because the younger pupils and those with the poorest spelling needed more of the lower order CPSS and little or no dictionary work to begin with.

3.3 The second problem to resolve

Remedial teachers consistently complained that when they taught how to correct a misspelling it inevitably re-appeared next time the pupil wrote the word. The student teachers in the clinics also reported this problem. The most favoured correction strategy they used was Look-Cover-Write-Check (LCWC) undertaken three times. In the Gillingham and Stillman [6] programme Bessie Stillman, the remedial teacher introduced her Simultaneous Oral Spelling (SOS) method. It involved saying the names of the letters of the correct spelling whilst writing the letters down in cursive. The pupil does this three times. It seems that LCWC was a diminished version of this. SOS was designed to make and stabilise the link between handwriting and spelling, the grapheme and phoneme.

The following protocol was developed for use with CPSS.

3.4 The 7-step protocol for using CPSS

i. Select **two** misspellings to learn in any one session.

ii. Identify the **area of error,** usually only one letter with help of the tutor or dictionary.

iii. Put a **ring round** the area of error and notice how much of the rest is correct.

iv. The student is taught (later selects) a **CPSS to** correct the misspelling; a reserve strategy is also noted where possible.

v. **Talk the strategy over** with the tutor and write the corrected spelling.

vi. **Check** the spelling to see if it is correct - the dictionary can be used again here.

vii. If correct the student covers up the spelling and writes the word three times from memory in **joined up/full cursive, naming** the letters - Simultaneous Oral Spelling (SOS). It is especially important to use the joined script at least **over the area of error** if full cursive presents a problem.

3.5 Why two strategies are needed to correct misspellings

Research by Kuczaj [43] found that the motor programmes for spelling words, particularly their bases and affixes were stored together in the brain. This meant that learning to write syllables and base words as cursive writing units during early learning was an important strategy that could contribute to spelling accuracy. It involves morphemes the smallest units of meaning and the word meaning in the lexicon (word memory store) is consistently associated with its motor memory (motoreme).

The posterior frontal lobe area (usually left hemisphere) organises and initiates the voluntary motor movements involved in forming the individual graphemes and syllables. These are stored in the motor memory linked with programmes in the cerebellum or "hind brain" and are available to be called up during writing. Over time and practice this process becomes automatic so that during essay writing we do not have to think about the details of the spelling or forming the letters. Rather like learning to play the piano.

The problem arises when as young writers or dyslexics we store incorrect spellings. In order to correct them we have to address the error both in the word memory store and in the motor memory store. The CPSS corrects the error in the lexicon and the SOS strategy is needed to correct it in the motor memory. As old memories are not deleted but persist they also will be called up when writing. The CPSS however gives the new spelling a higher profile and as the writer writes a sentence and the "problem" word comes nearer "warning bells" ring and the writer recalls the strategy, slows down and writes the correct version. Soon the writer is able to write the correct version without having to pause and recall the strategy. Eventually the correct version arises each time unless under stress when it may pop up again. On these occasions proof reading will clear it out.

LCWC may be useful in learning spellings but not in correcting them as it only deals with the motor programme. The neurology suggests that two strategies are needed if a spelling is to be corrected. One strategy is needed to correct the motor or handwriting programme already established. The second strategy needs to correct the spelling entry in the word memory store, the lexicon. The handwriting process thus connects spelling and meaning. SOS contributes to this through naming whilst writing is in progress.

The neurological significance of handwriting in learning to read was later established by James et al. [44]. Their research showed during fMRI scanning that when preliterate 5-year olds traced, printed or typed letters and shapes and then were shown images of these stimuli that a previously discovered "reading circuit" in the brain was activated during letter perception. This only occurred **after handwriting** not after tracing or copying that are frequently used in early years education.

The conclusion is that handwriting supports symbol-sound knowledge development in normal subjects and why multisensory phonogram training has been found to be effective. However in dyslexics, there appears to be a disruption in that neurological system possibly caused by a dissociation in the area of the left angular gyrus [45] so that very specific and often repetitive training is needed initially to overcome the barrier. This problem was identified as giving rise to an articulation awareness deficit [42] in dyslexics compared with reading and spelling matched controls. This meant that dyslexics initially had no concrete articulatory cues to link the abstract perceptual units [46] the sound and the symbol.

3.6 An early CPSS pilot study in elementary school

In this research project Parrant [47] tried the CPSS techniques with elementary school children. It showed effective results in 6 weeks with classes of 11 year olds (Year 6). The control class of 23 pupils and the experimental class of 21 pupils, including 7 with specific learning difficulties in reading and spelling were given a 100-word dictation pre and post intervention. Each week they worked on a set of common errors from the dictation. The control group was taught to use Look-Cover-Write-Check and write the word correctly three times. The experimental group tackled the same errors with CPSS, also writing the word correctly three times. Both groups' spelling improved but for the controls there was not a significant gain but the experimental groups' improvement was very significant ($p < 0.01$). Even the group with SpLD improved their spelling significantly ($p < 0.05$). The error rate of the experimental group for example dropped from 273 to 162.

Parrant also recorded a change to a positive attitude to spelling in the experimental group. They were more interested in spelling and more confident in their writing after the intervention. They had lost a "learned helplessness" in dealing with spelling that many pupils develop. This attitude change also occurred amongst the students in the clinics and they began to enjoy spelling.

3.7 A secondary school topic-based approach to strategic spelling

In her MA project Schaapkins [16] decided to test the value of introducing a small version of CPSS in Food Technology with Year 10 pupils. Pupils each year were given lists of technology words to learn but no specific techniques had been offered to help them study the words other than to tell them to memorise them.

The spelling list was: design, technology, temperature, coagulation, protein, carbohydrate, analytic, evaluation, hygiene, ingredients, manufacture, recipe, specification, research, vitamin, mineral, polysaccharides, whisk, hazard, nutrition.

There were two mixed ability classes and one served as the control group and the other as the experimental group. The experimental group was given copies of the 12 CPSS list for personal use and each word was syllabified when it was introduced to give them an example to follow. The post-test results showed no significant improvement in spelling accuracy in the controls but significant improvements and a lowering of spelling errors in the experimental group.

3.8 Comparison of the levels of spelling errors made by student teachers and year 7 s

An analysis of the types of spelling errors made by Year 4 undergraduate teacher education students in a 3-hour examination was undertaken. In 55 scripts there were 165 errors in total and 152 different errors. The estimated number of words was 3000 words per script making 165,000 words in total giving an error rate of 0.018% and a modest writing speed of 17 words per minute, taking into account that thinking time was involved. This compared favourably with previous error studies of 1.5% by Wing et al. [48] testing a cohort of 40 undergraduates writing an estimated 10,000 words.

The preponderance of errors of the B.Ed undergraduates fell into the linguistic/morphemic or higher order area rather than the lower order articulation and phonics areas. These higher order errors are not unexpected for an adult group and can be compared with the Year 7 results in **Table 3** below (p. 12).

Multiple errors of the same words' misspelling by an individual were only counted once.

The main difference between the Year 7 s and the undergraduates was that in developmental terms the Year 7 made more errors of a basic kind such as with articulation and phonics and in their grammatical knowledge.

Within the student group there were two who had been diagnosed as dyslexic at school and in their Year 3 examinations had made as many as 20 misspellings which had caused concern to their tutors and upset to the students. This was why they had opted to follow the Learning Difficulties course and had attended the clinics. In the final year examination their scripts showed no dyslexic-type errors. They in fact made no more than 3 and 5 misspellings and each of these was the slip of the pen or missing letter type that is common when essay writing at speed and that would not normally cause comment.

The spelling research resumed later when a suite of MA distance programmes was designed for Middlesex University, these included an MA SEN, MA SpLD and MA Gifted Education. On its resumption handwriting had also become a major concern in UAch and 10 and 20 minute handwriting speed tests were designed to investigate this aspect [2]. This provided the Year 7 data in **Table 2** below and the

Sequencing	**What the errors actually reveal about spelling knowledge**
bronwe (brown)	A typical visual recall error after Look and Say teaching plus phonics and long vowel "e" over-generalisation
filed (field)	Part phonic effort with long vowel sound error but visual recall of all the letters
berdy (buried)	Phonetic attempt, y added to deal with "ie" sound trace
colse (close)	Visual recall, lack of knowledge of "cl" blend
biult (built)	Visual recall, with "bi" use of phonetics
nigt (night)	Phonic structure but lack of knowledge of silent letters and origins
aronud (around)	Mix of phonic and visual recall needs diphthong knowledge
pepels (peoples)	Basic phonetic structure
"Bizarre"	
ckach (chase)	Mix of phonetic errors, long vowel sound correct, check articulation
takt (chased)	t, d. often used for ch. Lack of phonic knowledge except for vowel "a." Check articulation of words for spelling
janjoys (enjoys)	articulation error, and local dialect issue
coicens (cousins)	Outline phonetic structure with some visual recall and lack of phonic knowledge

Sequencing	**What the errors actually reveal about spelling knowledge**
oncl (uncle)	Vowel error and lack of knowledge of final stable syllable "-le"
evetchers (adventures)	Articulation errors with basic phonetic structure
haja (hair)	Phonetic structure plus local dialect emphasis
Omissions	
sise (since)	Lack of 'n' concealed by nasalified vowel
nity (ninety)	Lack of 'n' concealed by nasalified vowel
haging (Hanging)	As above
enharse (enhance)	As above
bscapering (scampering)	Articulation error as above
whet (went)	As above with "wh" digraph error
thigs (things)	As above also check articulation.
Concatenations	
favote (favourite)	All these errors show a lack of syllabification use and a need to articulate clearly in "citation mode" for spelling
deiced (decided)	
probl (probably)	
Basic phonics	
oncl (uncle)	Needs more help with short vowel sound knowledge and articulation
inuf (enough)	Basic phonetic structure, needs systematic synthetic phonics **support**
safen (Southend)	As above with articulation training and word structure knowledge
coules (colours)	Phonetic structure, needs systematic word building and synthetic phonics
thand (found)	Phonetic structure with th/f dialect confusion and lack of diphthong knowledge
moe (more)	Phonetic structure of local dialect
Reversals	
None	E.g. "was for saw" and "on for no" usually disappear in children's writing by about the age of 8 years.

Table 2.
Dyslexic errors using "traditional" categories from school C.

spelling data in **Table 3** below. The 6 types of error analysis in **Table 2** had been suggested by Miles [49].

The dyslexics in this case were the 4% of the School C cohort who had made the most misspellings and this turned out to be 10 or more misspellings per 100 words. At this age they were expected to make no more than 5 misspellings per 100 words [50].

As can be seen each error contains a wealth of information that could help a teacher intervene and make a difference to dyslexics' reading and spelling performance. It was decided that the CPSS programme could be used to summarise issues and suggest key interventions. However it would need an expansion of the category identified as Linguistic Rules to help teachers with rules they might not know having been brought up in a Look and Say teaching and learning era. There are of course many English teachers who have studied linguistics but the knowledge is not necessarily in the possession of Remedial teachers, Learning Support tutors or SENCos who on a day-to-day basis meet students who need this help.

Error type %	BEds	Cohort B	Cohort C	B + C
	N = 55	(N = 160)	(N = 251)	(Error %)
SYNTHETIC PHONICS				
Artic/Pronunciation/Syll	19 (Syll)	11.9%	12.9%	0.58%
Phonetic/Phonic	0	28.7%	29.1%	1.23%
MORPHEMICS				
Baseword/Origin	55	30.0%	19.6%	0.82%
Suffix/Pref/vowel rules	75	18.4%	17.2%	0.73%
Homophone	3	3.5%	9.5%	0.40%
Grammatical	0	9.7%	11.7%	0.49%
Total numbers of errors	152 (0.018%)	1953	2651	4.25%

Table 3.
Spelling error data, B Ed and Year 7 cohorts (20-minute test).

4. Case analysis studies and 15 linguistic rules (spells)

According to Hanna and Hanna et al. [51] it was possible to spell 85% of the English language with knowledge of phonics and some basic rules. These researchers found that it was possible to programme a computer to spell 17,000 basic words with some 300 rules and knowledge of how sounds were transcribed and represented by alphabetic symbols - phonics. But they were dealing with rules governing letter order and frequencies often called "surface rules" rather than with deep structure rules about word and syllable structure, morphemics and linguistics necessary in an opaque language.

Henry [52] in the USA suggested that with a knowledge of roots the rules governing only 14 words could teach all the spellings that an elementary school child might be expected to know. Her techniques were based upon different syllable structures but not a problem-solving approach and were laborious. However it did show that syllable structure and basic rules could contribute to correcting misspellings.

The collection of spelling error data in the speed writing research project made it possible to work out the most common linguistic errors that pupils made. It was the Linguistic rules in the CPSS that needed to be developed but with about a dozen not 300 rules. The list of rules had to be brief enough not to be daunting for someone unfamiliar with the subject and easy enough to remember for young students.

By this stage teacher education students, and teachers were testing out CPSS and undertaking case intervention studies and dissertations on the topic. Others were referring scripts for advice. It was the accumulation of error information from all these sources that enabled a list of 15 potential rules called "Spells" for the most common errors to be devised.

4.1 The "15 Spells" (for a barge trip)

1. **CUT** (cvc) short vowel, closed syllable. DOUBLING rule for adding suffixes - cut-t-ing, putting, running, bedding, hopping, sitting, in polysyllables - rudder, potter, kipper, cutter.

2. **HULL** (cvcc) short vowel and l-f-s rule. Must double l-f-s after a short vowel in single syllables till, hill, pill; off, boff, sniff; hiss, miss, (10 exception

words - if, gas, bus, yes, pal, nil – invent 2 sentences to remember and include them all).

3. **ROPE** (cvce) After long vowel sound in a closed syllable, silent/e/denotes long vowel sound. DROP silent/e/when adding suffixes: roping, hoping, riding.

4. **SAIL** (cvvc) "When two vowels go walking the first one does the talking, 'usually' rain, paint, cleats, load, tear." Bear Just ADD suffix - raining, painted, cleated, loads.

5. **COOK** (cvvc) book, look, took, hook, good, double/oo/short vowel sound, ADD rule, cooking MOON (cvvc) Long vowel sound/oo/in noon, cool, saloon, zoom, room, tool, ADD rule – zooming.

6. **LIST** (cvcc) short vowel followed by double consonants simply ADD rule applies - listing, rushed, missed, rusting, posted. Master, lasting, faster, bath - dialect change in south of England from short to longer/ar/sound.

7. **BARGE** (vowel r, –ge) r changes a in words large, are, art, mart; e softens g - ge.

8. **WHEEL** (wh- digraph) teach/wh/question words as a group why, who, where, what, which, when. (whether). Teach the 6 consonant digraphs ch, ph, ch, sh, wh and th voiced and unvoiced.

9. **LADEN** (cvc/ic/id/in) open syllables: these words follow the long vowel rule in open syllables – o pen, ba con, spo ken, la den, to ken. Exceptions are: cabin, robin, rapid, vapid probably pronounced with the long vowels once or an effect of vowel "i."

10. **WATER** (wa/or/and wo/ir/rules). W changes the vowel sounds of "a" and "o" - war, ward, walk, warm. Work, world, whorl, word, worm, worst.

11. **PAY** (cvy) CHANGE rule. Change y to i when suffixing. Instead of the regular form payed and sayed we change "y" to "I" and add "d" - paid, said, laid.

12. **ROUND** (diphthong/ou/ow sound is ah -oo or two sounds) ground, bound, found, sound, hound. Rouse, louse; row, cow; oi diphthong in oil, boil, toil. ow is also a digraph as in low, row, know.

13. **SIGN** (cv - gn, silent letters) Family words will help with detecting some silent letters - sign, signal; bomb, bombardment. Some letters were once pronounced knife, knight, knave, knitting perhaps from Norse.

14. **TABLE** - final stable common syllables e..g. "-le" and "-ly"; "-tion," "-sion" and "-cian," "-us" and "-ous."

15. **PAIR** "-air" and "-are" words. Pair, lair, fair, stair and pare, stare, ware, care.

Stress and unstressed syllables might replace "-air" words depending on the needs that emerge from the pupil's spellings but by the time they have worked through the 15 spells they will be able to investigate the problem and origins using the Spelling Detective Dictionary [53].

4.2 Development of the casework

Students on the 3 different MA programmes all undertook casework on the written scripts of key pupils in their schools or tutorial practices and demonstrated that they could use CPSS effectively. The casework showed that the programme was able to improve the spelling ability of the pupils and that it gave 2 years uplift in spelling most frequently in the less severe cases especially those without dysgraphia. It could often be achieved in a few months with only a three 10–15 minute tutorials per week. The pupils enjoyed the power it gave them to deal with their own chosen misspellings and said they looked forward to the sessions. This was after many of them had become disillusioned by the repeated attempts to help them and the boring nature previously of overtraining and rote learning.

Maia age 9 years 4 months after a year on CPSS tutorials [54].

- RA 10 years 4 months (2 years uplift in 1 year)
- SA 8 years 4 months (11 months uplift in 1 year).

Maia had problems using cursive writing and avoided using the SOS strategy and as Ridehalgh found this handicapped the spelling progress.

Natalie aged 15 was surprised that no one had thought to teach her the suffixing rules before. As the sessions progressed she gained in confidence and was enjoying studying spelling and getting very obvious benefit that she herself could see and experience. Her dyslexia tutor explained:

"Many of the students I work with have been following dyslexia spelling programmes with private tutors for years with little or no improvement in their ability to spell accurately when under pressure especially in a test or exam. When I first read about CPSS I was a little dubious as it seemed a time consuming way of teaching students correct spelling however I was desperate to find something which would work after years of repeatedly correcting the same errors."

As the CPSS became more widely known parents and teachers began to refer case example scripts for advice and information this was especially in the context of a pupil who was underachieving. Sometimes adults would refer themselves for advice following the increasing understanding of Dual and Multiple Exceptionality [55].

Figure 1 below shows the type of problem that teachers faced in determining interventions at the Orthographic stage. A typical CPSS analysis was offered as in the following case report. The pupil was asked to write a story or about a favourite topic in exactly 10 minutes as quickly as possible and not to worry about the spelling.

4.3 Case report "Alan"

Alan is in the late stage of the Alphabetic Phase and ready to move into the Orthographic Phase with CPSS help. He uses his phonic knowledge to create phonetic scaffolds onto which some orthographic mapping has taken place [34] and more can be assimilated.

4.3.1 The misspellings

wack (woke) downsters opend are (our) cousans knew(new) stokings and stockings chuweng (chewing) tine/time grand perants evaning are (our) preset are (our) shweets choclt wached filme wich 1 acloc.

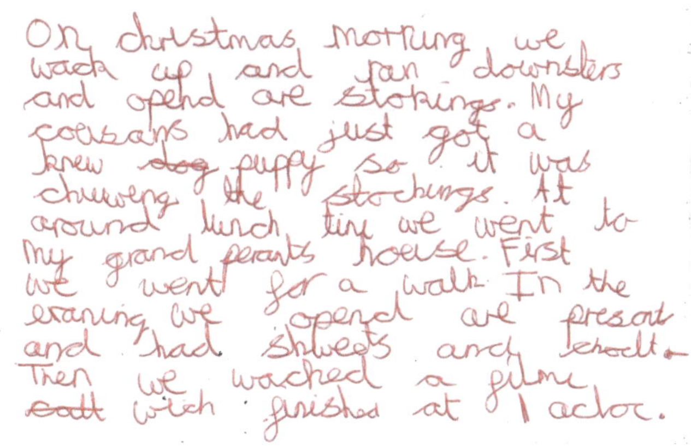
On christmas morring we
wsck up and ran downsters
and opehd are stokings. My
coeusans had just got a
knew dog puppy so it was
chuweng the stochings. At
around lunch tine we went to
my grand perants hoeuse. First
we went for a walk. In the
evaning we opend are presat
and had shweets and schoclt.
Then we wached a film
satt wich finished at 1 acloc.

Figure 1.
Handwritten script of a year 7 pupil. Half size.

There are two scribal errors where after letter “o” the link to “u” is formed as an “e” making “coeusans” and “hoeuse.” The “v” in evening is malformed or closed.

4.3.2 The handwriting

The script is rather large and round. It is mainly in cursive style and mostly with lead-in strokes. This indicates previous remedial training. The script shows mild coordination problems in that rivers of space run down the page and although there are lines to write on the script runs above and below it. Body size of letters and slope vary.

4.4 Correcting the misspellings

1. Ask Alan to **proof read** the script and to underline any errors and then write out the correct version to be checked with the dictionary.

2. **Check:** That he can hear and feel the difference between a long vowel and a short vowel sound. Long vowels “say their own names” e.g. A, E, I, O, U. Teach him to recognise these differences if necessary as the need arises during the following.

Below are example strategies that can be tried but **not all at once**. Select two words to work on in any one session to see how CPSS works. Then use the current written work and Alan’s own choices.

wsck (woke) Possibly planned to write “waked” here.

1. Articulate clearly for spelling. Note the **long vowel O** sound in “woke.”

2. In a one-syllabled word with the **long vowel** sound a silent “e” at the end tells us to make the long vowel sound (Do not call it magic “e” now) e.g. make, woke, lake, made, spoke, rode, tide, rude. Get him to generate some more and find them in a page of a book.

downsters – pronounce the word as he has written it and the target word “downstairs.”

Can he spell it correctly when pronounced correctly? Explain it is a compund word made up of "down" and "stairs," Generate some more compound words together and help him find some on a newspaper page.

opend – the word "open" is a **verb** or doing word. To change it to the past tense we must add "-ed" after the consonant. We just add a "d" when there is already vowel "e" present as in "close" and "closed." Collect some examples "mend-ed," "land-ed," "change-d."

are (our) – articulate the two versions "are" and "our." Note that "our" has the "ahoo" sound or diphthong. We use "ou" to denote the "ahoo" sound in words e.g. our, out, and in ground, sound, loud, found.

cousans – Over-articulate for spelling e.g. *cous* – ins, think of "in–laws."

knew(new) - discuss the meaning and origins of the two words. They are homophones.

The origin of knew is from Norse – kna – meaning to know. Related words are knowledge and knowing. To remember the family pronounce the now silent letter like the Norsemen did k-new to remember it. Cue articulate.

stoking and stocking: teach "c" "ck" and "k" rules.

1. Syllabify for spelling "stock" with suffix "– ing" added.

2. In one syllabled words with a short vowel and no other consonant before the last /k/use "–ck." Tell the story is of "kicking/k/and cushion consonant/c/." e.g. back, tack, ick, tick. Can he generate some more examples?

3. Use "c" in the middle of words – decoy, decay, recant.

4. When there is an extra consonant or an extra vowel before "kicking k" they protect the short vowel and the cushion is not needed e.g. leek, leak, seek, weak, mink, wink, sink.

chuweng – for the (u) sound we use "ew" at the end of one-syllabled words e.g. chew, knew, crew, flew, dew.

tine/time - Check that he articulates and can identify the different consonant sounds of "n" and "m." Describe together the different articulatory feel of these letters.

grand perants - this looks like a visual error, switching the position of "a" and "e." Over articulate "ar" and syllabify for spelling as in "pa – rent." Make a funny.

evaning – identify the Baseword – **"eve"** and its meaning, syllabify for spelling "eve – ning."and e-ven-ing.

preset – teach the –nt blend in words. It is difficult to detect the "n" before "d" and "t" because it nasalifies the preceding vowel. Hold nose whilst trying to say "bend," "went" and "present."

shweets – show the difference between shw- and sh- by getting him to articulate them.

choclt – articulate clearly and syllabify for spelling e.g. choc – o - late.

wached – the hard (ch) sound in words is represented by "tch" immediately after a **short vowel** sound e.g. watch, fetch, catch, witch, switch, after anything else we use "ch" e.g. lunch, munch, beach, beech, teach (exception is "which" because we already have "witch").

filme This is an over-generalisation of the long vowel rule. After short vowel sound the silent "e" is not needed because it only tells us to make the long vowel sound that is incorrect here for film.

wich – teach the "wh" digraph for all the question words. E.g. why, who, where, which, when, what. Try to aspirate the "wh" sound in these words as a cue.

acloc (one o'clock) articulate clearly (citation mode). The full version is "one of the clock" we put in the inverted comma to show the omission. Think of other examples e.g. do not; cannot; will not ask Alan to give the full versions of them as well.

4.5 Handwriting suggestions

To improve the fluency and form of the handwriting draw sets of double lines so that he writes the groups of 3 versions of his corrected spellings in between the lines.

See LDRP example below.

The rules are:

- The bodies of the letters should all be the same size as defined by the lines.
- All the bodies of the letters must sit on the bottom line and be the same size.
- All the "tails" of the letters must hang below the line.
- The "t" is a small letter.
- All the sticks must stand above the body line.
- All sticks and tails must be parallel to each other.

The ovoid sloping cursive is the fastest script. Left-handers may need to let their letters have a backward slope. Children in secondary schools who did not write at a speed of 15 words per minute were failing in all areas of the curriculum and had low self-esteem (**Figure 2**) [56].

4.6 An example of casework with an adult dyslexic

"John" aged 56 referred himself for advice about his misspellings after suspecting he had Dual and Multiple Exceptionality (DME) [55]. From school age he had severe writing and reading difficulties. Much later he discovered he was dyslexic with an IQ on WAIS (Wechsler Adult Intelligence Scale) of 132. (His scores on the test would be depressed by the dyslexia and would be likely to be 10 points higher in real terms). He had been a successful businessman and returning to academia was working on his PhD. His handwiting was almost indecipherable and he had to leave notes for people in print.

These are the examples given by "John" with the target CPSS discussed.

- typical or typicle? Final stable syllables –le, –al, –el; Family
- impact or empact? Prefixes – Articulation citation mode
- bureau or burreau? Short vowel rule
- recruit or recrute? Cue articulation
- vendor or vender – Both are regarded as correct just use one
- des or dis at the beginning? Meaning of prefixes

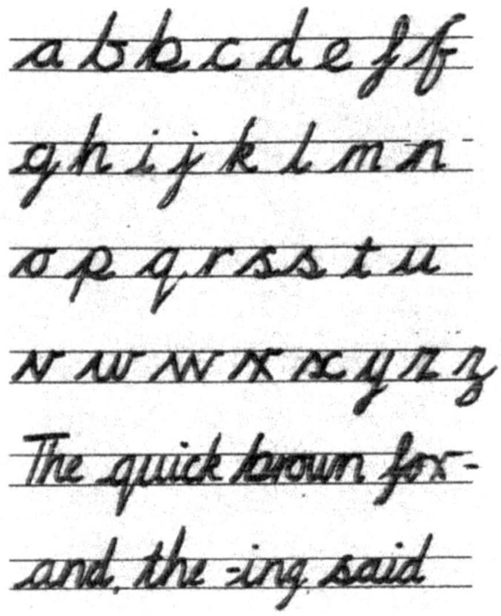

Figure 2.
LDRP ovoid cursive style.

- proposition – propo-propa-prope-propi? Basewords
- mitigation – miti- mita-mite? Meaning
- first – fist? Overarticulation
- relevant – rele-reli-rela? Origins
- decent or desent? Phonic rule
- deliberately- deliberatly? Suffixing Add rule

A special dictionary was compiled to help teachers correct pupil misspellings. The errors were those found in scripts from the 20 and 10-minute speed writing tests.

4.7 Examples to show the "Spelling Detective Dictionary" approach www.ldrp.org.uk

blurred
blured

1. identify the baseword "blur" and the closed syllable pattern (CCVC)
2. teach the DOUBLING rule that after the short vowel sound in a two syllabled word we must have two consonants to keep the short vowel pattern so we double consonant "r" (– VCCV -) blur - r - ed., blurring; occur, occurring, occurred

---

boarded
boaded boarded

1. identify the baseword "board" and its meanings such as a "plank of wood" and to go "on board" a ship or a boat
2. board and boat both have the vowel digraph "oa" in them, when a vowel is followed by consonant "r" it changes the usual sound it makes e.g. "oar" and "oa"
3. look for the "oars" on board the boats
4. check the articulation captures the final blend "-rd"
5. find five more words with the end blend "-rd" sword, ford, word, hard, nerd

____.

bodies
bobys, bodys

1. identify the base word "body"
2. clench the two fists with the thumbs up straight and put the knuckles together to form "bod" or "b d" showing where the ascenders should be
3. articulate (b - od) feeling the difference in the mouth for "b" and "d"
4. ask the pupil to describe the feel of these consonants in the mouth e.g "b" starts with lips closed
5. teach the CHANGE rule for suffixing plurals - after "y"we must change "y" to "i" and add the plural "es" - bod - i - es, babies, nannies.

____.

5. Recent writing and underachievement project

Concerns had been expressed by parents in Potential Plus UK about their children's writing and possible underachievement. This led to a new writing project. Any PPUK member could refer their child with High Learning Potential (HLP) and send a sample of handwriting using the 10-minute test.

Initially 30 families participated - 43 school age pupils and 7 adults. Later some schools also referred their problematic cases and made a total of 83 investigations.

In the PPUK 2016 sample there were 37 primary school-age pupils in Reception to Year 6; 3 in Year 7; 2 in Year 8 and one in Year 9. The statistical analysis focused upon the 40 pupils in Reception to Year 7 as follows:

- 8 girls and 32 boys took part in the study.
- 8 pupils (16%) were left- handed. This is above the 12% national average.
- Six handwriting factors: speed, style, form, fluency, legibility and coordination difficulties were reported upon.
- The number and nature of any spelling errors were analysed.

Of the 40 pupils only 8 had no identifiable spelling or speed and coordination handwriting problems except that in 7 cases suggestions were made that would improve legibility.

"Dyslexics" were those who made more than 10 misspellings per 100 words after the Reception year or wrote no decipherable words in Reception.

Speed problems were identified as cases where rate per minute was lower than the mean for the Year group (one word per minute faster than actual age) although the more able should be writing faster than other pupils.

Legibility was not scored but based on a Test of Handwriting Form and Legibility T-HFL interventions were suggested as appropriate and related to "body," size, ascenders and descenders, use of lines, letter formation and word space.

Of the whole group of 40:

- 8 were diagnosed with dyslexia (16%), only 2 had a formal diagnosis
- 4 had dyslexia and speed problems (50% of the dyslexics)
- 5 dyslexics had coordination difficulties (12.5% of the dyslexics)
- 13 had significantly slow speed, 25 per cent or more slower than the mean. (26%)
- 22 had handwriting/coordination difficulties (55%)
- 27 had some form of handwriting difficulty in speed or coordination (67.5%)
- 8 had both speed and coordination problems (16%)
- 28 had a speed 40 per cent or more slower than might be predicted from their high ability (70%).
- 32 of the group of 40 had a problem that would be detrimental to potential high achievement in school (80%).
- 7 used the more problematic quadruped or thumb over grip (17.5%), not the usual tripod flexible or rigid grips.
- Other problems such as weak grip and too firm a grip had to be inferred from pressure or lack of it on the scripts and reference to coloured photographs.
- Several adults and children reported pain in their writing hands after a few minutes of writing although this information was not specifically requested.

The conclusion from this sample is that in the majority of cases potential achievement was undermined by difficulties in handwriting and/or spelling. Handwriting difficulties were in the majority, two thirds of the sample. The distress that this creates in many such cases makes them vulnerable to nervous illness and withdrawal from school such is the disparity between their high ability and their writing accomplishment and its reception by the their teachers. If handwriting skill does not respond to intervention assistive technology should be introduced and this may be needed as soon as formal schooling begins in about 1% of cases. In relation to dyslexia a handwriting problem handicaps the remedial intervention strategies and contributes to the severe cases.

6. Conclusion

Although this research began with a concern about spelling problems in a wider group than just dyslexics a second problem emerged. This was a difficulty in handwriting and the large number of cases of potential underachievement it caused across the ability range that was going unobserved in schools. Neurological fMRI studies showed that handwriting was an essential component in both reading and spelling acquisition and development [44]. This meant that handwriting and spelling needed more attention in dyslexia remedial programmes following the approaches of the dyslexia pioneers using cursive and SOS training [25]. Government guidelines [57] on handwriting offer only a semi-cursive approach with 4 different places to start letters rather than one.

A further problem was revealed in the research and this was the case of very bright dyslexics with HLP who were identified late who read well but spellt poorly and often had problems with writing – the dysorthographics. Traditional SSP interventions were not relevant for them and they needed a strategic approach to spelling. This did work well.

For most of the 20th century, the belief was that English spelling was highly irregular and pupils did not use prior knowledge of previously learned words to help spell new words [58]. Because of these beliefs, spelling instruction in most classrooms was based on rote memorisation of assigned lists of words selected by the teacher or a spelling textbook that emphasised visual memorisation of the most common irregular sound/symbol correspondences [59]. These beliefs have been difficult to change and have become embedded in the limited approaches found in the UK government guidelines.

Because the strategies learnt by intending literacy teachers in England are limited to SSP they do not require them to be familiar with the stages in spelling development or understand how the English language system is organised. Research has shown however that spelling is not an exclusive process of rote memorising [60] and pupils do not learn spelling words in isolation instead they use prior knowledge and understandings to help make decisions and form concepts about how to spell new words.

Bear et al. [61] found that as children's knowledge of language, letters, sounds, and other phonological processes developed so did their ability to notice patterns within words. From basic letter-to-sound correspondences, to patterns associated with long and short vowels sounds, to structures within words associated with syllables and affixes, and finally, to Greek and Latin roots and stems, the child's brain looks for invariant patterns to help it spell efficiently. They suggested a hierarchical process in development. Although word pattern knowledge may develop in this way in non-dyslexics by implicit learning processes, dyslexics need specific help to learn the skills or at least get started on them as illustrated in the CPSS case example above.

A traditional spelling curriculum that assigns words based on content vocabulary, somewhat random spelling rules and synthetic phonics does not take advantage of the brain's capacity to learn through predictable patterns [62]. Word pattern theory has become a dominant theme in spelling research especially in the US and is relevant to the flexible CPSS approach described above for later phase dyslexics.

This wider research supports the view of spelling as a complex cognitive process intrinsically related to language, reading, and writing [34, 63] In support of this approach with dyslexics the International Dyslexia Association [64] stated that a spelling programme should not emphasise visual memory but instead, make the process of discovering the features of words more salient and allow students to become more efficient spellers.

Society, in general, values correct spelling above all other writing conventions and making anything beyond a few minor spelling errors is equated with ignorance and incompetence [65]. Helping dyslexics into the orthographic phase of development by giving them insights into word pattern structures and their linguistic rules can thus prevent them from becoming doubly disadvantaged. The CPSS system teaches dyslexics and other poor spellers key phonological, morphological and etymological information that good readers and writers pick up implicitly during reading and spelling.

Author details

Diane Montgomery
Middlesex University, London, UK

*Address all correspondence to: dmont507@aol.com

References

[1] DfE. Excellence for all Children. London: DfE; 1997. p. 15

[2] DfEE. The National Literacy Strategy. London: DfEE; 1998

[3] Peters ML. Spelling: Caught or Taught? London: Routledge and Kegan Paul; 1967

[4] Peters ML. Spelling: Caught or Taught? 2nd ed. London: Routledge and Kegan Paul; 1985

[5] BDA. 2020. Dyslexia. Available from: www.bda-dyslexia.org.uk

[6] Gillingham AM, Stillman BU. Remedial Training for Children with Specific Disability in Reading, Spelling and Penmanship Bath. Bath, England: Basic Books; 1956

[7] Hickey K. Dyslexia: A Language Training Course for Teachers and Learners Staines. Surrey: Dyslexia Institute; 1977

[8] Hickey K. In: Augur J, Briggs S, editors. Dyslexia: A Language Training Course for Teachers and Learners. 2nd ed. London: Whurr; 1991

[9] Naidoo S. Specific developmental dyslexia. In: Research Report of the Invalid Children's Aid Association (ICAA). London: Pitman; 1972

[10] Chall J. Learning to Read: The Great Debate. New York: McGraw-Hill; 1967

[11] Chall J. Stages in Reading Development. New York: McGraw-Hill; 1985

[12] Clark MM. Reading Difficulties in Schools. Penguin: Harmondsworth; 1970

[13] Ferreiro E, Teberosky A. Literacy before Schooling Exeter. NH: Heinemann Education; 1982

[14] Ridehalgh N. A comparison of dyslexia remediation programmes and an analysis of their effectiveness [MA SpLD dissertation] London: Middlesex University; 1999

[15] Vellutino FR. Dyslexia: Theory and Research. London: MIT Press; 1979

[16] Schaapkens T. An investigation into the feasibility of integrating cognitive process strategies into Food Technology lessons [MA SpLD dissertation]. London: Middlesex University; 2009

[17] Schiffman GB. Table to show percentage gains after 2 years of remedial intervention at different ages of intervention. In: Goldberg HK, Schiffman GB, editors. Dyslexia. Problems of Reading Disabilities. London: Grune and Stratton; 1972. p. 66

[18] Montgomery D. Identifying and remediating dyslexia in kindergarten and the foundation year. In: Learning Disabilities: Neurological Bases, Clinical Features and Strategies of Intervention. London: InTech; 2020

[19] DES. The Bullock Report. London: HMSO; 1975

[20] DfES. The Code of Practice (Revised). London: HMSO; 2001

[21] Cowdery LL, McMahon J, Montgomery D, Morse P, Prince-Bruce M. Teaching Reading through Spelling (TRTS) Vols 2A to 2F. Kingston: Learning Difficulties Research Project; 1983-1987

[22] Cowdery LL, Morse P, Prince-Bruce M. Teaching Reading through Spelling Series 1–7 Reprint. Wrexham: TRTS Publishing; 1994

[23] Cowdery LL. The Spelling Notebook (2F TRTS) Kingston: Learning

Difficulties Research Project Reprint 2007. Kent: Cambridge House; 1997

[24] Rutter ML, Caspi A, Fergusson D, Horwood LJ, Goodman R, Maughan B, et al. Sex differences in developmental reading disability. Journal of the American Medical Association. 2004;**9**(1):291

[25] Montgomery D. Dyslexia and Gender Bias. A Critical Review. London: Routledge Focus Book; 2018

[26] Montgomery D, editor. Able Underachievers. Chichester: Wiley; 2000

[27] Montgomery D. Spelling, Handwriting and Dyslexia. London: Routledge; 2007

[28] Montgomery D. Cohort analysis of writing in year 7 after 2, 4, and 7 years of the National Literacy Strategy. Support for Learning. 2008;**23**(1):3-11

[29] Frith U. Beneath the surface of developmental dyslexia. In: Patterson KE, Marshall JC, Coltheart M, editors. Surface Dyslexia. London: Routledge and Kegan-Paul; 1985

[30] Gentry J. Learning to spell developmentally. The Reading Teacher. 1981;**34**(4):378-381

[31] Read C. Children's Creative Spelling. London: Routledge and Kegan-Paul; 1986

[32] Rosencrans G. The Spelling Book. Teaching Children how to Spell. USA International Reading Association; 1998

[33] Bourassa D, Treiman R. Spelling in children with dyslexia: Analyses from the Treiman–Bourassa early spelling test. Scientific Studies of Reading. 2003; **7**(4):309-333

[34] Ehri LC. Acquisition of sight-word reading, spelling memory and vocabulary learning. The role of orthographic mapping. In: Keynote Lecture 11th International Conference of the BDA, 12–14 April. Telford UK; 2018

[35] Montgomery D. The contribution of handwriting and spelling remediation to overcoming dyslexia. In: Wydell NT, Fern-Pollak L, editors. Dyslexia - a Comprehensive and International Approach. Rijeka, Croatia: InTech Publication; 2012

[36] Allen BV. Logical Spelling. London: Collins; 1977

[37] Pollack J. Signposts to Spelling (Repr). London: Heinemann; 1981

[38] Moseley DV. From theory to practice. In: Brown GDA, Ellis NC, editors. Handbook of Spelling. Chichester: Wiley; 1994. pp. 459-479

[39] Spache GD. Characteristic errors of good and poor spellers. Journal of Educational Research. 1940;**34**(3):182-189

[40] Neale MD. 1958 Neale Analysis of Reading Ability Second Edition Windsor: NFER-Nelson. New ed. London: Macmillan; 1977

[41] Neale MD, Christophers U, Whetton C. Neale Analysis of Reading Ability Revised Edition. Windsor: NFER-Nelson; 1994

[42] Montgomery D. Spelling: Remedial Strategies. London: Cassell; 1997

[43] Kuczaj SA. Evidence for a language learning strategy in the relative ease of acquisition of prefixes and suffixes. Child Development. 1979;**50**:1-13

[44] James K, Engelhardt L. The effects of handwriting experience on functional brain development. Neuroscience and Education. 2012;**1**(1):32-42

[45] Geschwind N. Specialisations of the human brain. Scientific American. 1979; **231**(3):156-167

[46] Ehri LC. The development of orthographic images. In: U. Frith Cognitive Processes in Spelling. London: Academic Press; 1980. pp. 311-338

[47] Parrant H. An investigation of remedial approaches to children's spelling difficulties [unpublished SEN dissertation]. Kingston upon Thames: Kingston Polytechnic; 1986

[48] Wing AM, Baddeley AD. Spelling errors in handwriting, a corpus and distributional analysis. In: U. Frith Cognitive Processes in Spelling. London: Academic Press; 1980. pp. 251-288

[49] Miles TR. Dyslexia. The Pattern of Difficulties. 2nd ed. London: Whurr; 1993

[50] HMI. Report of her Majesty's Chief Inspector for Schools 1998–1999. London: HMCI; 1999

[51] Hanna PR, Hanna JS, Hodges RE, Rodori EH. Phoneme-Grapheme Correspondence as Cues to Spelling Improvement. Washington DC: US Office of Educn; 1966

[52] Henry MK. The decoding/spelling curriculum. Integrated decoding and spelling instruction from pre-school to early secondary school. Dyslexia. 1997;**3**: 178-189

[53] Montgomery D. Dyslexia-Friendly Strategies for Reading, Spelling and Handwriting. A Toolkit for Teachers. London: Routledge; 2017

[54] Morey K. Casework with an able dyslexic. Educating Able Children. 2001;**5**(1):27-30

[55] Montgomery D. Teaching Gifted Children with Special Educational Needs. Supporting Dual and Multiple Exceptionality. London: Routledge; 2015

[56] Roaf C. Slow hand. A secondary school survey of handwriting speed and legibility. Support for Learning. 1998; **13**(1):39-42

[57] DfE. National Curriculum, key stages 1 and 2. In: Framework for English and Mathematics. London: DfE; 2014

[58] Simonsen F, Gunter L. Best practices in spelling instruction: A research summary. Journal of Direct Instruction. 2001;**1**:97-105

[59] Robinson RD, editor. Readings in Reading Instruction: Its History, Theory, and Development. Boston, MA: Pearson; 2005

[60] Reed DK. Why Teach Spelling? Portsmouth, NH: RMC Research Corporation, Center on Instruction; 2012

[61] Bear DR, Invernizzi M, Templeton S, Johnston F. Words their Way: Word Study for Phonics, Vocabulary, and Spelling Instruction. 5th ed. Boston, MA: Pearson; 2012

[62] Dehaene S. Reading in the Brain. New York, NY: Viking, Dreyer; 2009

[63] Treiman R. Knowledge about letters as a foundation for reading and spelling. In: Joshi RM, Aaron PG, editors. Handbook of Orthography and Literacy Mahwah. NJ: Lawrence Erlbaum Associates; 2006. pp. 581-600

[64] International Dyslexia Association. Spelling. 2011. . Available from: https:// dyslexiaida.org/spelling/

[65] Moats LC. How spelling supports reading. American Educator. 2005;**29**: 12-43

Chapter 6

Mediating the Learning of a Student with Dyslexia in a Greek Supplementary School in the UK

Maria Rontou

Abstract

This paper's aim was to investigate a second language teacher's beliefs about teaching and learning and her practices in relation to a student with dyslexia from a sociocultural perspective. It first referred to studies on teachers' beliefs and practices, then the concepts of mediation, scaffolding and zone of proximal development were defined and studies on mediation and scaffolding were reviewed. The data from the interview with the teacher and the classroom observations were analyzed and compared. The study illustrated that the teacher's practices were not always consistent with her beliefs of how students with dyslexia learn better. Her teaching practice did not always have a theoretical concept behind it either. The observation of her lessons demonstrated though an effective use of multisensory methods, actions, objects and scaffolding to mediate a student's with dyslexia learning. In the end of the chapter suggestions for teachers of students with dyslexia in similar settings are given based on the data.

Keywords: teacher's beliefs, teacher practice, dyslexia, zone of proximal development, mediation, multisensory methods

1. Introduction

This paper's aim was to investigate a second language teacher's beliefs about teaching and learning and her practices in relation to a student with dyslexia from a sociocultural perspective. It first referred to studies on teachers' beliefs and practices, then the concepts of mediation, scaffolding and zone of proximal development were defined and studies on mediation and scaffolding were reviewed. The data from the interview with the teacher and the classroom observations were analyzed and compared. Although it was a small scale study and the conclusions cannot be generalized, the observation data along with the interview data demonstrate the usefulness of multisensory methods and collaborative learning for teaching foreign languages to the specific student with dyslexia and other students in similar settings.

1.1 Research on teachers' beliefs and practices

According to Borg (2015), teachers' beliefs influence teachers teaching practices, their actions and reactions to educational changes such as inclusion [1]. For this reason, this article investigates the relationship of a teacher's beliefs with her classroom practice in relation to the inclusion of a student with dyslexia.

After the 2000's research scholars begin to investigate teachers' beliefs and practices through the lens of the sociocultural theory focusing on beliefs as a complex system, and the connections between beliefs and change or actions [2]. Studies on teachers' beliefs and practice on dyslexia have been conducted with a variety of methods: surveys, interviews, narrative life history interviews, focus groups, observations.

Nijakowska (2000) conducted a survey study with 38 language primary and secondary teachers in Poland on teachers' knowledge and the support they offer to students with dyslexia [3]. Among other issues investigated whether teachers were familiar with the notion of multisensory teaching, if they apply any special methods of work with students with dyslexia and, if they give more time to students with dyslexia to complete a task when they need it. The findings showed inconsistencies between what teachers believed and knew and what they actually practiced: while 20 per cent of the teachers were familiar with multisensory teaching, only 15 per cent claimed that they had applied special methods and techniques with dyslexic students and even though 76 per cent admitted that children with dyslexia usually need more time to carry out an activity than other students, not more than 66 per cent allowed their dyslexic students more time when they need it to complete a task and only half of them did it during exams [3].

Kormos and Nijakowska (2016) conducted another survey study in order to investigate whether language teachers' self-confidence, self-efficacy and attitudes to using inclusive educational practices with dyslexic students are different before and after participation in an online training course. The study showed that EFL teachers tend to feel unable to use inclusive practices with students with dyslexia without training but after the training teachers' attitudes were more positive towards inclusion and their concerns were lower than before [4].

Nijakowska et al. (2018) conducted a more recent survey study in order to compare across different countries the beliefs of teachers of English as a foreign language (EFL) about their preparedness to include dyslexic learners in mainstream classrooms in Greece, Cyprus, and Poland and identify the training needs of teachers. The study showed that the teachers who had direct contact with students with dyslexia felt more prepared to include those students. There were similar findings among countries regarding the need for training which was indicated in the previous studies as well [5].

Tzanni (2018) also conducted a survey study exploring Greek EFL teachers' beliefs and practices related to differentiated instruction using an online questionnaire and quantitative analysis [6]. The study showed that although the EFL teachers had positive beliefs towards differentiation, in practice, they differentiated less than we might have expected which may happen because of lack of training or lack of preparation time [6]. This finding is similar to the inconsistency in teachers' beliefs and practices shown in Nijakowska (2000) [3].

Arapogianni (2003) conducted a small scale survey study with a different method than the previous studies, interviews with 8 secondary school teachers in Patras in Greece investigating the approaches used by teachers to support students with dyslexia in the classroom as well as their knowledge and training on dyslexia and their collaboration with other professionals [7]. Her study showed that the majority of the teachers did not know what to do to support students with dyslexia in the classroom as they did not have any training on dyslexia and had a lack of understanding about the nature of the students' difficulties. Because of their lack of knowledge they felt that they were not responsible for providing intervention. In this study I investigate a teacher's beliefs, knowledge and practice of teaching methods for dyslexia using interviews as Arapogianni (2003) did [7].

Schumm et al. (1994) have conducted research on general education teachers' beliefs, skills and practices in planning and making adaptations for mainstreamed students with learning disabilities. They first conducted a survey, as the studies mentioned before did, with sixty teachers in the U.S and then they conducted semi-structured interviews and classroom observations with twelve from the first sample. They investigated the relationship between teachers' beliefs, skills and practices and they found out that there are gaps between them. Although the teachers in this study were skilled in adapting course content and they considered adaptations as useful they did not actually do so because they were not practically able to do so because of lack of time [8]. This study showed inconsistency in teachers' beliefs and practices as in [3, 6] but unlike other studies, it used multiple methods of data collection.

Del Rosario (2006) also used a series of narrative interviews focusing on situations and events in order to investigate a high school English teacher's beliefs about teaching learning disabled students [9]. The study shows the importance of persistence and compromise in developing relationships with students.

Woolhouse (2012) conducted a qualitative study investigating the influence on teachers' identity of the training that they undertook in order to support students with dyslexia. The data were gathered through focus groups and narrative life history interviews conducted with teachers on a Specialist Dyslexia Training for Teachers Programme. The data suggested that the teachers who received training on dyslexia viewed themselves as distinct from other teachers in their schools and identified with the pupils they supported [10]. Aas (2019) conducted another qualitative study using content analysis of audio recordings of elementary school teachers' team meetings in order to investigate teachers' beliefs about student needs and teacher role and how these beliefs can challenge development towards a more inclusive practice. The study showed a general positive attitude of the school teachers towards inclusion but there were some aspects of teachers' beliefs that may prevent the development towards inclusive practice. These beliefs were: a limited view on learning focusing only on students' academic skills and not social skills, the idea of teacher centering disregarding learning that comes from collaboration and individualization which means that student needs were understood as individual problems that require time consuming adaptation [11].

This study investigated a teacher's beliefs and practices from a sociocultural perspective, using both interviews and observations as in Schumm et al's study (1994) [8] in the context of a Greek as a second language class with a student with dyslexia. The concepts of mediation, scaffolding and Zone of Proximal development which guided the analysis of the data in this study will be defined next.

1.2 Sociocultural theory

According to sociocultural theory, 'students need to be actively involved in the co-construction of knowledge through participation in a dialogue with teacher, texts and peers ...' [12]. Sociocultural theory is opposed to the empiricist idea of knowledge according to which students are treated as passive recipients of knowledge [12]. According to Vygotsky and Feuerstein, learning takes place through interaction with other people [13]. Therefore, it is through language that thinking develops and learning occurs [13].

According to Vygotsky and sociocultural theory, the human mind is mediated by symbolic tools, the most important of which is language [14]. Therefore, for Vygotsky, mediation is the use of symbolic tools in order to organize and control mental processes such as voluntary attention, problem-solving, planning and evaluation, memory and intentional learning [15] or to establish a relationship with others and with ourselves [14]. Language can be used to help learners move into their zone of proximal development [ZPD], that is to the layer of skill or knowledge which is beyond the learner's abilities [13].

Bruner expanded on Vygotsky and used the concept of 'scaffolding' to refer to this idea of a teacher or an adult supporting a child through dialog so that the child can carry out a difficult task [16]. Scaffolding can be done by checking what the students know and what they can do first and then by incorporating what they know and say into the discourse in order to move to the next level [16].

Mercer (1995) points out that in the scaffolding process both the teacher and the learner are actively involved in the construction of knowledge [16]. Therefore, the difference between the idea of mediating and the traditional idea of teaching as disseminating information is that mediation is concerned with empowering learners and helping them to acquire the skills that they need in order to learn more, to solve problems and become autonomous learners and independent thinkers [13]. Mediation, according to Feuerstein also involves sharing, co-operation among learners but also arecognition of their own individuality and uniqueness [13].

Co-operation among learners can take place with collaborative dialog which, according to Swain (2000) is 'problem-solving' and 'knowledge building' dialog [17]. 'Through saying and reflecting on what was said new knowledge is constructed' [17]. Mercer (1995) also claims that collaborative learning is very important because explaining something to a friend and arguing with someone helps you improve and revise your understanding [13].

Both Williams and Burden (1997) and Mercer (1995) argue that co-operation and sharing are ways of interacting that need to be taught to learners [13, 16]. According to Mercer (1995) learners should not be expected to make the rules they are expected to follow themselves. They need to know the rules, the rationale and principles of a collaborative activity [16].

1.3 Examples of the use of mediation/scaffolding in the literature

Beynon (2004) used the idea of mediation with non- reading adolescents in a multilingual and multicultural class of English as a second language in Johannesburg [18]. Beynon (2004) used the Multiliteracies approach to help these adolescents read. This is a way of mediating literacy by using a range of modalities - written and spoken language, sound, images, gestures and action - in order to make it accessible for each learner. Beynon (2004) argues that this approach allows both the teacher and the learner to be actively involved in the learning process and the construction of meaning. According to this approach, the teacher also 'mediates' her practice, adapts the curriculum and her instruction to meet the needs of each child and she takes into account the pedagogic history of each child. The students form collaborative groups in which the stronger students help the weaker. The students have to retell a story using their preferred modality, acting it out in small collaborative groups or drawing and painting it on paper and then they move on to learning to read the words they met in the story by using flashcards, games, dough. The fact that they have already met and acted out the words they try to read on flashcards and in the text of the story gives them meaning and a purpose for reading [18].

Donato's (1998) study addresses the role of collective scaffolding in the learning of French. Participants' knowledge of language such as the compound past tense formation of reflective verbs in French has been acquired through the process of collective scaffolding by all the participants [19]. Both Ohta (2000) and Swain (2000) also investigated the usefulness of collaborative dialog between adult learners of a foreign and a second language [17, 20]. Ohta (2000) found out that the collaboration and sensitive assistance from another learner can help a language learner become more independent and is useful for the internalization of L2 grammar while Swain's (2000) study has shown that it is useful for learning strategic processes as well as grammar [17, 20]. It would be interesting to investigate whether this can work with L2 learners.

De Guerrero and Villamil (2012) have also investigated peer revision scaffolding in an ESL writing classroom using qualitative methods and analyzing the interaction. The study showed that both students can be active partners and provide mutual scaffolding to each other [21].

Another study that investigated peer scaffolding was Lin and Samuel's (2013) qualitative study. The study examined the types of scaffolds used by students during peer response sessions and investigated how scaffolding facilitates learning. It was a case study that involved a group of six mixed-proficiency level students from a secondary school in Malaysia. Multiple methods were used; observation, interviews and fieldnotes. The study showed that the correction of errors in vocabulary and grammar as well as the use of questions were both effective scaffolds that helped weaker students progress in their writing skills. The implication of this study is that peer scaffolding can benefit students in the teaching and learning of writing [22].

Similarly, Khaliliaqdam (2014) conducted a case study based on Vygotsky's theory of scaffolding in the ZPD [23]. This case study attempted to examine the role of scaffolding via communicative activities in terms of development of basic speech on foreign language adult learners of EFL. The six students who participated in the study were asked to create the sentences with the help of the teachers. Then a series of pictures were given to them and they had to tell a story based on the pictures. During each scaffolding session, the adult experimenter negotiated meaning by asking questions and provided them the vocabulary needed in order to help them describe the pictures or illustrations. The analysis of this quantitative study shows that expert-novice group work created more learning opportunities than unassisted group work. This study also demonstrates the importance of purposeful interaction in making language scaffolding an effective tool for language development among adult foreign language learners [23].

Middleton (2004) investigated the ways in which teachers scaffolded and mediated the learning of children with specific learning difficulties in a special school. The researcher observed and analyzed qualitatively Mathematics and Guided Writing lessons. She found out that the teacher used tools to mediate students' learning: she used mathematical shapes like a cuboid and objects like a book or an A4 paper, and pointed to parts of them to demonstrate their properties and differences. She used her hands and some glasses to demonstrate the concept of symmetry. She also pointed to the board to elicit an answer and she gave a student a chart containing the answers in order to avoid giving him the answer [24].

The present study investigated the issues of mediation and scaffolding in the context of both a foreign language class and with a student with dyslexia, a combination which has not been addressed a lot by the literature.

1.4 Multisensory teaching

The teacher's knowledge and use of the direct multisensory structured approach is examined in this study. It is considered effective for teaching reading and spelling in the native language to children with dyslexia. The multisensory structured learning (MSL) style has been found effective for foreign language instruction as well [25–28]. The MSL approach teaches elements of the foreign language (the sound and spelling system, vocabulary and grammatical structures) through the auditory, visual, tactile and kinaesthetic pathways [29]. The presentation of new language with the use of as many modalities as possible benefit individuals with dyslexia.

A person with dyslexia learns how to read and spell words by hearing, seeing and pronouncing them [29]. When learning a new word, students repeat the word several times after the teacher (auditory channel), draw a picture to help memorization (visual channel) and act it out (kinaesthetic channel) [30].

2. The study

2.1 Aims

This study investigated a teacher's beliefs about how dyslexic students can learn better and compared her reported beliefs with her teaching practice, that is, the way she presented the new language and the way she mediated and scaffolded students' with and without dyslexia learning. The study also discussed her views on collaborative learning in relation to students with dyslexia and in relation to her practice.

2.2 The context

The study was conducted in a Greek Community school in the UK. There were seven students in that class aged 8–13 years who were bilingual in Greek and English and had Greek or Greek-Cypriot parents. The class was mixed ability and included two levels, five students at pre-intermediate level which is called 1B and two students at upper-intermediate level which is called 5A. The class was chosen as I was informed by the teacher that there was a student with an assessment of dyslexia aged 10 at the 1B level. The teacher had 11 years of teaching experience and was from Cyprus. She had a BA in primary Education from Cyprus and an MA in Inclusion from the UK and had attended two seminars on dyslexia in Cyprus.

2.3 Methods

I chose the approach of a case study, that is, a research strategy where the focus is on a case in its own right and taking its context into account and which involved multiple methods of data collection because I was interested in an in depth analysis of a teacher's views on pedagogy and her classroom practices [31]. I used two methods of data collection in order to compare between what the teacher said she believes and my perception of what she does: I first observed two of lessons in the same class and then I interviewed the teacher after the observations. The data were audio recorded and transcribed. Both the observations and the interview with the teacher were part of a wider study. I transcribed the questions from the interview which had to do with the teacher's beliefs about the teaching and learning of students with dyslexia and her ideas about collaborative learning which is a feature of mediation on which I would like to focus. I chose and transcribed one extract from the first lesson I observed and some extracts from the second lesson which show the scaffolding the teacher does with the student with dyslexia and other students in the class and how her ideas about teaching and learning are practiced. The interviews with participants were conducted in the Greek language and they were transcribed and translated into English. This process involved construction of meaning and interpretations by the transcriber and translator [32].

The selection of the schools was guided by convenience, that is, the accessibility of the school and the availability of individuals in them due to professional contacts [33, 34]. The headteacher had also given the researcher the information that there was a pupil with dyslexia in the class that was chosen. The teacher selected was the one who had a pupil with dyslexia in her classes and who agreed to participate in the study after being informed about its aims and procedure. The criterion for choosing the pupil was a dyslexia diagnosis and the parents' informed consent to participate in the study.

Since the student had not reached the age or maturity to be able to give informed consent I asked for the consent of her parents following BERA's guidelines [35]. The parents of the student with dyslexia were informed through a letter describing my study and their child's role in it and were asked to sign a consent form. The researcher made sure that the student with dyslexia did not suffer any psychological harm from the research [35]. For this reason the researcher did not sit near the student with dyslexia during the observation in order not to embarrass her and her diagnosis was not disclosed to other students in the class. Furthermore, in order not to identify the school and the participants, codes were used for the pupils (P, S1, S2) and the teacher (T) and the name of the name or location of the school was not disclosed.

Considering this was a small case study there is no generalizability of the conclusions as in quantitative studies. The findings can be applied in order to understand another similar situation [36]. The applicability of the findings from this case study to other foreign language classrooms depends on how far the case shares similar features with other foreign language classes, their teachers and other students with dyslexia. Such features may be class size, age of the students and the difficulties and abilities of other students with dyslexia [37].

2.4 The lessons

The first lesson I observed included the following activities for the pre-intermediate level: spelling from the previous lesson, students' reading the text from the previous lesson, exercises from the previous lesson, the teacher reading the new text and practice with exercises from the book and writing sentences with the new vocabulary.

The second lesson I observed included the following activities: spelling from the previous lesson, students' reading the text from the previous lesson, the teacher reading the new text, the teacher checking students' understanding of new vocabulary, the teacher reading the text again and the students repeating and translating the sentences and practice.

3. Analysis-discussion of data

3.1 Use of visual modality

The teacher believed that in the presentation of grammar it is better to show students with dyslexia a grammar rule with examples and signs like a smile under -o to show the letter omega (Ω), as this picture will remain in their mind:

T It is better to do, let us say what I imagine instead of telling them that the verbs that end in –o are always written with omega, it is better to show it to them … to make many verbs and in the end the –o to do it with a smile and tell them look. I think that this picture will stay in their mind more than the rule.

Extract 1: interview with teacher.

As extract 1 illustrates, the teacher believed that the use of the visual modality is particularly helpful for students with dyslexia in the presentation stage as she thought that it helps their memory. She said that she tries to use the visual modality, in the form of drawings in the activities they do as well. For example, in the second lesson I observed she asked the pre-intermediate level students to draw a picture of the sentences they wrote because she believed that they experience the new language better:

T Like two days ago ... that we learnt the in, under, on [that they had to] write a sentence but write next to it the picture as well, so that afterwards when they see it, let us say they had to write 'the glass is on the table' and make a picture, a table with a glass on it. I think that in this way they experience it better.

Extract 2: interview with teacher.

She also believed that this is useful for all the students not only the students with dyslexia:

Extract 3: interview with teacher.

T	**And this is so for all the children, not only the dyslexic students=**
M	=Yes
T	I mean the other children as well learn better in this way

The next extract from the second lesson I observed showed that she actually asked the students to make a picture of the sentences they would write:

Extract 4: lesson 2.

T	**... I'm gonna write these words that, in, on, in front of ok? And then you have to make your own sentences, for example what can you say about** μέσα?
S1	Το μωρό είναι μέσα στο κρεβάτι (*The baby is in the bed*)
T	Ok and then when you write these sentence which (**) you have to make a picture of the baby in the bed

This section demonstrated that the teacher believed that the use of the visual modality is helpful for students with and without dyslexia for memorizing new vocabulary which is in line with multisensory teaching [29]. She also practiced this idea in the second lesson when she asked the students with dyslexia to write a sentence in Greek and then draw a picture of it.

It should be mentioned though that in the first lesson the students were asked to make sentences with the new words they met but the teacher did not ask them to draw a picture which means that this kind of exercise may not be done consistently. Maybe the interview with the researcher lead the teacher to practice her ideas in the second lesson observed.

3.2 Use of multisensory methods

I also investigated whether the teacher used multisensory methods because they have proved to be effective with students with dyslexia learning foreign languages [25–28]. Ganschow et al. (1998) have suggested that the teacher should accompany oral language in the foreign language with a visual example when teaching students with dyslexia, for example, writing the foreign language words on an overhead [38].

I noticed in the first lesson I observed that the teacher corrected a student's pronunciation by saying a word correctly and writing it at the same time, that is, by using two modalities as Ganschow et al (1998) suggest [38]. I asked the teacher why and she said that it helps them:

M I saw that in phonology when you wanted to say that something is pronounced somehow you wrote it as well

T Yes because mm it helps them to see as well as to hear it

Extract 5: interview with teacher.

It seems though that she has not realized that this is multisensory teaching as earlier in the interview she said that she has not used multisensory methods:

M I say about multisensory methods that is do you use many [senses], apart from visual, to listen or first to listen then to see, then to write

T I think this would work but I have not used it

Extract 6: interview with teacher.

This section showed that the teacher in this study uses different modalities in her lesson for example, the visual modality along with the auditory one. She does not realize that this is multisensory teaching though as in the interview she said she does not use this method.

3.3 Use of actions

The teacher also used another modality, the kinesthetic one when she presented the new vocabulary: after she read the new text, she asked the student with dyslexia (P) and then two more students (S2 and S3) to do some actions in order to check if they and the rest of the class knew some words including the new vocabulary (on, in, in front). This is in line with multisensory teaching [30].

Extract 7: lesson 2.

15 **16**	**T**	**P** μπορείς να φτάσεις πάνω στην καρέκλα; (*P can you get on the chair?*) **Πού είναι η P;** (*Where is P?*)	**P gets on the chair** **To the rest of the class**
17	S1	Πάνω καρέκλα (*on chair*)	
18	T	()	
19	S1	Πάνω από το καρέκλα (*on the chair*)	
20 21 22 23 24 25	T	Πάνω στην καρέκλα (*on the chair*) ευχαριστώ κατέβα (*thank you get off*) S2, μπορείς να φτάσεις μπροστά από εκείνες τις καρέκλες; (*S2 can you get in front of these chairs?*) S2 μπροστά (4 δευτ) Ευχαριστώ (*S2 in front 4 secs. Thank you*). S2 τι σημαίνει μπροστά; (*S2 what does μπροστά mean?*)	S2 stands in front of the chairs
26	S2	In front	
27	P	In front (*)	

In extract 7 the teacher asked P in Greek to stand on the chair (line 15). In this way she checked if P understood the meaning of 'πάνω' in order to discover her ZPD and start the scaffolding process [15, 39]. Once P did what she was asked to do proving that she knew the word, then the teacher asked the rest of the class where P was in order to check if they could say 'Πάνω στην καρέκλα' (on the chair), checking their ZPD. Therefore, she tried to discover what the learners could do without help [40] A student attempted to answer (line 17) but she missed the article and in her second attempt she used the wrong article (το, line 19) so the teacher gave the correct answer in line 20. Then, she asked another student (S2) to stand in front of some chairs (line 22–23), she repeated μπροστά (line 24) and after he did it, she checked if he understood what μπροστά means. After this scaffolding process both S2 and P realized what μπροστά means (lines 26–27). The fact that the students were asked to act out the new vocabulary engaged them to think what it means and gave it meaning as happened in Beynon (2004) [18].

This section demonstrated the scaffolding process that the teacher in this study followed in order to help the student with dyslexia and the other students in the class understand and memorize the meaning of new vocabulary. She used the kinaesthetic modality that made the lesson more interesting and memorable for the student with dyslexia and the rest of the class.

3.4 Use of tools/objects

Extract 8: lesson 2.

Line	Speaker	Words said	Comments
1	T	Try and do sentences like you did here=	
2	P	=Yeah	
3	T	With these πά:νω (.) What does πάνω mean? (4 sec)	The T writes the word in P's notebook
4	P	Is it she?	
5	T	Άκου (.) η κασετίνα είναι πάνω στο τραπέζι *(Listen. The pencil case is on the table)*	The T puts the pencil case on the table
6	P	Em (3 sec) πά-	
7	T	Πάνω	
8	P	Oh on	
9 10 11 12	T	Ναι (3 δευτ) Κοίτα (.) Ο μαρκαδόρος είναι μέσα στην κασετίνα. *(Yes (3 sec) Look. The pen is in the pencil case)* Μέσα, κάτω. Η κασετίνα είναι κάτω από το τραπέζι *(in, under. The pencil case is under the table)*	The T puts the pen in the pencil case The T writes the words in P's notebook. She puts the pencil case under the table
13	P	Underneath	

In the dialog in extract 8 the teacher explained to the student with dyslexia (P) what she had to do during practice. She confirmed that the student knew what the words she had to use to make sentences meant. In line 3 she asked her what 'πάνω' (on) means and when she found out that the student did not know, she used objects as tools to mediate her learning and avoid giving the answer to the student as the teacher in Middleton's (2004) study did; she put the pencil case on the table while saying η 'κασετίνα είναι πάνω στο τραπέζι' [the pencil case is on the table] (line 5) [19]. The result of this process is that the student managed to give the correct answer in line 8. Then, the teacher went to the next word, μέσα (in), and demonstrated its meaning by putting the pen in the pencil case while saying 'Ο μαρκαδόρος είναι μέσα στην κασετίνα' [the pen is in the pencil case] (line 9). Then, she showed the meaning of 'κάτω' [under] by putting the pencil case under the table while saying 'Η κασετίνα είναι κάτω από το τραπέζι' [the pencil case is under the table] (lines 11–12). In this way, the student was able to give the meaning of 'κάτω' (line 13).

At the interview I mentioned to the teacher that I found the use of actions and objects effective and she answered that they knew those words but they needed to see what they heard in order to remember them (extract 9):

M I saw that, what I liked [was] that you showed them with actions=.

T A the 'on, under' yes because only in this way they can understand, because they know them but you have to connect what they listen to see it visually as well in order to remember it more.

Extract 9: interview with teacher.

Furthermore, the teacher avoided giving the meaning of the new words immediately and elicited them instead by asking the students to perform actions and by giving them visual examples with objects because she thought the students knew the words already as she said that she did in extract 10:

T ...if it is something they know I may not do it so explicitly, if it is something that I know that it is the first time they are taught it would be mooore=

M = Then you have to tell them.
T Yes
Extract 10: interview with teacher.

This section demonstrated the teacher's use of objects as tools when she tried to explain the meaning of the words used during the practice stage of the lesson. The teacher used the visual modality (showing the meaning with objects) along with the auditory one (listening to a sentence) in order to help students remember the meaning of the words she had already taught. It has to be mentioned though that in the first lesson observed there was no use of actions, tools or the visual modality. One reason may be that the new vocabulary of the second lesson (words for location) was easier to demonstrate visually or kinesthetically, with actions and objects.

3.5 Collaborative learning

The issue of collaborative learning for dyslexic students will be discussed next because paired learning, with spelling partners and peer tutoring have been reported by SENCOS to be effective in assisting dyslexic students [41]. Working on speaking tasks in small groups without having to worry about making errors, and without the pressure of having to perform in front of a large audience is advisable for students with dyslexia who also need a lot of planning time before they start a task [30]. Collaborative dialog and peer scaffolding between L2 learners has also been proved to be useful [17, 19–23].

The teacher told me at the interview (extract 11) that she would place the student with dyslexia next to a good student in order to help her which means that she thought that the collaboration between the student with dyslexia and another student would be beneficial.

T I would put her to sit with a child who first of all would not make fun of her and would help her that is with a good student, so that s/he would give her some help and I do not think that there would be a comparison, only to help her.

Extract 11: interview with teacher.

In practice though she did not interfere about where the student with dyslexia would sit and with whom in any of the lessons I observed and in the first one she stressed that the students should do an exercise by themselves (extract 12). She encouraged them to ask questions only to her:

Extract 12: lesson 1.

Speaker	Words said	Comments
T	You have to do (the reading) by yourselves. Thirty eight. Each one will do this exercise alone. Ok? You have to read (*) and write. You have an example. So (.) check you know the colors. If there are any words you do not know ask me	*Stressed word*

At the interview I asked the teacher to explain why she asked the students to work alone (extract 13, lines 39–40) and she answered that in the specific class I observed the work was sometimes done only by one student and the rest copied (line 42). For this reason, she did not consider collaboration useful if it meant copying. She preferred them to do the exercise by themselves so that she knew they have all understood it (lines 42–43). This is in agreement with Aljaafresh and Lantolf's (1994) argument that help from the expert to the novice should be contingent, that is, it should be offered only when it is needed, it should be kept to the minimum and should be withdrawn when it is not needed any more [39]. Therefore, this teacher probably thought that the students were able to do the task independently. This teacher may have been influenced by the idea that it is more important that students acquire academic skills than social skills found in Aas' study [11].

She mentioned though that in some other cases she encourages collaboration by asking students to help a weaker student or to listen to a 'good' student (lines 45–46).

Extract 13: interview with teacher.

39 **40**	M	**=When you did exercises you told them do the exercises by yourselves which means that you did not want them to help each other**
41 42 43	T	Ah because in some cases one person does it, in the specific class I have, and then all the others copy. You know in order to know what each one has understood=
44	M	=Mmm
45 46 47 48	T	There are cases though that I say help let us say this person or listen for what let us say S4 will say who is the best [student] but there are cases that I know that they will copy from each other so there is no point, is there?

I observed though that even though the teacher did not encourage the students to help each other in the first lesson, the student with dyslexia (P) asked the student sitting next to her for help in the same lesson; she asked what a word meant. I mentioned this to the teacher Line 49 who asked me whether S3 told P the answer or whether she helped her Line 52 which means that she distinguished between giving the answer and students helping each other.

Extract 14: interview with teacher.

49	M	**Perhaps with P, I just saw that she worked with S3 and that this helped her.**
50	T	S3 with P yes
51	M	Perhaps sitting together helps
52	T	Mmm You saw that she didn't tell her [the answers] she helped her
53	M	I saw that she worked alone but when she wanted to ask what does this mean=
54	T	Yes
55	M	She asked her let's say instead of being ashamed of asking you=
56	T	=Mmm
57	M	It is better to ask the other student=
58	T	=Yes
59	M	Of course you should know=
60	T	=yes yes
61	M	Not to copy, to watch what's going on
62	T	Yes yes

One could argue though that this teacher chose the easy solution of not letting the students work in pairs or groups instead of training them on how to do so. Both Williams and Burden (1997) and Mercer (1995) argue that co-operation and sharing are ways of interacting that need to be taught to learners [13, 16]. Mercer (1995) argues that learners should not be expected to make the rules they are expected to follow themselves [16]. They need to know the rules, the rationale and principles of a collaborative activity [16].

It has to be mentioned though, that pair and group work was something not very common in Greek primary school classrooms until recently as class teachers considered behavior management more important than collaboration and they thought that learning should come from the teacher which are ideas that also were found in Aas study (2019) [11]. Previous research in a Greek state and a private school has shown that Greek teachers do not encourage group or pair work unless the exercise asks for it because they think it does not work [42]. This may be the case in Cyprus where the teacher in this study comes from and where she has worked for eight years.

When I suggested that it's better for the student with dyslexia to ask her partner what something means instead of asking her and being embarrassed (58–60), the teacher agreed (line 61). She also agreed with my suggestion that she should monitor them and make sure they do not copy (lines 62–65) but we cannot know why she agreed, because she was convinced or just to please me.

This section showed that the teacher in this study considered beneficial the collaboration between a student with dyslexia and a stronger student but in practice in the lessons observed she did not encourage collaboration between the students in this class. This happened because she did not want weak students to copy from stronger students and she wanted to know what each one understood. On the other hand, she agreed that the collaboration in order to ask for the meaning of a word would be useful for the student with dyslexia who would want to ask this question in front of the class. Asking for and providing information have been reported as scaffolds that peers use in peer scaffolding to help each other [22].

4. Suggestions for teachers

Multisensory methods have proved to be effective for the improvement of students with dyslexia skills in reading, writing, listening, phonology and spelling in a foreign language [25]. The teacher in this study also agrees that multisensory methods help students' memory and uses them without realizing she does so. Provided that there is lack of training and practice on dyslexia support in different countries [3, 5–8] and the right training on special educational needs changes teachers' attitudes towards inclusion and students with disability [4, 10] language teachers need to be trained on how to support students with dyslexia. For example, language teachers at primary schools or language teachers of young learners like the teacher in the study can be trained on the use multisensory methods, for example, the use of cards with vocabulary and pictures, color-coding, drawings in order to make practice more interesting and help memorization of new vocabulary and grammar [30, 43]. Language teachers can also use the kinesthetic modality by asking the students to move in the classroom or mime actions in order to help them memorize the new language or by using tools to demonstrate the new language as the teacher in this study did [29]. Collaborative learning would also be effective for students with dyslexia as they would not be ashamed to make mistakes in front of the class [29]. Pair or group work and peer scaffolding would be effective provided that the students are taught the rules they need to follow and they are monitored and assisted by the teacher in order to avoid cases in which the students with dyslexia copy the answer from their partners as the teacher in this study mentioned [16].

5. Conclusion

This paper has investigated a foreign language teacher's beliefs about learning and teaching and the actual application or not of them in the classroom, that is, the way she mediated a dyslexic student's learning but also the learning of the rest of the class. Although it was a small study including only two lesson observations which means that conclusions cannot be generalized, the study illustrated that the teacher's practices were not always consistent with her beliefs of how students with dyslexia learn better. She might practice what she believes but not in all the lessons as happened with the use of visuals and actions which may depend on the lesson taught. This finding is similar to Nijakowska's (2000), Tzanni' s (2018) and Schumm et al's (1994) findings [3, 6, 8]. She also did things that she had not thought why or without having a theoretical concept of them like the use of multisensory methods. She also thought that collaborative learning is useful for students with dyslexia (extract 13) but she did not encourage it in all her classes and all the lessons if she thought it would not work. The lesson observations though demonstrated an effective use of multisensory methods, actions, objects and scaffolding that lead the student with dyslexia and the rest of the students to understand the new vocabulary.

These findings have implications for teachers' training. Language teachers of students with dyslexia may need to be trained on multisensory methods and on how to use them in class and on how to apply collaborative learning in the form of pair or group work and peer scaffolding in their classes.

Acknowledgements

I would like to thank the teacher of Greek at the Greek Community school as well as the students of this class for their participation in this study.

Conflict of interest

"The author declares no conflict of interest."

Appendix

Speakers:

T	teacher
M	me

Students referred:

P	student with dyslexia
S1	student 1
S2	student 2

Transcription conventions:

(.) brief pause (less than 2 seconds) (Graddol, Cheshire and Swann 1994)

(2 secs) timed pause (longer than 2 seconds)

M	... τι ξέρεις για τη δυσλεξία;
T	Μμμ. Λοιπόν δυσλεξία,

DOI: http://dx.doi.org/10.5772/intechopen.94267

overlapping speech (Graddol, Cheshire and Swann 1994).

(*)	Inaudible one word
(**)	Inaudible more than one word (Edwards and Westgate 1987)
....	omitted speech
=	no pause between speakers (French and French 1984 in Edwards and Westgate 1987)

Author details

Maria Rontou
University of Peloponnese, Department of Political Science and International Relations, Hellenic Open University, Greece

*Address all correspondence to: rontou.maria@ac.eap.gr

References

[1] Borg, S. Researching teachers' beliefs. In B. Paltridge & A. Phakiti (Eds.), *Research methods in applied linguistics: A practical resource*. London: Bloomsbury; 2015. p. 487-504.

[2] Gao, Y. Language Teacher Beliefs and Practices: A Historical Review. *Journal of English as an International Language. 2014; 9*, 40-56.

[3] Nijakowska J. Dyslexia - Does it mean anything to a foreign language teacher? In L Peer. and G Reid, editors. *Multilingualism, Literacy and Dyslexia: A Challenge for Educators* London: David Fulton Publishers Ltd; 2000. p. 248-256.

[4] Nijakowska J, Tsagari D, & G., S. English as a foreign language teacher training needs and perceived preparedness to include dyslexic learners: The case of Greece, Cyprus, and Poland. Dyslexia. 2018; 24(4): 357-379.

[5] Kormos, J., and Nijakowska J. Inclusive practices in teaching students with dyslexia: Second language teachers' concerns, attitudes and self-efficacy beliefs on a massive open online learning course. *Teaching and Teacher Education.* 2017; *68*, 30-41.

[6] Tzanni, V. (). Exploring Differentiated Instruction in TESOL:The Teachers. Beliefs and Practices in Greece. Research Papers in Language Teaching and Learning. 2018; 9 (1), 149-165.

[7] Arapogianni, A. Investigating the Approaches that Teachers in Greece Use to Meet the Needs of Children with Dyslexia in Secondary Schools [Unpublished MA dissertation]. University of Birmingham, Birmingham; 2003.

[8] Schum, J. M., Vaughan, S., Gordon, J and Rothlein, L. General education teachers' beliefs, skills, and practices in planning for mainstreamed students with learning disabilities. Teacher Education and Special Education. 1994.17: 22-37.

[9] Del Rosario, B. Narrative study of a high School English teacher's beliefs about students identified as having a disability. International Journal of Inclusive Education. 2006 10(6), 645-655.

[10] Woolhouse, C. Reflective practice and identity construction: the particularities of the experiences of teachers specialising in dyslexia. Reflective Practice. 2012. 1-14.

[11] Aas, H. K. (2019). Teachers talk on student needs: exploring how teacher beliefs challenge inclusive education in a Norwegian context. International Journal of Inclusive Education. DOI: 10.1080/13603116.2019.1698065

[12] Wells G. Language and Education: Reconceptualizing Education as Dialogue. Annual Review of Applied Linguistics. 1999. 19: 135-155.

[13] Williams M., and Burden R. Psychology for Language Teachers: A Social Constructivist Approach. Cambridge: Cambridge University Press; 1997.

[14] Lantolf J. P. Sociocultural Theory and Second Language Learning. Oxford: Oxford University Press; 2000.

[15] Lantolf J. P. Sociocultural theory and second language learning. Modern Language Journal. 1994; 78(4): 418-420.

[16] Mercer N. The Guided Construction of Knowledge: Talk Amongst Teachers and Learners. Clevedon: Multilingual Matters; 1995.

[17] Swain M. The output hypothesis and beyond: Mediating acquisition through

collaborative dialogue. In J. P. Lantolf, editor. Sociocultural Theory and Second Language Learning. Oxford: Oxford University Press; 2000.

[18] Beynon, A. Tinker, Tailor, Teacher, Text: Using a Multiliteracies Approach to Remediate Reading. In M. R. Hawkins, editor. Language Learning and Teacher Education. Clevedon: Multilingual Matters Ltd; 2004.

[19] Donato, R. Collective Scaffolding in Second Language Learning. In Vygotskian Approaches to Second Language Research, edited by James P. Lantolfand Gabriela Appel, 33-56. Norwood, N.J.: Ablex; 1998.

[20] Ohta A. S. Rethinking interaction in SLA: developmentally appropriate assistance in the zone of proximal development and the acquisition of L2 grammar. In J. P. Lantolf, editor. Sociocultural theory and second language learning. Oxford: Oxford University Press; 2000.

[21] De Guerrero, M. C. M., & Villamil, O. S. Activating the ZPD: Mutual Scaffolding in L2 Peer Revision. The Modern Language Journal. 2012; 84(1): 51-68.

[22] Lin, S., & Samuel, M. Scaffolding during Peer Response Sessions. Procedia-Social and Behavioural Sciences. 2013; 90, 737-744.

[23] Khaliliaqdam, S. ZPD, Scaffolding and Basic Speech Development in EFL Contex. Procedia- Social and behavioral Sciences. 2014; 98, 891-897.

[24] Middleton V. Defining Scaffolding in the Context of Specific Learning Difficulties [Unpublished EdD thesis]. Open University; 2004.

[25] Sparks R., Artzer M., Patton J., Ganschow, L., Miller K., Hordubay D.J. and Walsh G. Benefits of Multisensory Structured Language Instruction for at-risk Foreign Language Learners: A Comparison Study of High School Spanish Students. Annals of Dyslexia. 1998; 48: 239-270.

[26] Schneider E. Multisensory Structured Metacognitive Instruction: An Approach to Teaching a Foreign Language to at-risk Students at an American College. Frankfurt am Main: Peter Lang Verlag; 1999.

[27] Sparks R. L. and Miller K. S. Teaching a foreign language using multisensory structured language techniques to at-risk learners: a review. Dyslexia. 2000; 6: 124-132.

[28] Crombie, A., & McColl, H. Teaching modern foreign languages to dyslexic learners: A Scottish perspective. In L. Peer & G. Reid, Editors., Multilingualism, Literacy and Dyslexia. London: David Fulton; 2000. p. 115-152.

[29] Nijakowska, J. Dyslexia in the Foreign Language Classroom. Bristol: Multilingual Matters; 2010.

[30] Kormos, J., & Smith, A. M. Teaching Foreign Languages to Learners with Specific Learning Differences. Bristol: Multilingual Matters; 2012.

[31] Robson, C. Real World Research: A Resource for Social Scientists and Practitioner-Researchers. 2nd ed. Oxford: Blackwell; 2002.

[32] Marshall, C. and Rossman, G. B., *Designing Qualitative Research* (5th ed.). London: Sage; 2011.

[33] Cohen, L., Manion, L., & Morrison, M. Research Methods in Education. London: Routledge; 2007.

[34] Fine, G. A., & Shulman, D. Lies from the field: ethical issues in organizational ethnography. In S. Ybema, D. Yanow, H. Wells & F. Kamsteeg, editors, Organizational Ethnography: Studying the

Complexities of Everyday Life. London: Sage; 2009. p. 177-195.

[35] BERA. Revised Ethical Guidelines for Educational Research. 2004.

[36] Denscombe, M. The Good Research Guide for Small-Scale Social Research Projects (4rth ed.). Maidenhead: Open University Press; 2010.

[37] Stake, R. E. The Case Study Method in Social Inquiry. Educational Researcher. 1978; 7(2): 5-8.

[38] Ganschow L., Sparks R, and Javorsky J. Foreign language learning difficulties: an historical perspective. Journal of Learning Disabilities. 1998; 31: 248-258.

[39] Aljaafresh A., and Lantolf J. P. Negative feedback as regulation and second language learning in the Zone of Proximal Development. Modern Language Journal. 1994; 78: 465-483.

[40] Lantolf J. P., and Aljaafresh A. Second language learning in the zone of proximal development: A revolutionary experience. International Journal of Educational Research. 1995; 23: 619-632.

[41] Hunter-Carsch M. Learning support in the secondary school: needs analysis and provision for dyslexic students. In M. Hunter-Carsch and M. Herrington editors. Dyslexia and Effective Learning in Secondary and Tertiary Education. London: Whurr Publishers; 2001. p. 12-37.

[42] Rontou M. Issues in Grammar Teaching [Unpublished MA dissertation]. University of Warwick, Coventry; 2003.

[43] Ganschow, L., Sparks, R. and E. Schneider. Learning a foreign language: challenges for students with language learning difficulties. *Dyslexia, 1.* 1995; 75-95.

Chapter 7

Visual-Motor Perception and Handwriting Performance of Students with Mixed Subtype Dyslexia

Simone Aparecida Capellini, Larissa Sellin, Ilaria D'Angelo, Noemi Del Bianco, Catia Giaconi and Giseli Donadon Germano

Abstract

This study aimed to characterize and compare the visual-motor perception and handwriting performance of students with mixed dyslexia and students with good academic performance. Twenty-six schoolchildren of both sexes participated in this study, aged 9 to 11 years and 11 months old, from fourth and fifth grades of an elementary school in municipal public schools, from an average socioeconomic level, divided into two groups: Group I (GI) composed of 13 students with a multidisciplinary diagnosis of mixed developmental dyslexia and Group II (GII) composed of 13 students with good academic performance from a municipal school and matched according to gender, education, and age to GI. All students in this study were subjected to the application of the following procedures: Developmental Test of Visual Perception III—DTVP-III, Dysgraphia Scale and writing analysis by NeuroScript MovAlyzeR 6.1 software. The results were analyzed statistically using the following tests: Mann-Whitney test, Wilcoxon signed-rank test, and Friedman test, aiming to verify intragroup and intergroup differences for the variables of interest in the DTVP-III, the Dysgraphia Scale, and the measures of handwriting speed and pressure by the MovAlyzeR software. The results were analyzed statistically at a significance level of 5% (0.050). The results showed that there were statistically significant differences between GI and GII in the parameters of the Dysgraphia Scale, floating lines, irregular spaces between words, junction points, sudden movements, and dimension irregularities. GII showed a superior performance in relation to GI in the variables analyzed with the DTVP-III in visual-motor integration, reduced motricity perception, and general visual perception. There was no statistically significant difference between GI and GII in the variables analyzed by the MovAlyzeR software. The results of this study allowed us to conclude that students with mixed dyslexia present a lower performance profile than the students with good academic performance in general visual perception, reduced motricity visual perception, and visual-motor perception skills, which may be the cause of the quality of dysgraphic writing characterized by floating lines, irregular spaces, junction points, sudden movements, and dimension irregularities.

Keywords: dyslexia, evaluation, handwriting, visual motor perception skills

1. Introduction

According to Reid [1], dyslexia refers to differences in individual processing, in which they are characterized by difficulties in the beginning of literacy, affecting the acquisition of reading, writing, and spelling. In addition, there are failures in cognitive, phonological and/or visual and memory processes, information retrieval, speed processing, time management, coordination, and automation [2].

Developmental dyslexia, according to Galaburda and Cestnick [3], is presented as a condition that manifests near the age of 3, in which the child demonstrates a delay in verbal development. For the author, dyslexia is considered to be phonological and occurs due to damage in the region of the upper temporal gyrus and temporo-parietal regions, while visual dyslexia is associated with parieto-occipital regions.

Dyslexia can manifest itself through three subtypes, in which the phonological subtype is due to a dysfunction in the region of the upper temporal gyrus and the temporo-parietal regions, thus causing changes in auditory processing. Some authors indicate that the decrease in the auditory information processing capacity may be the basis of the problems manifested in this subtype [4].

Regarding prevalence, there is a variation of 6–17% of the school-age population [5]. In addition, dyslexia has a high probability of hereditary issues, in which the chances of being predominant in males are two to three times higher [6, 7]. They may also present deficits in fine motor skills, which cause changes in letter and spelling in copy tasks [8], difficulty in bimanual coordination, and manual dexterity that would justify the occurrence of dysgraphia in this population [9].

For there to be precision in the form of letters, it is necessary to use fine motor skills, visual perception, visuo-motor integration, maturity, and integration of cognition [10], making the development of writing a demanding process, long and complex [11]. The acquisition of handwriting requires that there is a combination of coordination of visuo-motor skills with motor, cognitive, and perceptual skills, being tactile-kinesthetic, organization in space, and time [11].

Mathes and Denton [12] also mentioned that there is a combination of biological and environmental phenomena in learning to write in which they involve motor, sensory-perceptual, and socio-emotional integrity. Schirmer et al. [13] described that the acquisition of written language, as well as oral language, involves several brain regions, among them the parieto-occipital area, in which there is the primary visual cortex, the main responsible for the processing of graphic symbols and areas of the parietal lobe that are responsible for visual–spatial issues of the spelling, information that is recognized and decoded in the Werneck area, in which it is responsible for the understanding of the language and for the written expression it is necessary to activate the primary motor cortex and Broca's area.

Thus, in order to make use of handwriting, representations are needed to assist the visual memory of each letter, the recognition of the features that make up each letter and the ability to reproduce features in a motorized way while respecting order and direction [14]. Visual perception is a system that is concerned with the identity of the object, as well as with the location in space, where it is directly linked with action systems [15]. Changes related to fine motor function can cause failures in the development of writing skills [16]. These changes affect the student's performance, influencing the quality and quantity of learning in the classroom, also relating the student's motivation and self-esteem. With this, the cause of changes in fine motor coordination is noticeable, which is mainly responsible for the writing layout (graphics/calligraphy) since it is one of the skills learned with more difficulty.

Those manifestations might be related with dysgraphia. Dysgraphia is referred to as a difficulty in written expression, in which the individual can present an appropriate intellectual novel and receive appropriate instructions for the acquisition of handwriting during the literacy process. When submitted to the practice of writing during his academic training and, even so, he has the inability to produce an understandable and acceptable writing, it is called as dysgraphia [17].

In Brazil, there is a scarcity of procedures for evaluating handwriting; those that exist are available only for research purposes, in which, it is impossible for the education and health professional to use them, such as the Dysgraphic Scale [18]. Although there are international studies investigating the perception-visual-motor relationship, reading and writing in the population of students with dyslexia [16, 19], these studies are restricted in Brazil, thus making it difficult to establish the perception visual-motor profile of this population.

The need to investigate and understand the perceptual-visual-motor performance of these students with dyslexia is linked to the fact that many of the handwriting errors are identified as spelling errors in which they may actually be covering up errors of calligraphic nature, such as the poor shape of letter in which it triggers unintelligible handwriting [19].

Thus, the aim of this chapter was to characterize and compare the visual motor perception and handwriting performance of students with mixed subtype dyslexia and students with good academic performance.

2. Method

This project was approved by the Research Ethics Committee of the Faculty of Philosophy and Sciences of the São Paulo State University "Júlio de Mesquita Filho" (UNESP), Marília, São Paulo, Brazil, under the protocol number 3.098.493.

Twenty-six students, of both sexes, participated in this study, aged 9 years to 11 years and 11 months, from the fourth and fifth grade levels of an elementary school, with average socioeconomic level, divided into two groups: Group I (GI): composed of 13 students with a multidisciplinary diagnosis of developmental dyslexia of the mixed subtype; and Group II (GII): composed of 13 students with good academic performance, paired according to sex, education, and age group with GI.

The GI students were assessed by an interdisciplinary team from Investigation Learning Disabilities Laboratory, Department of Speech and Hearing Sciences, São Paulo State University "Júlio de Mesquita Filho" (UNESP), Marilia, São Paulo, Brazil, following criteria [20, 21]. As inclusion criteria, the presentation of the Free and Informed Consent Term signed by the parents or guardians was considered and they were not submitted to any speech therapy, pedagogical or psychopedagogical intervention. Failure to meet at least one of the criteria described above would automatically exclude students from the sample in this study. The GII students in this study were selected at a public school indicated by their teachers for having good academic performance in Portuguese and Mathematics. From this indication, students were submitted to the application of the School Performance Test—TDE [22]. Only schoolchildren who achieved average to superior performance were included in the GII of this study. The exclusion criterion for GII was the presence of sensory deficits (hearing and/or visual impairment), cognitive or physical, according to aspects described in the school record. Excluded from this study were students who had already undergone some type of speech therapy remediation or who did not write in cursive.

The students were evaluated individually and submitted to the procedures:

- *Dysgraphic Scale* [18]: students were asked to write a dictation using a 2B pencil and sheet without lines and guidelines. Capitalized writing was performed, as the GI students were unable to execute the cursive letter. The evaluated items were floating lines; descending and/or ascending Lines; retouched letters; irregularity of dimension; poor forms; and total for handwriting under dictation. The punctuation is made by the sum of the number of mistakes made. The procedure is validated for the Brazilian population.

- *Visual Perception Development Test III—DTVP III* [2]: the procedure is validated for students aged 4 years to 12 years and 11 months. The protocol consists of a battery of five subtests being eye-hand coordination (EH), coping (C), figure-ground (FG), visual closure (VC), and form constancy (FC). The composite score generated allows the classification in relation to the general visual perception (GVP, composed by the somatory of all subtests), motor-reduced visual perception (MRVP, composed by the subtests figure-ground, visual closure and form constancy), and visual-motor integration (VMI, composed by the subtests coping and eye-hand coordination). The students were classified according to the composite scores. The students were classified according to the composite scores, being "very poor" (1), "poor" (2), "below average" (3), "average" (4), "above average" (5), "superior" (6), and "very superior" (7).

- *Analysis of writing by* the *NeuroScript* MovAlyzeR *Software*: the writing analysis procedure was performed by a software that analyzes the movement performed through a graphics tablet, which is used to interpret the movements generated by a pen, providing data of inclination, speed, acceleration, and pressure of the pen. In addition, it is used to process handwritten images, being able to record and segment the writing, descent, elevation, and pauses of the pen.

The data obtained were analyzed statistically in order to compare the intragroup and intergroup results. The IBM SPSS Statistics program (Statistical Package for the Social Sciences), version 25.0, was used to obtain and analyze the results.

The results were analyzed statistically using the following tests, the Mann-Whitney test, Wilconxon signaled test, and the Friedman test, aiming to verify the intragroup and intergroup differences studied for the variables of interest in DTVP III, the Dysgraphic Scale, and the analysis of the speed and pressure measures of writing by the MovAlyzeR software aiming to characterize and compare the performance between the groups. The results were analyzed statistically at a significance level of 5% (0.050). The level of significance (p-value) is marked with an asterisk. Descriptive analysis of the data was performed by obtaining the values of mean, standard deviation, and p-value.

3. Results

With the application of the Mann-Whitney test, it was possible to observe that there was a statistically significant difference in the comparison between GI and GII in floating lines, irregular space, junction point, sudden movements, and dimension irregularity, demonstrating that the group of students with good performance academic (GII) had a lower score in the cited parameters when compared with the group of students with mixed dyslexia GI (**Table 1**).

In the qualitative analysis of the Dysgraphic Scale, it was possible to observe that 100% of the students of GI presented quality of dysgraphic writing, whereas, 100% of the students of GII did not present quality of dysgraphic writing.

Table 2 shows the mean value, standard deviation, and p-value of the comparison between GI and GII in the gross score subtests of DTVP-3.

Parameters	Group	Mean	Standard deviation	p-Value
Floating lines	I	1.38	0.51	0.002*
	II	0.62	0.51	
	Total	1	0.63	
Descending and/or ascending lines	I	0.77	0.26	0.144
	II	0.58	0.34	
	Total	0.67	0.31	
Irregular space	I	0.85	0.24	0.002*
	II	0.39	0.36	
	Total	0.62	0.38	
Retouched letters	I	1.23	0.73	0.294
	II	0.92	0.76	
	Total	1.08	0.74	
M, N, U, and V curvatures and angulations	I	0.08	0.19	>0.999
	II	0.08	0.19	
	Total	0.08	0.18	
Junction points	I	1	0.58	0.001*
	II	0.15	0.38	
	Total	0.58	0.64	
Collisions and grips	I	2.04	0.8	0.268
	II	1.5	1.22	
	Total	1.77	1.05	
Sudden movements	I	1.23	0.73	0.002*
	II	0.31	0.48	
	Total	0.77	0.77	
Dimension irregularity	I	1.39	0.65	0.006*
	II	0.58	0.64	
	Total	0.98	0.75	
Poor shape	I	0.92	0.19	0.076
	II	0.69	0.38	
	Total	0.81	0.32	
Total	I	10.89	1.71	<0.001*
	II	5.81	1.56	
	Total	8.35	3.05	

(p-value < 0.05).

Table 1.
Distribution of mean values, standard deviation, and p-value when comparing GI and GII performance.

Referring to **Table 2**, it was possible to analyze that all subtests showed a statistically significant difference. According to the visual-motor coordination subtest, GII showed a superior performance in relation to GI. In the copy subtest, it is possible to observe that GII performed better than GI. In the figure-ground subtest, it is possible to observe that GII performed better than GI. In the visual closure subtest, it is possible to observe that GII showed a superior performance in relation to GI. In Form constancy subtest, it is possible to observe that GII performed better than GI.

Subtests	Group	Mean	Standard deviation	p-Value
VMC	I	140.31	24.2	
	II	181.69	7.17	<0.001*
	Total	161	27.41	
CO	I	27.54	5.36	
	II	41.46	6.96	<0.001*
	Total	34.5	9.35	
FG	I	49.23	8.31	<0.001*
	II	59.54	3.41	
	Total	54.38	8.14	
VC	I	11.08	3.59	<0.001*
	II	17.62	3.12	
	Total	14.35	4.69	
FC	I	38.62	7.48	0.001*
	II	47.62	2.53	
	Total	43.12	7.14	

Caption: VMC—visual-motor coordination; CO—copy; FG—figure-ground; VC—visual closure; and FC—form constancy.

Table 2.
Distribution of mean, standard deviation, and p-value for GI and GII in the gross score subtest.

Table 3 shows the mean value, standard deviation, and p-value of the comparison between GI and GII in the subtest Description of Terms.

Referring to **Table 3**, the subtests visual-motor coordination, visual closure, and constancy of form did not present a statistically significant difference. In the subtest visual-motor coordination, it is possible to observe that GII presented a superior performance in relation to GI. In the copy subtest, it is possible to observe that GII performed better than GI. In the figure-ground subtest, it is possible to observe that GII performed better than GI. In the visual closure subtest, it is possible to observe that both groups showed similar performance. In the form constancy subtest, it is possible to observe that GII presented a superior performance in relation to GI. **Table 4** shows the mean value, standard deviation, and p-value of the comparison between GI and GII in the somatory of terms.

According to **Table 4**, all subtests showed a statistically significant difference. It is possible to observe that in the visual-motor integration subtest, GII presented a superior performance in relation to GI. In the Motor-Reduced Visual Perception subtest, GII showed a superior performance in relation to GI, as well as in the general visual perception subtest, in which GII also presented superior performance in relation to GI. **Table 5** shows the mean value, standard deviation, and p-value of the comparison between GI and GII in the subtest description of terms.

According to **Table 5**, all subtests showed a statistically significant difference. It is possible to observe that in the visual-motor integration subtest, GII presented a superior performance in relation to GI. In the reduced visual perception to the motor subtest, GII showed a superior performance in relation to GI, as well as, in the general visual perception subtest, in which GII presented superior performance.

In this analysis, the Wilcoxon Signed Posts Test was applied in order to verify possible differences between the subtests in the groups.

Subtests	Group	Mean	Standard deviation	p-Value
VMC	I	4	0	0.149
	II	4.31	0.75	
	Total	4.15	0.54	
CO	I	4	0	<0.001*
	II	6	1.35	
	Total	5	1.39	
FG	I	4	0	0.033*
	II	4.54	0.88	
	Total	4.27	0.67	
VC	I	3.92	0.28	>0.999
	II	3.92	0.28	
	Total	3.92	0.27	
FC	I	4.08	0.28	0.056
	II	4.62	0.87	
	Total	4.35	0.69	

Caption: VMC—visual-motor coordination; CO—copy; FG—figure-ground; VC—visual closure; and FC—form constancy.

Table 3.
Distribution of mean values, standard deviation, and p-value of GI and GII in the subtest description of terms.

Subtests	Group	Mean	Standard deviation	p-Value
VMI	I	50.62	3.95	0.002*
	II	80.85	21.61	
	Total	65.73	21.66	
MRVP	I	50.54	6.39	<0.001*
	II	78.77	16.17	
	Total	64.65	18.77	
GVP	I	48.08	8.98	<0.001*
	II	82.77	14.46	
	Total	65.42	21.26	

Caption: VMI: visual-motor integration; MRVP: motor-reduced visual perception; and GVP: general visual perception.

Table 4.
Distribution of mean values, standard deviation, and p-value of GI and GII in the visual motor integration subtest.

Table 6 shows the mean, standard deviation, and p-value for the speed and pressure subtests in Attempts 1 and 2 of GI.

According to **Table 6**, it is possible to observe that there was no statistically significant difference. In the speed subtest, Attempt 1 and Attempt 2 had similar average values. In the pressure subtest, it is possible to observe that in Attempt 1, there was a higher average in relation to Attempt 2. **Table 7** shows the values of mean, standard deviation, and p-value for the speed and pressure subtests in trials 1 and 2 of GII.

Subtests	Group	Mean	Standard deviation	p-Value
VMI	I	4	0	<0.001*
	II	5.46	1.13	
	Total	4.73	1.08	
MRVP	I	4	0	<0.001*
	II	5.08	1.04	
	Total	4.54	0.91	
GVP	I	4	0	<0.001*
	II	5.23	1.01	
	Total	4.62	0.94	

Caption: VMI: visual-motor integration; MRVP: motor-reduced visual perception; and GVP: general visual perception.

Table 5.
Distribution of mean, standard deviation, and p-value for GI and GII in the subtest description of terms.

Subtests	Mean	Standard deviation	p-Value
T1-Speed	0.74	0.39	0.6
T2-Speed	0.75	0.38	
T1-PRE	79.17	41.06	0.463
T2-PRE	77.32	40.59	

Caption: Speed; PRE: Pression T1—Attempt 1, T2—Attempt 2.

Table 6.
Distribution of mean values, standard deviation, and p-value in the GI subtests.

Subtests	Mean	Standard deviation	p-Value
T1-Speed	0.74	0.31	0.753
T2- Speed	0.68	0.23	
T1-PRE	102.19	34.87	0.695
T2-PRE	95.73	29.98	

Caption: Speed; PRE: Pression T1—Attempt 1, T2—Attempt 2.

Table 7.
Distribution of mean values, standard deviation, and p-value in attempts at GII.

According to **Table 7**, it is possible to observe that there was no statistically significant difference. In the speed subtest, Attempt 1 had a higher average than Attempt 2. In order to verify a possible difference between both groups in the subtests of interest, the Mann-Whitney test was applied.

4. Discussion

Based on the data obtained, it was observed that all students with mixed dyslexia (GI) presented the quality of dysgraphia writing in relation to the group with good academic performance (GII) regarding the Dysgraphia Scale procedure [18].

In the variables of DTVP III, visual-motor coordination, copy, background figure, form constancy, and visual closure, GI presented a lower performance in relation to GII, as well as in the variables of visual motor integration, reduced visual perception to the motor and general visual perception. In the analysis of the NeuroScript MovAlyzeR Software, there was no statistically significant difference between the groups studied.

According to the literature, the presence of dysgraphia in students with dyslexia suggests the existence of changes in the tracing of letters in tasks involving copying, and manual dexterity [23].

Studies have shown that students with dyslexia present changes in motor skills, involving difficulty in bimanual coordination, manual dexterity, and fine motor skills, justifying the occurrence of dysgraphia [9, 24, 25].

Regarding the variables studied in the Dysgraphia Scale [18], students with mixed dyslexia presented an inferior performance in floating lines, irregular space, junction point, sudden movements, and dimension irregularity. Students with dyslexia had a predominant score in retouched letters and junction points, considering that they were due to changes in the skills of discrimination, memory, visuo-spatial relationship, and form constancy.

Concerning the perceptual-visual-motor function, according to Brow and Rodger [26], there is a combination of the visual-motor, motor, cognitive, perception-visual skills (eye-hand coordination) position in space, spatial relationship, figure-ground, and form constancy. Therefore, students with dyslexia are prone to show manifestations of visual perception changes due to dysfunctions in the brain areas responsible for visual-spatial perception, which is responsible at the time of writing [19].

In this study, it was proven that students with dyslexia showed changes indicating deficits in visual-motor perception, in addition to presenting an inferior performance in visual-motor coordination skills, position in space, copy, visual closure, visual motor speed, and constancy in a way when compared to the group with good academic performance.

Visual-motor perception skills are related to handwriting, that is, graph-motor actions and also reading skills. These skills depend on the recognition of details, visual-spatial organization, and spatial relationship between integration figures of the parts of a whole, assigning meaning to the shapes of the letters and thus affecting the graph-motor performance [27–29].

Thus, it is considered that the difficulty in performing the skills of visual-motor perception and visual perception in these students compromise the performance of handwriting, and dysgraphia may occur as described in the literature [28].

There are technologies that assist in writing and analyzing handwriting, aiming to estimate parameters for movements performed in the motor act of writing. A study of Costa [30] analyzed through the Neuro Script MovAlyzeR software the number of segments, reaction time, and pressure of students and preschoolers. With regard to pressure, preschoolers showed less pressure when compared to students, also registering lower values in the pressure of the pencil grip. The study of Barrientos [31] states that the pressure exerted at the time of writing has a progressive increase according to age in the copy tasks in students with learning difficulties, and students without learning difficulties tend to have less pressure at the moment of writing.

The fact that there was no statistically significant difference between the variables studied (speed and pressure) in the comparison between the groups of this study raises some hypotheses such as the size of the studied sample of students with mixed dyslexia, requiring the continuation of the study, due to the fact that be a study limitation or the lack of handwriting practices in the academic grade of elementary school in our country, making different profiles of students with or without specific learning disorders do not differ in terms of the parameters analyzed.

The hypothesis of this study was partially confirmed since the measures of visual-motor perception and quality of writing were fundamental for the differentiation of handwriting in students with mixed dyslexia and with good academic performance; however, the analysis of writing by the software used in this study did not allow stem differentiation.

The establishment of the handwriting profile of students with mixed dyslexia is extremely important for the discussion of the subtype, especially for the investigation of whether it has a perceptual-visual-motor profile and different writing quality than students with good school performance, thus allowing to characterize this population both for the performance of the differential diagnosis and for the performance of interventions in the clinical and educational context, taking into account the fact that Speech Language Pathology is the area that investigates the changes in information processing and, consequently, its impact on the acquisition and in the development of reading and writing and can help the teacher's understanding of handwriting alteration.

The teachers' lack of knowledge about the perceptual-visual-motor performance of students with mixed dyslexia causes confusion about the nature of the writing error, causing spelling errors to be confused with handwriting errors, for example, the poorly drawn letters that cause the writing of an unintelligible letter or word. Thus, it is necessary to use perceptual-visual-motor assessment procedures, so that educational intervention programs are designed in order to reduce the impact of poorly written letters on the spelling of students with dyslexia, more specifically students with mixed dyslexia.

5. Conclusion

The results of this study allowed us to conclude that the students with mixed dyslexia in this study presented an inferior performance compared to the students with good academic performance in relation to the skills of visual-motor coordination copy, figure-background, visual closure, and constancy of form, characterized by changes in general visual perception, visual perception of reduced motricity, and visual-motor perception.

In the intragroup analysis of the GI, it was observed that the students with mixed dyslexia had a similar visual-motor perception performance between them, showing a statistically significant difference only in the subtests gross score and scalar score. In the GII, students with good academic performance showed a superior performance in most of the subtests studied, with a statistically significant difference in gross score, percentile of rank, scalar score, description of terms, visual-motor integration, reduced visual perception to motor, perception general visual, and scalar score. From the intergroup analysis, GII showed a superior performance in all studied subtests.

In the Dysgraphia Scale, it was possible to observe that all of the group of students with mixed dyslexia presented writing considered dysgraphic characterized by floating lines, irregular space, junction point, sudden movement, and irregularity of dimension.

With regard to the analysis of writing using the MovAlyzeR software, it was possible to verify that this instrument did not allow the differentiation between the groups of this study in the variables of speed and pressure.

At the end of this study, we concluded that it was possible to characterize and compare two different populations of students and, in addition, to observe the aspects that make them distinct from the evaluation of handwriting. It is clear that there is still a lack of studies that identify, along with other procedures, what characteristics students with difficulty regarding proficiency in handwriting present, specifically students with the diagnosis of dyslexia and its subtypes.

Thus, future studies should be carried out with an aim of investigating whether the characteristics evidenced in this study may or may not be associated with changes in the final motor function, because only then it will be possible to plan appropriate guidelines and strategies for the students diagnosed with mixed dyslexia to overcome their handwriting difficulties.

Author details

Simone Aparecida Capellini[1,2*], Larissa Sellin[1], Ilaria D'Angelo[2], Noemi Del Bianco[2], Catia Giaconi[2] and Giseli Donadon Germano[1]

1 São Paulo State University "Júlio de Mesquita Filho" - UNESP, Brazil

2 Università di Macerata - UNIMC, Italy

*Address all correspondence to: sacap@uol.com.br

References

[1] Reid G. Dyslexia: A Practitioner's Handbook. Hoboken, Nova Jersey, EUA: John Wiley & Sons; 2016

[2] Hammill DD, Pearson NA, Voress JK. Developmental Test of Visual Perception: DTVP-2. Austin, TX: PRO-ED; 1993

[3] Galaburda AM, Cestnick L. Dislexia del desarrollo. Revista de Neurologia. 2003;**36**(1):3-9

[4] van Setten ER, Hakvoort BE, van der Leij A, Maurits NM, Maassen BA. Predictors for grade 6 reading in children at familial risk of dyslexia. Annals of Dyslexia. 2018;**68**(3):181-202

[5] Fletcher JM, Lyon GR, Fuchs LS, Barnes M. Learning Disabilities: From Identification to Intervention. New York: The Guilford Press; 2007

[6] Liederman J, Kantrowitz L, Flannery K. Male vulnerability to reading disability is not likely to be a myth: A call for new data. Journal of Learning Disabilities. 2005;**38**(2):109-129

[7] Pennington BF. Diagnosing Learning Disorders: A Neuropsychological Framework. New York, USA: Guilford Press; 2008

[8] Gomes TVB, Ugrinowitsch H, Marinho NFS, Benda RN. Efeitos da prática mental na aquisição de habilidades motoras em sujeitos novatos. Revista Brasileira de Educação Física e Esporte. 2012;**26**(3):511-521

[9] Crawford SG, Dewey D. Co-occurring disorders: A possible key to visual perceptual deficits in children with developmental coordination disorder? Human Movement Science. 2008;**27**(1):154-169. DOI: 10.1016/j.humov.2007.09.002

[10] Stevenson NC, Just C. In early education, why teach handwriting before keyboarding? Early Childhood Education Journal. 2014;**42**(1):49-56

[11] Yu NY, Chang SH. Characterization of the fine motor problems in patients with cognitive dysfunction—A computerized handwriting analysis. Human Movement Science. 2019;**65**:71-79

[12] Mathes PG, Denton CA. The prevention and identification of reading disability. In: Seminars in Pediatric Neurology. Vol. 9, No. 3. Philadelphia, USA: WB Saunders; 2002. pp. 185-191

[13] Schirmer CR, Fontoura DR, Nunes ML. Distúrbios da aquisição da linguagem e da aprendizagem. Jornal de Pediatria. 2004;**80**(2):95-103

[14] Schickedanz JA. Much More than the ABCs: The Early Stages of Reading and Writing. Washington, DC: NAEYC; 1999

[15] Jeannerod M. Motor Cognition: What Actions Tell the Self (No. 42). New York, USA: Oxford University Press; 2006

[16] Feder KP, Majnemer A. Handwriting development, competency, and intervention. Developmental Medicine and Child Neurology. 2007;**49**(4):312-317. DOI: 10.1111/j.1469-8749.2007.00312.x

[17] Rosenblum S, Aloni T, Josman N. Relationships between handwriting performance and organizational abilities among children with and without dysgraphia: A preliminary study. Research in Developmental Disabilities. 2010;**31**(2):502-509. DOI: 10.1016/j.ridd.2009.10.016

[18] Lorenzini MV. A scale to detect dysgraphia based on the Ajuriaguerra

scale [Master in Special Education dissertation]. São Carlos, SP, Brazil: São Carlos Federal University; 1993

[19] Wuang YP, Su CY. Rasch analysis of the developmental test of visual-motor integration in children with intellectual disabilities. Research in Developmental Disabilities. 2009;**30**(5):1044-1053

[20] American Psychiatric Association. DSM-5: Manual Diagnóstico e Estatístico de Transtornos Mentais. Porto Alegre, Brazil: Artmed Editora; 2014

[21] Germano GD, Reilhac C, Capellini SA, Valdois S. The phonological and visual basis of developmental dyslexia in Brazilian portuguese reading children. Frontiers in Psychology. 2014;**5**:1169. DOI: 10.3389/fpsyg.2014.01169

[22] Stein LM. TDE - Teste de Desempenho Escolar: Manual para Aplicação e Interpretação. São Paulo, SP: Casa do Psicólogo; 1994

[23] Nicolson RI, Fawcett AJ. Dyslexia, dysgraphia, procedural learning and the cerebellum. Cortex. 2011;**47**(1):117-127

[24] Getchell N, Pabreja P, Neeld K, Carrio V. Comparing children with and without dyslexia on the movement assessment battery for children and the test of gross motor development. Perceptual and Motor Skills. 2007;**105**(1):207-214

[25] Jefferies E, Sage K, Ralph MAL. Do deep dyslexia, dysphasia and dysgraphia share a common phonological impairment? Neuropsychologia. 2007;**45**(7):1553-1570

[26] Brown T, Rodger S. Validity of the developmental test of visual-motor integration supplemental developmental test of visual perception. Perceptual and Motor Skills. 2008;**106**(3):659-678

[27] Falk TH, Tam C, Schellnus H, Chau T. On the development of a computer-based handwriting assessment tool to objectively quantify handwriting proficiency in children. Computer Methods and Programs in Biomedicine. 2011;**104**(3):e102-e111

[28] Racine MB, Majnemer A, Shevell M, Snider L. Handwriting performance in children with attention deficit hyperactivity disorder (ADHD). Journal of Child Neurology. 2008;**23**(4):399-406

[29] Ratzon NZ, Lahav O, Cohen-Hamsi S, Metzger Y, Efraim D, Bart O. Comparing different short-term service delivery methods of visual-motor treatment for first grade students in mainstream schools. Research in Developmental Disabilities. 2009;**30**(6):1168-1176

[30] Costa BIM, et al. A relação entre o desempenho motor e o desempenho visuo-motor, em crianças entre os 4 e os 6 anos [Dissertação de Mestrado]. Évora, Portugal: Universidade de Évora; 2019

[31] Barrientos P. Handwriting development in Spanish children with and without learning disabilities: A graphonomic approach. Journal of Learning Disabilities. 2017;**50**(5):552-563

Chapter 8

Understanding the Socio-Emotional Impact of Dyslexia in the Inclusive Classroom

Trevor O' Brien

Abstract

Much of the literature pertaining to children's experiences of dyslexia points to low self esteem and low self-concept as compared with typically developing peers (i.e. those without dyslexia). While the specific difficulties associated with dyslexia may present challenges for those children, the author outlines how external forces such as the environment, relationships and teacher understanding may contribute to (or alleviate) such negative self perceptions. While children may learn and process information differently, negative feelings are often compounded by a teacher's lack of knowledge regarding this different way of learning in the inclusive classroom. In order to develop truly inclusive practices in schools, it is imperative that contextual issues impacting children are understood and that this understanding is utilised to improve outcomes for all children, including those with dyslexia. It is also contended that children should be at the centre of this process and their views on how they learn best must be considered paramount.

Keywords: dyslexia, self esteem, self concept, teacher understanding, multi-sesnsory

1. Introduction

With a chapter focusing on affective issues relating to dyslexia, it is necessary to begin by considering how dyslexia has been constructed. The author adopts the view that dyslexia is socially constructed and the impairments experienced by students results in disabling children, due to a lack of teacher understanding and environmental issues [1]. This disabling may result in children having a lower sense of identity, particularly in terms of self-esteem and self-concept. If dyslexia is socially constructed, then these constructs may need to be identified in order to address the socio-emotional issues impacting young people. These issues, as they relate to dyslexia, are discussed in detail. It is argued throughout that teacher understanding of dyslexia is a critical consideration when aiming to support all children, including those with dyslexia. Listening to the views of children is considered important in this regard. The author concludes by providing the reader with some key insights in improving support in the inclusive classroom, with a focus on the imperative of a multi-sensory approach to teaching and learning.

2. The social construction of dyslexia

While the term dyslexia emphasises literacy difficulties, there is little consensus on a definition, with some favouring that the term should no longer be used and even argue against the very existence of dyslexia [2]. Although controversy surrounds the word and differing views exist, it is contended that dyslexia does exist, although it is socially constructed [3]. The identification of dyslexia along with labelling, assessments and interventions have all been a result of powerful social forces at particular times in history [4]. These forces which have helped to shape dyslexia have emanated from political, cultural and social pressures to adapt to what society considers important [5]. Often catering for the needs of the masses [4], those who do not conform to certain standards, including literacy, are particularly disadvantaged or "disabled". Children with dyslexia are one such group. It is not argued that these children do not face challenges as a result of their impairments in literacy but this impairment is often regarded as a disability due to society's lack of understanding of difference and of the full human experience [1]. This human experience is central to the lives of all children with dyslexia, particularly regarding how they perceive themselves as young people [4]. When children begin to view themselves as "lesser" as a result of their impairments and their self-esteem and self- concept are impacted, it may be timely to identify the factors which contribute to this and to seek to improve the outcomes for a group which have already become marginalised.

It is fortunate that the social model of disability has replaced the medical, within child, model as the latter often serves to reinforce negative views of self-worth and self-esteem, resulting in a decreased sense of wellbeing [4]. This model which is tied up with assessments and specialist intervention often ignores the inclusive approach which is about viewing children's difficulties as differences between individuals. That is not to say that specialist intervention is not necessary at certain times but perhaps the focus should shift to exploring ways to serve the needs of all children where possible, including those with dyslexia [6]. Moreover, the move away from the deficit model to an inclusive model allows more for the possibility of change as educational experiences are often determined by proactive and well planned interactions by adults [7].

The cultural influence in terms of how dyslexia is understood and contextualised is important and some studies have demonstrated how these cultural and structural biases, which focus on children's difficulties rather than differences, may result in "othering" young people, causing a reduction in self-esteem and self-worth [8, 9]. Understanding how dyslexia has evolved and is indeed a product of social construction [3] may assist practitioners and policy makers to fully comprehend the implications of these social pressures. In a literacy dominated society which, since the Industrial Revolution, has been closely linked to productivity and worth [4], it is clear that those with differences in these key areas would be at a disadvantage [3]. Therefore, the argument can be made that it is only when the construction of dyslexia and all it entails are interrogated, can we reach a point where all children's needs are met resulting with an increase in self-concept and self-esteem. Socio-cultural theory suggests that a person's identity and how they view themselves strongly depends on what society deems to be important [8] so, perhaps, it is indeed important to view difference and diversity as critical, which will have an impact on strategies and interventions which can be best used to serve the needs of a range of children in schools.

3. Socio emotional issues

In this section affective factors such as self-esteem and self-concept, as they relate to dyslexia, are discussed. In order to examine the relationship between dyslexia and socio emotional issues, the terms need to be defined. Burden defines self-efficacy as the level of confidence one experiences when completing a particular task [8] whereas self- esteem may be regarded as "a measure of how far an individual's perceived self-image lives up to their ideal self" ([7], p. 37). While the two are often considered synonymous, there are differences which need to be clarified.

Much of the research in special education highlights the fact that children with special needs often view themselves in a negative way, resulting in lower levels of self-esteem and self- concept [10]. In fact, strong evidence has emerged that these affective factors are relevant to children with dyslexia and often impact students' wellbeing [7, 8, 10–15]. In a study by Polychroni et al. [16], it was also found that children with dyslexia demonstrated lower levels of self-concept in literacy and mathematics compared with other children without dyslexia. The children (n32) in the research completed self-reported measures, which showed lower self-confidence in these areas and also the fact that students were less likely to read for enjoyment. This is hardly surprising if the specific impairments associated with dyslexia are not fully understood or addressed. In other studies, it is reported that children with dyslexia in mainstream schools had significantly lower self- esteem compared with those without dyslexia and, interestingly, children with dyslexia in a special setting had higher self-esteem that those with dyslexia in a mainstream setting [10]. These findings are congruent with more recent studies ([14, 15, 17–21]). If socio-emotional elements are lower in mainstream settings, it can be argued that it is the contextual and environmental domains which are responsible for this and not the specific impairments associated with dyslexia. However, if socio-emotional issues as they relate to dyslexia are contextual, then it cannot be assumed that all children with dyslexia will have lower self-esteem than their typically developing peers at all times. It may indeed depend on the quality of support they are provided with, including the use of appropriate resources and teacher understanding at a particular time. There may now be an opportunity for practitioners to consider the socio-emotional benefits of special settings in order to provide an appropriate and educationally rewarding experience for all children, including those with dyslexia [14, 15]. Novita [22] examined the impact of dyslexia on wellbeing and also found that there was indeed a correlation between lower levels of self- esteem and self-concept in the group as compared with classmates without dyslexia. These are referred to as the "secondary symptoms" of dyslexia. Children also exhibited higher levels of general anxiety and lower self-esteem in certain school contexts but not in the general living environment [22]. Novita argues that it is indeed the context or the setting that cause these secondary symptoms, which again raises an important issue for practitioners both in terms of understanding and provision.

4. Teacher understanding

While the research has shown that many children with dyslexia have a negative experience in school, questions need to be asked why this is the case. It has already been argued that these experiences are often impacted by external factors, such as the way teachers understand dyslexia. While a simplistic approach cannot be applied to a complex issue, there is a growing body of research which highlights the positive effect of teacher understanding and positive student-teacher relationships on children's self-confidence [8, 12, 14, 15, 23]. While this may be the case, the opposite is also true. Children's self-esteem may be negatively impacted when they are treated unfairly by teachers or when they are bullied by teachers or other children [12, 14, 15]. In fact, the critical role of teachers is highlighted in much of literature [12, 14, 15, 24]. The European Agency for Development in Special Needs Education [24] note the imperative of teacher understanding in meeting the needs of all learners. The agency contends that it is vital to view learner difference as normal and that all teachers need to be able to listen to views of children in order to appreciate learner diversity. It also acknowledges the pivotal role teachers play in fostering self-esteem in young people by understanding their key challenges and, it is only when learner diversity is fully understood, can teachers appropriately plan and execute interventions and strategies which may benefit all children. The impact of teacher understanding of difference has the potential to include all children and assist them in reaching their potential. The opposite is also true; when children are unfairly treated and ostracised due to learner differences, this may cause a reduction in self-esteem and feelings of disconnectedness.

In Glazzard [12] study, children reported feeling humiliated and ostracised when unfairly treated and reported that certain teachers did not really understand them. Incidents of teachers bullying children were provided, where teachers used to shout at children and use names such as "stupid". There were also accounts of teachers encouraging class mates to laugh at a particular child. This lack of understanding, on the teachers part, of the difficulties associated with dyslexia, is noteworthy. In the same study, it was reported that the exclusion felt by some children severely impacted their self-esteem as teachers refused to accept their spelling difficulties. Many children with dyslexia will have difficulties with tasks which contain too many words and the speed it takes to process information. Teacher understanding of these issues is imperative and one needs to be mindful of the anxiety it may cause a child when they are unable to access a particular task. A teacher in this study used the word "rubbish" in relation to the child's efforts, which undoubtedly had a negative impact on their self-esteem and self-concept [12].

Another study which highlighted the importance of teacher understanding when working with children with dyslexia is that of O′ Brien [14, 15]. Children reported being told to sit at the back of the class when they were unable to attempt a particular task and being quite upset. In this study, the students highlighted the school context which impacted their self- esteem and wellbeing, with one student commenting that they liked attending a special school because, unlike in the former, mainstream school, they did not get stressed due to the teachers' understanding of their impairments. It is important to note, that while students self-worth was negatively impacted by negative experiences, they were also able to identify positive contributions from teachers, which contributed to their sense of well-being. This support and understanding was welcomed by the children who needed additional assistance. Children made reference to increased self-esteem, self-confidence and the fact that teachers gave freely of their time when striving to support children in accessing tasks [12, 14, 15]. In the case of O′ Brien [14, 15] study, the children mentioned the lack of pressure applied by the teachers in the special setting. This pressure to keep up is often cited as a difficulty for children with dyslexia. If learner difference and learner diversity are understood, it is probable that children's educational experiences would be improved and that, consequently, their levels of self-concept and self-esteem may increase. The important and positive attitudes of teachers cannot be underestimated and these attitudes have the potential to include, affirm and motivate children.

Teachers who understand dyslexia are cognisant of the challenges with phonological awareness, working memory and rapid naming. It appears that students appreciate the use of explicit teaching techniques, the slower pacing of work and re-teaching of certain concepts [3]. The importance of direct and explicit teaching is highlighted by some authors as key when striving to meet the needs of children with dyslexia [25]. However, it must be stated that strategies which could be employed to support the needs of children with dyslexia could indeed be used to support all children [6, 26]. In other words, evidence based strategies used to work with students with dyslexia could be utilised with all students, thereby fostering self-esteem. Understanding the differences in way children learn is a key principle in effective pedagogy and understanding the different ways children with dyslexia learn is no exception.

According to some studies, it is noteworthy that the words teachers use are considered important and impact self-esteem and self-concept [7, 12, 14, 15]. Therefore, the language of inclusion is also worth noting as words matter and have the power to include or, indeed, exclude [27]. Adopting a person first approach (eg person with dyslexia as opposed to a dyslexic person) may appear trivial but educators have the power to communicate messages though language which may impact feelings of self-worth and self- concept. These messages may be communicated without teachers being aware of them so perhaps there may be an opportunity for educators to reflect on the language used when aiming to support the needs of all children.

While it is not intended to address the contested and topical issue of labelling in detail in this chapter, it should be noted that many children value the label as it helps them and their teachers to understand the associated challenges. The label of dyslexia has drawn much debate in recent times [2] but it is clear that children have reported that having such a label may impact how they view themselves. Riddick [7] asked children how they felt about having dyslexia and some of the responses included the ways it helped them to understand why they could not keep up with their peers and also that they no longer considered themselves "thick" having received the diagnosis.

Riddick's findings are in line with Glazzard [12] who reported that most students in the study stated that their self-esteem had increased when they received an official diagnosis of dyslexia. This may also have aided teachers' understanding of the students' related impairments.

Like in Riddick's study, the students no longer perceived themselves as "thick" with responses involving issues of bullying and feelings of alienation before the diagnosis. Children were in agreement that the label changed the way they viewed themselves and they considered the label as almost empowering. These children's views regarding the label is a useful way for teachers to understand the students' perspective, even if teachers are not in agreement with labelling in general. Children's views highlight the importance of teacher understanding, the relationships between children and teachers and how these have the potential to affect how children view themselves. Children's wellbeing appears to be positively impacted by having the label of dyslexia. However, as mentioned, the general issue of labelling is contested and not clear-cut so perhaps a robust discussion on this should be left for another time.

Finally, in a section on teacher understanding, it is important to note that teachers are well educated professionals who perform an exemplary job in often difficult conditions. Therefore, the differences associated with dyslexia can often be addressed by adopting interventions which are evidence based and are informed by the views of children. In doing so, the psychological harm to children with dyslexia may be reduced and the deficiencies in self-esteem and self-concept may be addressed [4]. This leads to the next section which interrogates the issue of student voice in education.

5. Student voice

There has been a growing body of research in special education which focuses on eliciting the views of children on issues which matter to them [28]. It is argued that this process of listening to students should aim to transform practice or impact change in some way [29] as without change, there may no point in the process to begin with. Moreover, promising to listening to children without actually hearing what they have said has the potential to further increase isolation and disconnection [23]. It should also be acknowledged that the invitation to children to speak about topics which are important to them is now a fundamental human right and not just something considered commendable [14, 15, 30].

Eliciting the views of students may be regarded as a powerful way to include students in decision making processes [31] and to ultimately improve outcomes for all children. Inviting children' participation may provide an opportunity to give ownership to participants and to increase children's sense of worth [28]. Researchers and practitioners do, however, need to be mindful of avoiding over interpretation of children's words or "adulterating" what they have said [32]. Are these really the child's views or is this what I have interpreted as their views? This process requires careful consideration of the sensitive power dynamics which exist between children and adults, particularly when discussing topics which may be of a highly personal or sensitive nature. When formulating questions, it may be beneficial to consider "how do I listen to children?" and "how do I speak to children?" [33, 34]. These reflections may help researchers to be aware of their own biases and their potential to lead questions. As children with dyslexia may already be considered part of a marginalised group, it is especially important to be aware of how I position myself in relation to children and how they position themselves in relation to me. Children's wellbeing needs to be a critical consideration, especially when they are speaking about affective issues such as self-esteem and self-concept. Much of the research regarding dyslexia and socio emotional issues is conducted from purposefully listening to children's stories and experiences [7, 10–12, 14, 15]. However, some studies have examined the relationship between groups of children with reading difficulties and those without such difficulties, ignoring "within group" issues. In doing so, the differences between the children in the group is not always clear [7]. Although commonalities exist between children with dyslexia, there must be a continued effort to listen to individual voices, which will more accurately inform policy and practice.

6. Multi-sensory learning in the dyslexia friendly classroom

This section will focus on the importance of creating a dyslexia friendly classroom by adopting a multi-sensory approach to teaching and learning. The benefits of such an approach have been documented in the literature and may serve to address affective factors associated with disabilities, including dyslexia [25, 35–40]. While it is not contended that this is a panacea for all children with dyslexia, a multi-sensory approach may alleviate some negative feelings associated with dyslexia and may indeed improve the sense of connection with peers. As children learn in different ways depending on the context as well as individual learning profiles [40], resources should be presented in a multi modal manner where children choose ways to access particular tasks. The adoption of a Universal for Design for Learning (UDL) approach gives children this flexibility when attending to tasks.

Giving the child a level of autonomy may reduce anxiety and enable them to understand and process the task in hand in their own way and in their own time.

This element of choice is critical to support children who may have difficulty with print rich resources, as an accompanying visual representation may help them to scaffold the task (or make connections) with prior knowledge. Children with dyslexia are able to access tasks more effectively if the task is multi-sensory [41] and Smith and Barr [39] recommend using a "connective pedagogy" which helps students to make connections between what is presented in school and what they have experienced in their outside environment. While a multi-sensory approach is advised for students with dyslexia, this should not be confused with the promotion of various learning styles, which have largely been discredited.

While educational research does not support the idea of learning styles [38], there is still overwhelming support among teachers that teaching to a child's learning style improves learning [37]. However, it appears that the opposite may actually be the case. As it has no basis in educational research, teaching to a child's dominant learning style could lead to a decrease in effort and performance [38]. Although Reid [42] emphasises that children with dyslexia should be aware of their own style of learning, perhaps a broader understanding is required; that children are aware of the various ways they learn in different situations and at different times [36–38, 43]. As mentioned, it may be preferable to provide opportunities where children are able to make sense of various tasks presented to them in a multi-modal manner [40].

Reid [42–44] asserts that all learners with dyslexia can be taught to read initially through their learning style and maintains that children construct knowledge in their own ways according to the dominant style of learning. It should be acknowledged that children do indeed learn in different ways but perhaps this could be attributed more to their interests, backgrounds and abilities rather than to learning styles [43]. There is also a contention that children with dyslexia may learn better when their learning style is understood [42–46]. As there is significant research addressing specific differences associated with dyslexia, what is needed is attention to the differences associated with dyslexia rather than a blanket approach to learning styles, which is in effect placing children in categories [43]. Also, there may be a danger that children who are labelled as having one dominant style may be reluctant to take on tasks which they may perceive to include other learning styles, which may result in a loss of self-esteem and self-efficacy [37].

Even a proponent of learning styles such as Mortimore [46] offers a word of caution when it comes to matching learning styles to teaching methods as there are so many constructs of learning styles and "very little agreement" (p. 145). What does seem to be agreed upon is that all children learn differently and external factors may account for this. There is also the belief that if one does not agree with learning styles theories, then they are propagating that all children are the same, which is not true [43]. It is not disputed that children do learn differently at particular times [35–38, 43]. However, this is determined by other factors such as the environment, interest, subject and previous knowledge rather than an innate learning style [36]. Some children may learn visually in one context while kinesthetically in another [36, 43]. This learning "preference", rather than style may be understood by identifying the actual differences between children [36–38, 43] and this preference for learning should not be confused with a learning style [35]. The strategies which teachers use may indeed influence how a child engages with the subject and Reid [42] considers it "logical" to appreciate individual learning styles when planning these strategies. However, others have put this logic to the test and have been unable to find any support for the connection between learning styles and effective teaching [35–38, 43]. In fact, there does not appear to be any evidence to prove that teaching tailored to individual learning styles improves learning [38]. What is important, however, is that practitioners understand how all children learn in different ways and in different contexts, which may require a return to the originators of educational theory, such as Piaget and Rousseau [36, 38].

It is considered necessary to find effective teaching and learning strategies for students with dyslexia who experience such a complex variety of learning differences [47]. However, rather than focusing on one mode of learning for each child, it may be beneficial to consider their prior knowledge and issues from the environment as these may be more indicative of how new information should be presented [38]. Furthermore, to incorporate a multi-sensory approach for all children may be more effective in terms of including all children [40]. This may be more appropriate, as meaning and understanding are constructed in different ways and not as a consequence of teaching to one sensory domain [37]. When this multi-sensory approach is used, children may be more likely to access tasks presented to them, which may result in improved self- esteem and self-efficacy.

7. Conclusion

In this chapter, the social construction of dyslexia has been briefly discussed as it is important to appreciate the origin of disability and how it has evolved over time. It has been argued that this construction has, in some way, contributed to negative self-perceptions that children with dyslexia have reported. The key topics of self-esteem and self-efficacy have been considered, with an acknowledgement of the lower levels of these affective factors for children with dyslexia compared with their peers without dyslexia. It has also been acknowledged that children who attended special settings were happier and felt more included than they had in mainstream schools. This presents teachers and researchers with an opportunity to explore the key benefits of specialised settings when planning effective provision. The centrality of teacher understanding, as discussed in the literature, provides the reader with some insights when reflecting on the important nature of student-teacher relationships. It is contended that listening to children on matters which impact them is a useful way to support this understanding and to increase children's feelings of self-worth. While there are several evidence based interventions which could be used to support children with dyslexia, the chapter concludes with a section on the cruciality of a multi-sensory approach to teaching. This may help children to benefit from tasks, ultimately leading to a more rewarding and fulfilling experience for all children, including those with dyslexia.

Author details

Trevor O' Brien
Mary Immaculate College, University of Limerick, Limerick, Ireland

*Address all correspondence to: trevor.obrien@mic.ul.ie

References

[1] Oliver M. *Understanding Disability: From Theory to Practice*. Basingstoke: Macmillan; 1996

[2] Elliott GJ, Grigorenko EL. *The Dyslexia Debate*. Cambridge: Cambridge University Press; 2015

[3] O' Brien T. Exploring the social construction of dyslexia. LEARN. 2018;**40**:97-105

[4] Armstrong, D. and Squires, G. (2015). *Key Perspectives on Dyslexia*, London: Routledge.

[5] Hughes R. The social model of disability. British Journal of Healthcare Assistants. 2010;**4**(10):508-511

[6] Florian L, Rouse M. The inclusive practice project in Scotland: Teacher education for inclusive education. Teaching and Teacher Education. 2009;*25:594-601*

[7] Riddick B. *Living with Dyslexia*. London: Routledge; 2010

[8] Burden R. Is dyslexia necessarily associated with negative feelings of self-worth? A Review and Implications for Future Research. *DYSLEXIA*. 2008;**14**:188-196

[9] Cooper P. Like alligators bobbling for poodles? A critical discussion of education, ADHD and the biopsychosocial perspective. Journal of Philosophy of Education. 2008;**42**(3-4):457-474

[10] Humphrey N. Teacher and pupil ratings of self-esteem in developmental dyslexia. British Journal of Special Education. 2002;**29**(1):29-36

[11] Armstrong D, Humphrey N. Reactions to a diagnosis of dyslexia among students entering further education: Development of the 'resistance–accommodation' model. British Journal of Special Education. 2008;**36**(2):95-102

[12] Glazzard J. The impact of dyslexia on pupils' self-esteem. Support for Learning. 2010;**25**(2):63-69

[13] Glazzard J, Dale K. Trainee teachers with dyslexia; personal narratives of resilience. Journal of Research in Special Educational Needs. 2012;**13**(1):26-37

[14] O' Brien T. Affective issues impacting children with dyslexia in a special school in Ireland. Journal of Research in Special Educational Needs. 2019a;**19**(4):315-324

[15] O' Brien T. Developing an inclusive pedagogy - listening to the views of children *with Dyslexia*. REACH. 2019b;**32**(1):50-60

[16] Polychroni F, Koukoura K, Anagnostou I. Academic self-concept, reading attitudes and approaches to learning of children with dyslexia: Do they differ from their peers? European Journal of Special Needs Education. 2006;**21**(4):415-430

[17] Casserly AM, Gildea A. A review of a reading class placement for children with dyslexia, focusing on literacy attainment and pupil perspectives. European Journal of Special Needs Education. 2015;**30**(3):304-322

[18] Casserly AM. The socio-emotional needs of children with dyslexia in different educational settings in Ireland. Journal of Research in Special Educational Needs. 2012;**13**(1):79-91

[19] McPhilips T, Shevlin M. Evaluating the teaching and learning experience for the child with dyslexia in special and mainstream settings in Ireland. Support for Learning. 2009;**24**(2):63-72

[20] Nugent M. Services for children with dyslexia – The child's experience. Educational Psychology in Practice. 2008;**24**(3):189-206

[21] Nugent M. Comparing inclusive and segregated settings for children with dyslexia –parental perspectives from Ireland. Support for Learning. 2007;**22**(2):52-59

[22] Novita S. Secondary symptoms of dyslexia: A comparison of self-esteem and anxiety profiles of children with and without dyslexia. European Journal of Special Needs Education. 2016;**31**(2):279-288

[23] Mitra D. Student voice in secondary schools: The possibility for deeper change. Journal of Educational Administration. 2018;**56**(5):473-487

[24] EADSNE, 2015. Empowering Teachers to Promote Inclusive Education. Literature Review. Odense, Denmark. Retrieved on 10th August 2020 from: https://www.european-agency.org/sites/default/files/Empowering%20Teachers%20to%20Promote%20Inclusive%20Education.%20Literature%20Review.pdf

[25] Rose J. Identifying and Teaching Young People with Dyslexia and Literacy Difficulties; *An independent report from Sir Jim Rose to the Secretary of State for Children, Schools and Families*. Nottingham: DCSF Publications; 2009

[26] Mitchell D. *What Really Works in Special and Inclusive Education. Oxon: Routledge*; 2008

[27] Freire P. *Pedagogy of the Oppressed*. New York: Herder and Herder; 1972

[28] Rudduck J, McIntyre D. *Improving Learning through Consulting Pupils*. London: Routledge; 2007

[29] Fielding M. Transformative approaches to student voice: Theoretical underpinnings, recalcitrant realities. British Educational Research Journal. 2004a;**30**(2):295-311

[30] Lundy L. "Voice is not enough" conceptualising article 12 of the United Nations convention on the rights of the child. British Educational Research Journal. 2007;**33**(6):927-942

[31] Mitra D. Youth as a bridge between home and school: Comparing student voice and parent involvements as strategies for change. Journal of Education and Urban Society. 2006;**38**(4):455-480

[32] Flynn P. The Learner Voice Report. Embedding Student Voices in Education Discourse: Curricular co-construction and development. Dublin: NCCA; 2018

[33] Billington T. Working with autistic children and young people: Sense, experience and the challenge for services, policies and practices. Disability and Society. 2006a;**21**(1):1-13

[34] Billington T. *Working with Children*. London: Sage Publications; 2006b

[35] Kirschner P. Stop propagating the learning styles myth. Computers and Education. 2016;*106:166-171*

[36] Krank M. Commentary: Learning styles and higher education: A tool for inclusion or exclusion? Journal of College Reading and Learning. 2001;*32(1):58-59*

[37] Newton P. The learning styles myth is thriving in higher education. Frontiers in Psychology. 2015;*6:1908), 1*-1908), *5*

[38] Olsen J. The myth of catering to learning styles. Science and Children. 2006;*44(2):56-57*

[39] Smith R, Barr S. Towards educational inclusion in a contested society: From critical analysis to creative action. International Journal of Inclusive Education. 2008;**12**(4):401-422

[40] Westwood P. *Inclusive and Adaptive Teaching*. Oxon: Routledge; 2013

[41] Reid G. *Dyslexia and Inclusion*. Oxon: Routledge; 2013

[42] Reid G. *Dyslexia: A Practitioner's Handbook*. West Sussex. John Wiley and Sons; 2009

[43] Riener, C. and Willingham, D. (2010). The Myth of Learning Styles. Retrieved on 20th March 2017 from: https://www.researchgate.net/profile/Cedar_Riener/publication/249039450_The_Myth_of_Learning_Styles/links/0046353c694205e957000000.pdf

[44] Reid G. *Learning Styles and Inclusion*. London: Sage Publications; 2005

[45] Exley S. The effectiveness of teaching strategies for students with dyslexia based on their preferred learning styles. British Journal of Special Education. 2003;**30**(4):213-220

[46] Mortimore T. Dyslexia and learning style – A note of caution. British Journal of Special Education. 2005;**32**(3):145-148

[47] Mortimore T. *Dyslexia and Learning Style*. West Sussex: John Wiley and Sons; 2008

Chapter 9

Potential Logographic Dyslexics Identified via Self-Reporting during a Questionnaire Survey in Taiwan

Ying-Fang Sun and Pei-Shan Liao

Abstract

According to the patterns of difficulties of the dyslexics that have been reported in Western societies, a questionnaire in traditional Chinese was developed to carry out initial screening among Taiwanese. The questionnaire includes 30 items with four-point scales and 7 open-ended questions. Of the 2133 copies distributed, a total of 1599 questionnaires were collected which gives a 75.0% response rate and 1442 were completed. The mean of 30-item scores collected from 1442 participants is 87.99 ± 11.9. Among these participants, 9 self-reported potential logographic dyslexics have been identified. The individual scores of 30 items of the nine subjects were at least 1 SD to 4.5 SD lower than that of their counterparts. There are two potential logographic dyslexics families show genetic influence. Since there is no standard test for dyslexics, we developed a 30-item questionnaire that can be completed in 15-20 minutes on average. The questionnaire may serve as a low cost, initial screening tool and allows the potential probands to self-report while the formal diagnosis is not available.

Keywords: Chinese, logographic, questionnaire, dyslexia, self-report

1. Introduction

Dyslexia was listed by World Health Organization (WHO) in International Classification of Diseases 11th Revision (ICD-11) as Symbolic dysfunctions, code as MB4B.0 [1], and also documented by The American Psychiatric Association on The Diagnostic and Statistical Manual of Mental Disorders (DSM) 5th edition [2]. The disorder has complicate patterns that can be observed in reading, spelling, and writing behaviors [3]. It is linked to the acquisition of cognitive and learning skills [4]. Despite the above disadvantages, some dyslexics show talents [3, 5–7], visuospatial strengths [8, 9], creative thinking [10] and the way to develop coping strategies [11]. For example, Albert Einstein was described as "*a late talker who was not only a mathematical genius, but also a self-admitted dyslexic*" Brain 123: p.2377 [12, 13].

Dyslexia may happen together with autism [14] and/or attention deficit hyperactivity disorder (ADHD) [15]. The proband has normal intelligence but seems to be a spectrum with different severities [16]. These primary syndromes may lead to long term disease, such as anxiety, and social problems later on.

In terms of the origin, studies on twins confirmed the involvement of gene/genes in dyslexia [17]. Researchers proposed that the genotypes cause the functional changes of the brain and generates the cognitive and perceptive deficits in dyslexics [18]. The predominant opinions agree that genes [19–21] and brain [16] are two areas to focus on [22]. The potential risk loci located on chromosome 1, 2, 3, 4, 6, 11, 12, 13, 15, 17, 18, and X [19]. Apparently, it is polygenetic. The left posterior temporo-parietal cortex, left occipital-temporal cortex and left inferior frontal gyrus are brain regions involved [16, 23, 24]. In addition, cerebellum might play a role [23–25]. It could happen across languages [26] and writing systems [16, 26]. For example, the brain activation is similar for Mandarin and English users with dyslexia [27]. However, the definitions of dyslexia used by different research groups vary, due to disagreement in its diagnosis criteria [28–30].

Recently, dyslexia was suggested as a coping response to environmental challenges [31]. In 2016, the prevalence of dyslexia was estimated to be 5-17% in the United States [32], however, no definitive answer has been found [33]. Since the clear mechanism for dyslexia remains unknown, the proposed theories for dyslexia have not reached consensus.

Previous studies have examined dyslexia in Taiwan from different perspectives. However, few has examined the strength of the affected individuals, despite that they may or may not be diagnosed with dyslexia. In order to identify the at-risk, we develop a questionnaire in traditional Chinese logographic characters for initial screening. This questionnaire allows self-report of symptoms, which is a reliable means [34–36] and non-costly. It might distinguish the affected from the non-dyslexics as well.

2. Methods and procedures

Based on the 20-item English version of the adult dyslexia checklist from The British Dyslexia Association [37, 38], a questionnaire in traditional Chinese characters with 30 items on a four-point scale (1 = often, 2 = sometimes, 3 = seldom, and 4 = never) was developed (appendix 1). Among the 30 items, the first seven items are related to reading, followed by items 8 to 11, which examine the sense of directions. Items 12 to 14 investigate writing ability and items 15 to 20 are associated with the numerical competency. Items 21-26 describe the individual behavior characteristics. The defective cerebellum hypothesis of dyslexia is assessed via item 27. The strength of the dyslexics is applied in item 28, which is less emphasized in previous studies. The clinical signs of fatty acid deficiency are exploited in item 29. The last item, item 30, examines if a heritable aspect to any dyslexia that is identified. The profiles for dyslexic difficulty patterns described by T.R. Miles [3] were adopted in items 1, 3, 4, 5, 9, 10, and 11. In addition to the 30 items, we incorporated seven open-ended questions that allowed the participants to self-report any related symptoms explicitly in written traditional Chinese.

3. Results and discussions

1. The frequency and mean of 30-item scores in the questionnaire survey

The questionnaire was self-administered and 2133 copies were distributed to 20 groups; mostly different levels of schools, during July to December, 2009. A total of 1599 questionnaires were collected with a response rate of 75.0%, and of which 164 questionnaires were dropped from analysis due to missing data. Response values of the 30 items were added, with a lower score indicating a higher chance of being affected by dyslexia. The mean score for the 1442 completed questionnaires was 87.99, with a standard deviation (SD) of 11.9 (**Figure 1**). Among these respondents, the scores ranged from 36 (the most affected) to 120 (the least affected).

The participants can be classified based on the standard deviation around mean value of the 30 items. Among them, 233 had a score lower than 76, approximately 16.1% of the 1442 participants. The number of participants with a score of 2 SD below the mean value was 55, which is approximately 3.7% of the 1442 participants.

2. Identifying potential logographic dyslexics via self-reporting

The potential logographic dyslexics were identified by self-reporting either by themselves or by their family members. Interestingly, self-reported cases or proxy are all female. The phenomenon is in accord with the findings from the article [39] which found that the females have more positive altitude. The demographic characteristics of these individuals are presented in **Table 1**. We have documented the available information on these five potential probands, denoted as D1 to D5 in **Table 2**, and their offspring as carefully as possible since a standard test has not yet available for the adult dyslexics [40].

When compared D1's score of the 30 items, which was 83, with those at the same gender, similar age and education level (which was 91.67 ± 5.51), the former is found to be about 1.5 SD lower (**Table 2**). The score of 30 items of the gender, age matched subjects was 93.8 ± 9.33, which was 1SD higher than D1's score. In other words, the evaluation result of D1 based on the 30-item questionnaire is poor than the average of those with similar characteristics.

As described by his wife on March 6, 2010, *D1 cannot concentrate on what he is reading, becomes distracted very easily and cannot comprehend the meaning of context. He is very impatient when writing things, although his hand writing is readable. He loves arts, however, has never pursued it as a career. He was born as a left handed but was forced to change as a right hander at age of 2-3 years old.*

For the case *D2, reported by his mother, the thirteen-year-old boy was diagnosed as having "reading disability" by Kuan-Tu hospital several years ago. He fell asleep while conducting MRI scanning. Described by his mother, he cannot concentrate on the text that he is reading, and is unwilling to write the traditional Chinese characters. He becomes more energetic in the evenings than that in the mornings. He is right handed.*

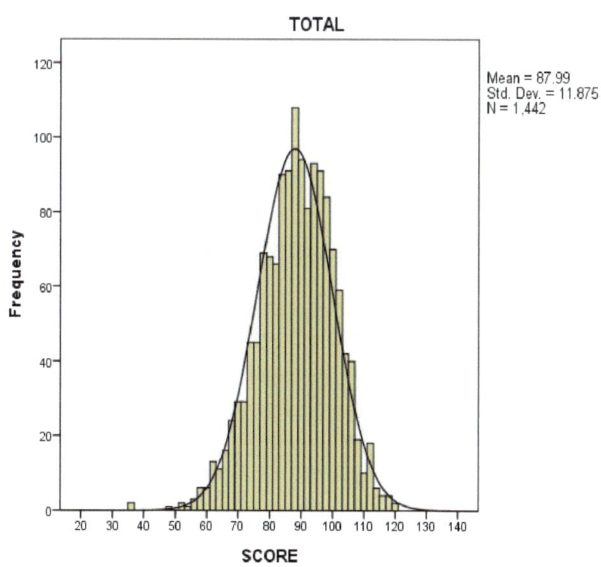

Figure 1.
The frequency and mean of the 30-item scores for all completed questionnaires.

ID No	Age	H (cm)	W (kg)	BMI	Hand	Edu. level	30-Item score
M1	19	175	60	19.6	R	C	90
M2	23	175	65	21.2	R	C	100
M3	43	182	85	25.7	R	M	117
M4	45	170	65	22.5	R	M	83
M5	52	173	70	23.4	R	H	116
M6	53	170	69	23.9	R	Ph	96
M7	69	166	61	22.1	R	Ph	96
M8	89	178	72	22.7	R	C	104
Mean ± SD	**40.7 ± 20.2**	**172.3 ± 4.7**	**66.4 ± 7.9**	**22.4 ± 2.5**			**90.6 ± 13.2**
F1	14	150	40	17.8	R	J	90
F2	23	164	68	25.3	R	M	96
F3	25	158	46	18.4	R	M	80
F4	39	163	62	23.3	R	M	93
F5	43	166	78	29.3	R	C	99
F6	51	150	46	20.4	R	Ph	88
F7	53	157	51	20.7	R	M	73
F8	56	162	65	24.8	R	C	103
F9	59	157	60	24.3	R	Ph	99
Mean ± SD	**40.4 ± 15.3**	**158.2 ± 6.3**	**56.9 ± 10.8**	**22.7 ± 3.8**			**88.6 ± 15.6**
D1	57	175	72	23.5	L + R	C	83
D2	13	165	72	26.4	R	J	77
D3	58	146	53	24.9	L/R	M	49
D4	61	165	60	22.0	R	C	+

***H:** Height **W:** Weight.*
***Hand:** Handedness was determined by filling out a structured form with 13 questions. L + R: Was a left hander and switched into right handed during schooling. L/R: Ambidextrous, use both right and left hands in daily life. R-L: A right hander but become left handed after impairment of the right hand.*
***Edu. level:** Education level **H:** high school **M:** master **J:** junior school **C:** college **Ph:** PhD.*
S: The scores of 30 items in a questionnaire survey conducted in July–December in year 2009.
+: Could not complete the 4-page long questionnaire.

Table 1.
Demographic characteristics of potential logographic dyslexics.

Some Chinese characters were replaced by phonetic symbols or English at the answers of the questionnaire that he submitted.

As a comparable group to D2, the mean of the score obtained from 30 items for 34 male junior school students is 95.59 ± 8.9 (**Figure 2**) which was 2 SD higher than D2's score of 77 (**Table 2**). The mean of scores from 30 items of the gender and age matched participants was 89.33 ± 12.07, which was 1 SD higher than that of D2.

For the case *D3, a high achieving, self-reporting female subject with a master degree. She found that reading is difficult and was medically diagnosed as having compensated learning disability, dysorthographia*. *That is a particular form of dyslexia* [41] and *logographic processing disorder diagnosed by a medical neurologist (stationed at Changhua Christian Hospital in 2009, personal communication, unpublished data upon request). Some of her hand writing was difficult to recognize and was criticized as lazy and stupid when she was young.*

ID	Gender	Age	Education level	Mean scores of the 30 items		
					Subjects matched with gender, age and education	Subjects matched with gender and age
D1	Male	57	College	83	91.67 ± 5.51	93.80 ± 9.33
D2	Male	13	Junior school	77	95.59 ± 8.92	89.33 ± 12.07
D3	Female	58	Masters	49	80.60 ± 6.58	90.04 ± 11.35
D3-1	Daughter 1 of D3	19/ 29	High school	74	87.33 ± 13.19	86.87 ± 10.94
D3-2	Daughter 2 of D3	19/ 29	Junior school	64	70	86.87 ± 10.94
D4	Female	61	College	+	78.75 ± 13.89	83.14 ± 13.06
D4-1	Daughter 1 of D4	34	Masters	50/75	90.62 ± 11.59	86.29 ± 14.49
D4-2	Daughter 2 of D4	NA	Masters	NA	NA	NA
D5	Female	61	College	+	78.75 ± 13.89	83.14 ± 13.06

+ ***D4** and **D5** as two potential logographic dyslexics had great difficulty in completing the 30-item questionnaire.*
***NA**: not applicable.*

Table 2.
The 30-item score of the potential logographic dyslexics identified via self-reporting.

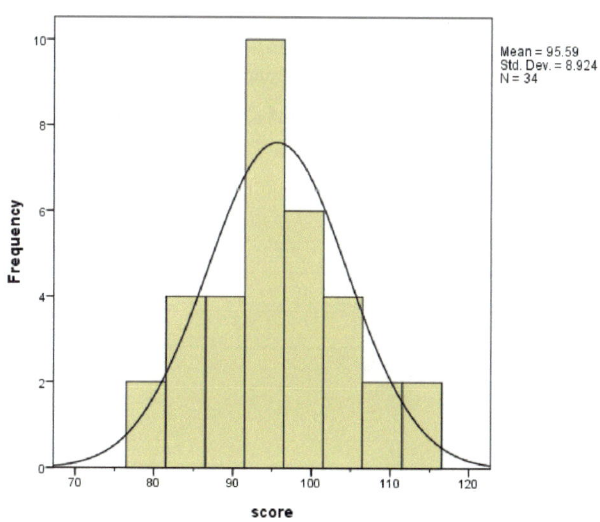

Figure 2.
The frequency and mean of the 30-item scores for junior high school participants.

She had a hard time keeping up with her classmates of the same age and had to spend an extra year at junior high school. She hates to recite, or write but appreciates arts and music. She has never learned to ride a bicycle due to balance problems, which is a sign of a defective cerebellum [42] *and is related to dyslexia* [43, 44]. *She was late on the day scheduled for MRI scanning though she did not mean to be. That indicated an impaired sense of time estimation, which is one of the symptoms of a typical dyslexic* [42]. *She also mentioned that she does better in the night times for schooling than that in the day times. Therefore, she had to attend night schools instead of going to regular schools operating in day times.* Her two daughters (D3-1, D3-2) also experienced difficulties at school, specifically, reciting multiplication table, (reported by her mother, D3), which is a symptom of dyslexia [3]. D3-1 graduated from junior high school and the other, D3-2 did get high school diploma. Both were between 19 and 29 years old. This implies a genetic basis for the problems in this family. D3 showed a tendency to use two hands together and had a good taste in terms of design and art.

The mean of scores of the participants matched with gender, age and education level was 80.6 ± 6.58, which was about 4.5 SD higher than D3's score (49). The mean of scores of the participants matched with gender and age is 90.04 ± 11.35, which was about 3.5 SD higher than that (equals to 49) of the D3 (**Table 2**). When compared with the average score of 1442 participants, namely, 87.99 ± 11.9, D3's score was 3 SD lower.

For the case D3-1, the average of 30-item score of the participants matched with gender, age and education level and those with gender and age are 87.33 ± 13.19 and 86.87 ± 10.94, respectively, which were both 1 SD higher than that of the D3-1 (74). Similar patterns were found for the case D3-2. Her score (64) was about 2 SD lower

Description	Evidences, Tests	Subjects
Advantages of dyslexics (strengths)		
1. Imaginative writing creative writing	p.146 p.147	S192, S204, S237, S128, S46
2. Good at chess	p.144	S62, S118, S179
3. Gifted musically	Flute, "my sight reading is a bad point, eventually my fingers remember" p.145	S72, S74, S193, S147, S112, S241
4. Gifted in art and craft	p.146	S171, S199,
5. Remarkable drawing	p.146	S46, S54, S150, S179
6. Carving, woodwork, pottery, drawing	P.146	S123, S257, S120, S112, S199
7. A fine analytical mind able to accept, understand and implement new concepts	p.31	S95
8. Assembling the parts of a radio, a dyslexic person can perfectly well do in sequence	p.96	
9. Function more effectively when dealing with three dimensions than when dealing with two	p.230	
10. High score on the Advanced Raven's Matrices	p.228 total 48 adult dyslexics	norms for university students is 21 ± 4; three were of 30 or above and seven were between 25 and 29
11. Very strong at processing for sentence meaning	p.139	S59, S75, S83, S99
12. Unusual powers of creativity	p.189	Albert Einstein, Thomas Edison, WB Yeats

Table 3.
The strength of Dyslexia summarized from 1993 TR Miles.

than the average score (86.87 ± 10.94) of the participants matched with gender and age (**Table 2**).

D4 held a college degree in art and performance. She was also a talented singer but could not even complete the questionnaire that normally required 15-20 minutes on average. She is a mother of two daughters (D4-1 and D4-2) and was reported by her elder daughter, D4-1.

For the case *D4-1, the score of 50 was given by the subject and she claimed that it was based on her conditions before the age of 22. Her score at the time of completing the questionnaire was 75. Her score is 1.3 SD lower than the average score of the participants matched with gender, age and education level (90.62 ± 11.59), and was 1 SD lower than those matched with gender and age (86.29 ± 14.49) (**Table 2**). She was labeled as lazy and stupid at early schooling though she has talents in music and singing.*

Not until she went to the United States and obtained a master degree, she regained her confidence. She recalled that 22 years old is a turning point for her life. We are not sure how and when the compensation processes occurred for a person who uses both logographic (i.e., Chinese) and phonological language system (i.e., English) simultaneously. The brain organization is related to the compensatory process, specifically the right hemisphere [45]. As she was pregnant at the time of data collection, we cannot scan her brain with MR. We do not know whether she had adopted any strategies while she was in the United States.

The case *D5 was a 61 years old female with a college degree, and was an excellent art teacher in a primary school. She is constantly bothered by her problems and does not know why. She struggled through schooling and had to spend one more year at junior school. She has no sense of time with numerical difficulties and becomes confused about directions. She has talents in arts such as paper sculpture and knit weaving. She states her disadvantages and talents in Chinese characters at the questionnaire that she submitted.* The unusual balance of the skills was described by the book written by T.R. Miles [3] (p.189, p.237), see **Table 3**.

She could not complete the 4-page long questionnaire as normally done in about 15-20 minutes. Having problems with filling in forms is one of the symptoms of dyslexia [46]. Among the subjects from whom we received questionnaires, four females had a college degree and were 61 years old. Their average score of the 30 items was 78.75 ± 13.89, see **Table 2**.

Overall, our self-report cases support the involvement of genes and brain for dyslexia. The disorder did have a biological origin though the nature is unmasked. Each individual of these 9 logographic potential dyslexics possesses unique behavior, in agreement with the statement that "no typical phenotype could be claimed as dyslexia" [16]. In other words, the form and degree of dyslexia varied.

Each of our cases revealed specific symptoms of dyslexia. Case D1 has deficits of reading skills, which is probably related to ADHD [15]. Also, both of D2 and D3 are more energetic in the evening than in the daytime, in addition to reading and writing impairments. This may be related to hypothalamic–pituitary–adrenal (HPA) axis [4]. The two daughters of case D3 both experienced difficulties for schooling, suggesting that the genes are involved [20, 21]. D3 could not learn to ride a bicycle supports the cerebellum theory for dyslexia [23–25].

Although D4 and D5 could not finish the questionnaire and hate to deal with forms, D4 is a talent singer, and D5 is a great art teacher. These talents [5–7] documented in previous research had never been noticed when they were at school. D4's elder daughter D4-1, after suffering from schooling, was sent to the USA, where she found confidence. This is a typical compensated case, probably related to brain organization specifically in the right hemisphere [45]. Again, the cases of D4's family, as well as D3 's family, demonstrated the involvement of genes for dyslexia.

4. Conclusions and future work

It is found that the 30-item questionnaire allowed us to identify the potential logographic dyslexic probands. It should be noted that self-reporting cases are all females or identified by a female family member of the potential logographic dyslexics. The genetic influence was implied from the two potential dyslexic families of D3 and D4. More importantly, our data suggested that some of the dyslexics may carry gifted talents, which has never been recognized by local educators and teachers before. When reading and writing difficulties are found in students, along with observable focusing or balancing problems, educators are encouraged to employ this tool for initial screening on potential dyslexics and lend them necessary support. Future work should concentrate on the validity and reliability of the questionnaire for group screening [47]. A qualitative multiple case study of the potential logographic dyslexics is suggested.

Acknowledgements

We value the contributions of all the participants who completed the questionnaire for the dyslexia research. Our deep and sincere thank you to all the potential logographic dyslexics for their sharing while they have been struggling constantly. The author received scholarship from Center for Survey Research, RCHSS, Academia Sinica for the development of the questionnaire and data collection.

Author details

Ying-Fang Sun[1*] and Pei-Shan Liao[2]

1 Keelung Municipal Badou Elementary School, Keelung, Taiwan ROC

2 Research Center for Humanities and Social Sciences, Academia Sinica, Taipei, Taiwan ROC

*Address all correspondence to: ysun564988@hotmail.com

References

[1] WHO, *https://icd.who.int/browse11/l-m/en#/http%3a%2f%2fid.who.int%2ficd%2fentity%2f724140102 20200822.*

[2] Diagnostic and statistical manual of mental disorders, fifth edition (DSM-5). *Washington DC*. In: *The American Psychiatric Association*. 2013

[3] Miles TR. *Dyslexia: The pattern of difficulties 2nd ed. Whurr publishers*. London. ;*303*:1993

[4] Zakopoulou V et al. *Linking early life hypothalamic-pituitary-adrenal Axis functioning, brain asymmetries, and personality traits in Dyslexia: An informative case study*. Frontiers in Human Neuroscience. 2019;**13**:327

[5] von Károlyi C et al. *Dyslexia linked to talent: Global visual-spatial ability*. Brain and Language. 2003;**85**(3):427-431

[6] Chakravarty A. *Artistic talent in dyslexia--a hypothesis*. Medical Hypotheses. 2009;**73**(4):569-571

[7] Lifshitz Ben Basat A, Fostick L. *Music-related abilities among readers with dyslexia*. Annals of Dyslexia. 2019;**69**(3):318-334

[8] Winner E et al. *Dyslexia and visual-spatial talents: Compensation vs deficit model*. Brain and Language. 2001;**76**(2):81-110

[9] Attree EA, Turner MJ, Cowell N. *A virtual reality test identifies the visuospatial strengths of adolescents with dyslexia*. Cyberpsychology & Behavior. 2009;**12**(2):163-168

[10] Everatt J, Steffert B, Smythe I. *An eye for the unusual: Creative thinking in dyslexics*. Dyslexia. 1999;**5**(1):28-46

[11] Kannangara CS. *From languishing Dyslexia to thriving Dyslexia: Developing a new conceptual approach to working with people with Dyslexia*. Frontiers in Psychology. 2015;**6**:1976

[12] Habib M. *The neurological basis of developmental dyslexia an overview and working hypothesis*. Brain. 2000;**123**:2373-2399

[13] Witelson SF, Kigar DL, Harvey T. *The exceptional brain of Albert Einstein*. Lancet. 1999;**353**(9170):2149-2153

[14] Huang M et al. *Two autism/Dyslexia linked variations of DOCK4 disrupt the gene function on Rac1/Rap1 activation, Neurite outgrowth, and synapse development*. Frontiers in Cellular Neuroscience. 2019;**13**:577

[15] Cui X et al. *Visual search in Chinese children with attention deficit/hyperactivity disorder and comorbid developmental Dyslexia: Evidence for pathogenesis from eye movements*. Frontiers in Psychology. 2020;**11**:880

[16] Richlan F. *The functional Neuroanatomy of developmental Dyslexia across languages and writing systems*. Frontiers in Psychology. 2020;**11**:155

[17] Olson RK. *Dyslexia: nature and nurture*. Dyslexia. 2002;**8**(3):143-159

[18] Galaburda AM et al. *From genes to behavior in developmental dyslexia*. Nature Neuroscience. 2006;**9**(10):1213-1217

[19] Sun YF, Lee JS, Kirby R. *Candidate genes for dyslexia by an In Silico approach*. Asian Journal of Health and Informaiton Sciences. 2009;**4**(2-3):81-92

[20] Nishiyama KV, Satta Y, Gojobori J. *Do genes associated with Dyslexia of Chinese characters evolve neutrally?* Genes (Basel). 2020;**11**(6)

[21] Bieder A et al. *Rare variants in dynein heavy chain genes in two individuals with situs inversus and developmental dyslexia: A case report*. BMC Medical Genetics. 2020;**21**(1):87

[22] Mascheretti S et al. *Neurogenetics of developmental dyslexia: From genes to behavior through brain neuroimaging and cognitive and sensorial mechanisms*. Translational Psychiatry. 2017;**7**(1):e987

[23] Pernet CR et al. *Brain classification reveals the right cerebellum as the best biomarker of dyslexia*. BMC Neuroscience. 2009;**10**:67

[24] Sun YF, Lee JS, Kirby R. *Brain imaging findings in dyslexia*. Pediatrics and Neonatology. 2010;**51**(2):89-96

[25] Starowicz-Filip A et al. *The role of the cerebellum in the regulation of language functions*. Psychiatria Polska. 2017;**51**(4):661-671

[26] Paulesu E et al. *Dyslexia: Cultural diversity and biological unity*. Science. 2001;**291**(5511):2165-2167

[27] Hu, W., et al., *Developmental dyslexia in Chinese and English populations: Dissociating the effect of dyslexia from language differences.* Brain, 2010. **133**(Pt 6): p. 1694-1706.

[28] Thomson M. *The definition of dyslexia*. Dyslexia. 2002;**8**(1):53-54

[29] Fletcher JM. *Dyslexia: The evolution of a scientific concept*. Journal of the International Neuropsychological Society. 2009;**15**(4):501-508

[30] Stein J. *What is developmental Dyslexia?* Brain Sciences. 2018;**8**(2)

[31] Kershner JR. *Dyslexia as an adaptation to cortico-limbic stress system reactivity*. Neurobiol Stress. 2020;**12**:100223

[32] Ozernov-Palchik O, Gaab N. *Tackling the 'dyslexia paradox': Reading brain and behavior for early markers of developmental dyslexia*. Wiley Interdisciplinary Reviews: Cognitive Science. 2016;7(2):156-176

[33] Wagner RK et al. *The prevalence of Dyslexia: A new approach to its estimation*. Journal of Learning Disabilities. 2020;**53**(5):354-365

[34] Snowling M et al. *Validity of a protocol for adult self-report of dyslexia and related difficulties*. Dyslexia. 2012;**18**(1):1-15

[35] Tamboer P, Vorst HC, Oort FJ. *Identifying dyslexia in adults: An iterative method using the predictive value of item scores and self-report questions*. Annals of Dyslexia. 2014;**64**(1):34-56

[36] Tamboer P, Vorst HC. *A new self-report inventory of dyslexia for students: Criterion and construct validity*. Dyslexia. 2015;**21**(1):1-34

[37] Turner M. *Psychological Assessment of Dyslexia Chapter 11. Whurr Publishers*; 1997

[38] Vinegrad M, Revised Adult Dyslexia Checklist A. **Educare**. 1994;**48**:21-23

[39] Gwernan-Jones R, Burden RL. *Are they just lazy? Student teachers' attitudes about dyslexia*. Dyslexia. 2010;**16**(1):66-86

[40] Nicolson RI, Fawcett AJ, Miles TR. *Feasibility study for the development of a computerized screening test for dyslexia in adults*. In: *Report No.OL176*. 1993

[41] Fersten E et al. *Dynamics of blood flow velocity in middle cerebral arteries in dyslexic persons*. Neurologia i Neurochirurgia Polska. 1999;**33**(5):1099-1108

[42] Nicolson RI, Fawcett A, Dean P. *Time estimation deficits in developmental dyslexia: Evidence of cerebellar involvement*. Proceedings of the Biological Sciences. 1995;**259**(1354):43-47

[43] Raberger T, Wimmer H. *On the automaticity/cerebellar deficit hypothesis of dyslexia: Balancing and continuous rapid naming in dyslexic and ADHD children*. Neuropsychologia. 2003;**41**(11):1493-1497

[44] Rochelle KS, Talcott JB. *Impaired balance in developmental dyslexia? A meta-analysis of the contending evidence*. Journal of Child Psychology and Psychiatry. 2006;**47**(11):1159-1166

[45] Chiarello C et al. *Neuroanatomical and behavioral asymmetry in an adult compensated dyslexic*. Brain and Language. 2006;**98**(2):169-181

[46] Brachacki GW, Nicolson RI, Fawcett AJ. *Impaired recognition of traffic signs in adults with dyslexia*. Journal of Learning Disabilities. 1995;**28**(5):297-301, 308

[47] Wolff U, Lundberg I. *The prevalence of dyslexia among art students*. Dyslexia. 2002;**8**(1):34-42

Chapter 10

An Ecocultural Perspective on Learning Disability: Evaluation of Familial and Cultural Factors and Presentation of an Integrated Model

Suzan Cen-Yagiz and Berna Aytac

Abstract

Ecocultural theory defines culture as a broad context that includes the tasks, goals, beliefs, values, and resources of society. According to ecocultural theory, culture shapes families' resources, routines, goals, and parenting practices. In turn, these characteristics of family ecology and parenting determine child development. Ecocultural theory is one of the modern approaches that examine the adaptation of children with disabilities and their families. This chapter aims to outline the relationship between cultural values and families' support resources, and their influence on adaptation of the families and their children with learning disability (LD) within the framework of ecocultural theory. Previous studies supported that cultural values determine public knowledge, awareness, beliefs, and attitudes about LD. This chapter outlines both the detrimental and positive effects of the public knowledge, beliefs, and attitudes on families' support resources. Also, families' diversified support resources are detailed, and their differential influences on family and child development are elaborated. In the chapter, an integrated model is presented based on findings of previous empirical studies and ecocultural perspective. The model might enhance a culturally sensitive understanding of the experience of families and children. This chapter can also guide researchers in developing more comprehensive and effective intervention programs for the target group.

Keywords: ecocultural theory, learning disability, family support resources, cultural values, causal beliefs

1. Introduction

Learning Disability (LD) is a biologically originated, neurodevelopmental disorder including difficulties across the academic domains of mathematics, reading and writing [1]. Children with LD face different developmental outcomes due to both biological (e.g., neurocognitive and adaptive deficits associated with a significant disturbance of the white matter in the right hemisphere) [2], and environmental factors (e.g., attending to special education) [3]. In other words, the development of the child with LD is also affected by the contextual factors [4]. There are several

IntechOpen

studies investigating the effect of contextual factors such as family functionality and school environment on the development of children with LD [5–7]. However, there is a scarcity of studies differentiating the effects of different levels of contextual factors such as familial factors and cultural factors [8].

Ecocultural theory offers a wide theoretical perspective combining the effect of these factors on development of children with neurodevelopmental disorders like LD [9–11]. According to ecocultural theory, family's practices, activities, and resources of support are organized and shaped by the characteristics of the culture (e.g., culture values); in turn influencing child developmental outcomes, such as child daily living and communication skills, and developmental status of children with disabilities [11, 12]. In the chapter, the effect of familial and cultural factors in determining the family practices and development of children with LD are examined within the perspective of ecocultural theory.

At the cultural level, the role of cultural values in determining family social support resources is evaluated. At the familial level, the association between family social support resources and the adjustment processes of parents and children is covered. It has been thought that investigation of these factors in the light of ecocultural perspective would (1) contribute to develop an understanding of contextual effects on child development, (2) guide future studies and researchers in developing more comprehensive and effective intervention programs for the target group.

In the chapter, the definition of LD is presented and the importance of evaluating LD within a contextual perspective is discussed. Subsequently, the link between culture, family and child development is addressed in the history of developmental psychology. In the following parts, the basic assumptions of ecocultural theory, contextual factors and associations among these factors along with studies about LD are summarized. Finally, in the scope of the chapter, an integrated model is presented based on findings of previous empirical studies and ecocultural perspective.

2. Learning disability (LD)

According to DSM5 [1], individuals with learning disability (LD) demonstrate cognitive abnormalities, impairments in verbal and nonverbal information processing of brain, and/or disruption in processing abilities of individuals. These impairments in development of the brain result in difficulties in the acquisition and use of academic skills such as reading, writing, reasoning, and/or mathematical abilities [1]. Five to fifteen percent of school-aged children in the world exhibit low performance on some of these skills [1, 13].

The subtypes of LD have been defined in DSM 5 as; (1) reading disorder "dyslexia", (2) writing disorder "dysgraphia" and mathematics learning disorder "dyscalculia" [1]. While one of the subtypes of the expressed disorder is observed in children with mild LD (e.g., dyslexia), the severity of the difficulty increases if children experience difficulties in more than one academic area (e.g., dyslexia and dyscalculia together). Children with severe LD were more prone to demonstrate an increased number of social skill deficits, hence they reported more problem behaviors compared to children with mild or moderate LD [14–16]. Within the scope of the chapter, previous studies including children experiencing problems in at least one of the subtypes of LD are covered.

3. Culture, family and child development

The earlier studies of human development have been argued to be based on the perspective where the genetic influences are dominant [17, 18]. However, when anthropologists (e.g., Malonowski Trobia Islands) began to study culture in the 1920s with World War I, cultural and contextual influences also started to dominate explanations of human development (e.g., ecocultural models). In those years, Vygotsky was one of the foremost theoreticians emphasizing the indispensable role of sociocultural factors for elementary nature of human development as well as biological processes. He defined human development especially cognitive and language development by integrating cultural and hereditary influences [17]. According to Vygotsky, the life-span development (ontogenetic) should be examined within the framework of both genetic/evolutionary changes (phylogenetic) and the cultural context/historical times (e.g., symbols, technology, values, norms) in which the individual is living. Vygotsky claimed that it is not possible to separate these levels from each other because interaction between these levels also determines the structure of human development [17].

Vygotsky's emphasis on the importance of cultural-historical effects in understanding human development had also influenced the views of many developmental theorists [17]. Many developmental theorists' precious works have led to the accumulation of knowledge in terms of elaboration of contextual factors [19–21]. They examined the differential roles of contextual factors such as distal (e.g., values, beliefs, social politics, welfare, child-rearing customs) and proximal process (e.g., physical and social context of children living, parenting practices, families' support resources). Inspection of the theories indicated that these distal process shape the family environment that plays an active role in the development of the child. In other words, child development is embedded in the context in which the child lives. However, these contextual developmental theories generally focused on examining the characteristics of cultural and familial factors on development of children with typical development. Ecocultural theory suggests examining the role of contextual factors on the development of both children with and without developmental disabilities. Taken together, evaluations presented in the chapter aimed to incorporate examining the role of familial and cultural factors on development of children with LD within the perspective of ecocultural theory.

4. Ecocultural theory

The term ecocultural or ecological/cultural refers to the physical and social characteristics of the environment surrounding the families [12]. Thus, the theory defines culture as a broader context that includes societal tasks, goals, believes, values, resources, and traditions. These factors constitute the cultural trajectory of families and their life, activities, parenting practices, relationships, support resources, etc. [9–10, 22]. Each family organizes its daily activities, routines, and resources. Since the main goal of development is to ensure and maintain individuals' well-being, for example, families' resources are equally distributed concerning the needs of members within the family [9, 22]. According to the ecocultural theory, the activities, routines, and resources of the family help the child to internalize cultural values and beliefs. Through this way, the child can participate and adapt to the culture where s/he is living, which in turn linked with child's well-being [11].

4.1 Culture, family and disability in ecocultural theory

The previous studies investigating children with disabilities and their families were criticized for including mostly univariate variables, distal measurements of family characteristics, and being pathology-oriented [12]. However, the new social and ecological views trivialized old approaches, conceptualized the disability as a multidimensional issue and guided the development of comprehensive applications for children and their families [12, 23, 24]. Ecocultural theory is one of these new approaches that integrates family ecology, members and culture into one ground for the children with developmental disabilities [19, 24].

Individuals with disabilities are seen passive, and disability is seen as only medical or social issue in medical and social models. However, ecocultural theory takes explanatory model as its basis. In explanatory model, the meaning of developmental disabilities in a cultural context is shaped by cultural values, beliefs, meanings and tools in which individuals are embedded [25, 26]. Therefore, the explanatory model provides an extensive perspective for researchers on individuals' and families' understanding and experiences related to disability within different social contexts (e.g., schools, social services, institutions, etc.). Although this theory takes the perspectives of professionals in this field into consideration, it emphasizes families' perspectives more, especially for children with disabilities. According to ecocultural theory, professionals in this field should analyze the risks (necessities) and opportunities (supports) of the family, and how family interprets and perceives these factors [12]. For example, Kellegrew [27] found that mothers of children with disabilities who considered to send their children to a regular preschool seemed to be more focused on their children's self-care and social skills. On the other hand, mothers whose children were attending to a special education center showed greater interest in their children's academic skills or school works. Also, one of these mothers stated that she did not have to worry because her child was learning self-care skills in the special education center. Professionals in this field should assess the parents' internalized beliefs in terms of child-rearing as it seems that they shape the family's practices, which in turn influence child development. As a whole, families' values, goals, support resources, and practices are dynamic processes that interact with each other rather than passive processes seen in other models. It can be speculated that professionals in this field could design integrative intervention programs for families by assessing both ecological characteristics of families and their perception about the disability.

4.2 Ecocultural theory and learning disability

Ecocultural theory captures many disabilities and discusses the effects of familial and cultural characteristics on the developmental outcomes of children; LD is one of them. Although, ecocultural theory assumes that LD is a neurobiologically originated problem, it also stresses that the assessment process of the LD can be influenced by the cultural characteristics such as values, goals and beliefs [4]. For example, ecocultural perspective argues the diagnosis criteria of LD in different contexts. To explain, literacy and academic achievement are the main goals of the families for their children in western countries. Therefore, academic abilities in reading, writing and mathematics are taken as the diagnosis criteria of LD. On the other hand, in agricultural societies, criteria of intelligence or competence of a child is whether s/he is doing a task independently or/and behaving appropriately according to his/her developmental age group [4]. Diagnosis criteria for LD could change due to ecological characteristics (e.g., resources, services), customs in child rearing, the nature of individuals' early experience of literacy and learning process, expectancy concerning child development etc. Inspection of cultural differences pinpoints the necessity of providing culturally sensitive assessment and intervention services to these children [4].

In recent years, the effects of the relationships between the different individual and contextual factors on developmental outcomes of children with LD have also started to attract researchers' attention more [8]. One of the reasons for this is that different contextual characteristics of individuals have divergent consequences on the adaptation processes of children and families. Another point is that interventions based on the improvement of children's abilities and environmental conditions (e.g., cognitive schemas, family resources) are seen to have positive effects on the adaptation processes of children and families [28, 29]. As a result, the evaluations of contextual factors and the presented model within the scope of the ecocultural theory would provide a comprehensive perspective for future studies.

4.3 Contextual factors in ecocultural theory

The relationship between culture, family resources, and child development was emphasized and analyzed for children with developmental disabilities in ecocultural theory [12, 23]. However, integrating the role of these factors on the development of children with LD was mainly overlooked. We aim to outline these factors within the scope of ecocultural theory and with previous findings of studies in LD. At the cultural level, we detailed the role of cultural values on families' support resources. In the context of the family, specific support resources are examined since families' specific support resources are emphasized to have different roles on families' adaptation process and child development [23].

4.3.1 Cultural values

According to ecocultural theory, parenting practices and families' daily activities are influenced by cultural values [12, 22]. Values are described as the concepts that guide and explain people's desirable actions, such as cognitive, emotional, and motivational processes [30, 31]. Link of the values with different cultural interests have been guided researchers to study relation of values with family processes or parenting behaviors. The individualistic and collectivistic values are the cultural parameters that has been used to determine the tendency of societies or/and individuals [32]. Collectivistic values are mostly related with social harmony, dependency, compliance and maintaining close ties [32]. On the other hand, in individualistic cultures, individuals tend to strive for autonomy, openness to change, self-direction and independence [32]. Since individualistic and collectivistic values have significant effects on families and parenting practices, we presented the findings based on individualistic and collectivistic cultural values in the chapter.

4.3.2 Cultural values and social support resources

There have been many studies examining the role of support resources in families with children with LD. However, there are limited cross-cultural studies that aim to elaborate the process of determining these resources. The existing studies indicated that there is a link between familial support resources and cultural values. Families have more chance to attain social and educational support resources in individualistic cultures, compared to collectivistic cultures [33–35]. Also, families achieve a greater chance of social inclusion in individualistic cultures. To explain, competence and autonomy are believed to be essential aspects of the self in individualistic cultures [30]. Therefore, people who score higher on individualistic values might believe more in the role of providing help to people with disabilities for improving their autonomy and self-competence. This belief might lead to a decrease in their desire for social distance towards these families and children in daily life [36, 37]. Regarding collectivistic cultures, for example, Taiwanese families reported that they have limited social support resources and social networks, and they have also less interaction with their close relatives [38]. On the other hand,

Fatimilehin and Nadirshaw [37] found that Asian and African families received more support compared to British families. The contradictory findings about collectivistic cultures could be explained with vertical and horizontal collectivism [33]. In horizontal collectivism, each member has equal status in the group [39]. Emphasizing equality might lead to increase tolerance and acceptance of families of children with disabilities. On the other hand, in vertical collectivism, there are differences between status of the group members, namely hierarchy [39]. People with mental health problems are believed to violate social harmony or negatively influence families' reputation in these collectivistic cultures [40]. These thoughts lead to feelings of shame, fear and blame, which in turn linked to increased social distance and negative relationships with people with disabilities [41]. The dominance of hierarchy among group members in Thailand compared to other African countries also supports these findings [42]. The principle of equality between members in collectivistic cultures increases the likelihood of individuals being accepted and supported within the group, independent of their cognitive functionality [37].

In addition, studies indicated that cultural values may have indirect effects on social support resources. In this context, researchers claimed that beliefs about the causes of LD play a significant role in explaining the relationships [37, 38, 43, 44]. Belief is the mental representation of people about what is right or wrong [45]. These mental representations might be based on scientific or non-scientific knowledge [46]. Recently, efforts to generate a comprehensive understanding of public responses to disabilities resulted in assessing the role of beliefs about causes of disabilities on families in various cultures. Based on lay people's causal attributions of disability, researchers have defined some basic causal beliefs in the literature; biomedical (e.g., genetic mutations), environmental (e.g., lack of daytime occupation), supernatural/fate (e.g., being punished by God), adversity (e.g., suffering abuse as a child) [47]. The scientific evaluations of the disability (biomedical) decreased people's anxiety levels and stigma hence increasing their skills for providing effective social support. On the other hand, non-scientific attributions to the causes of disabilities result in higher endorsement of social distance by increasing negative reactions such as anger and anxiety [36]. Regarding cultural differences, studies indicated that individuals scored higher on collectivistic values tended to attribute disability to religious and environmental causes, and report less biomedical causes of the disability in comparison to people scored higher on individualistic values [37, 48]. Similarly, in collectivistic cultures, families emphasized that their relatives strongly believe the child's diagnosis is a God's plan of punishment for their past wrongdoings [38]. They also expressed these beliefs as the source of perceived stress, stigma, and social distance. In turn, stigma and social distance had adverse effects on families' help-seeking behaviors and their attainment to support services.

Parents' own non-scientific beliefs might also negatively influence their professional and educational help-seeking behaviors [49]. To illustrate, parents' beliefs about the role of self-discipline, an imbalance between body fluids and organs, and supernatural influences on disabilities shaped their understanding about LD and their help-seeking behaviors in China. These beliefs were linked with parents' preferences for searching religious (e.g., seeing a religious person) and lifestyle (e.g., diet to balance foods and drinks) interventions instead of professional, educational and rehabilitation services. In all, causal beliefs determine families' and public reactions to disability, which in turn linked with their help-seeking behaviors for attaining professional and social support resources [49, 50].

When the link between cultural values and beliefs examined, it was seen that there were also cross-cultural differences in terms of the meanings attributed to success and failure. Given that LD are described with academic failure, such references to success and failure may also change public attitudes towards families of children with LD. In general, while people attribute success to intrinsic factors (e.g., abilities) and failures to external factors (e.g., bad luck) in individualistic cultures, in collectivistic cultures, it is the opposite. These attributions to failures result in parents to be seen as responsible for children's failure in academic settings in collectivist cultures. Similarly, parents often blame themselves for the failure of their children that lead to decrease families' information-seeking behaviors [49]. In addition, social and interdependent motives for success and failure in collectivistic cultures are argued to be linked with emphasizing less the role of personal effort on change and development [30]. For example, parents believed that failures of their children were the result of unsuccessful parent–child relationship instead of their children's lack of abilities in China [49]. Therefore, mothers give more priority to focus on improving their close relationship by applying parental control for children's academic success [49]. On the contrary, mothers scored higher individualistic values were believing more in the significance of early development in childhood and motivated their children about personal effort or practice for the achievement [48]. Researchers have also found that attainment of children in support resources in different contexts (e.g., home, school) and their academic success decreased, when parents overlooked the role of effort on achievement [51]. In spite of the considerable amount of information accumulated in previous within-culture studies, future studies could enhance our understanding about assessing the cross-cultural differences in terms of the differential role of cultural values on attributions to LD.

In sum, according to ecocultural theory, each culture constructs their own ecological characteristics such as values, beliefs and attributions, and this ecology influences the families' support seeking behaviors, child rearing practices and child development. Inspection of the values, attribution and beliefs contributed to our understanding of how they shape families' daily routines, activities, and relationships [10, 52, 53]. In the context of LD, we believe that causal beliefs and attributions to failure and success might have mediator roles between cultural values and families' support resources. On the other hand, instead of the role of cultural values, researchers discussed the role of education, technology and developmental level of countries in determining public knowledge, attitudes and beliefs about disabilities. Both lay people and families in collectivistic countries reported that they have less knowledge about disabilities, and they have limited chances to get information from professionals [37, 47]. When the participants' educational and knowledge level controlled, the cross-cultural differences in terms of negative attitudes and non-scientific beliefs of disabilities disappeared across groups in previous studies [33, 54]. As a result, it is argued that cross-cultural differences might decrease with the improvement in educational, technological and informational innovations of the cultures. Future studies might examine cultures with a range of ecological factors, from values and beliefs to educational and technological development of the countries.

4.3.3 Family social support resources

Based on the ecocultural theory, Nihira and colleagues [23] formed twelve ecocultural factors (e.g., integration into non-disabled networks) via home interviews of families of children with disabilities; predicting 30–60% variance of the child developmental outcomes. Children usually need help in academic, behavioral and social domains. More commonly, special education and specific education techniques are used for the improvement of academic abilities. LD, with its diagnosis and treatment process, is an impairment that affects an individual's life-span development. With disability, child's necessities, families' needs, well-being, resources, activities, routines and qualities are also influenced [55]. Previous studies demonstrated that families of children with LD perceive the disability as a source of stressor and experience more stress than families of children without disabilities [2]. Since Hastings [56] proposed that stressful parents developed certain parenting behaviors (e.g., using more control), these parenting behaviors tended to reinforce the child's problem behaviors. Social support resources are linked with higher quality of care, especially by reducing stress levels of caregivers and maintaining their well-being [57–59]. In other words, these ecocultural support resources provide a protective context for the families and children [23]. This linkage forms the basic assumption of the ecocultural theory.

In the LD literature, the relation between total social support score and child outcomes was mainly studied instead of specific support resources. It was seen that the studies mainly overlooked the differential effects of specific support resources on child problem behaviors [8]. Thus, differently from previous studies, the effects of specific support resources were evaluated separately as indicated in the ecocultural theory. Given the importance of these ecocultural factors on the development, the current study covers seven of these factors (e.g., socioeconomic status, multiple service usage), and these resources are conceptualized under four support resources (e.g., financial, informational support) (see **Table 1**). In addition to these resources, emotional support to family support resources also added based on previous work [8].

4.3.3.1 Informational support

Multiple service usage (accessibility and utilization of services), variety and amount of formal and instrumental help (support received from professionals, programs or partners), and the use of information from professionals (information-seeking for child prognosis and well-being) are described as *informational support*. Families of children with LD reported that they did not receive sufficient information and support from professionals [38, 49, 59]. Therefore, they have difficulties in understanding the diagnosis and they concern about the prognosis [38, 52]. Lack of information about the diagnosis and prognosis might negatively influence families' help-seeking behaviors for attaining in educational and psychological services [43, 52].

Informational support was argued to motivate parents in guiding their children for academic achievement. For example, groups of mothers with and without familial risk for dyslexia (having parent or close relative with dyslexia in family history) were examined in a longitudinal study in terms of their causal attributions concerning their children's success and failure. For the group of children with familial risk of dyslexia, researchers found that mothers tended to attribute their children's success less to

Ecocultural Support Resources	Families Support Resources
1. Family socioeconomic status 2. Parent's occupation or employment status	Financial support
3. Connectedness of family (e.g., spousal relationship)	Intimate relations support
4. Supplemental help for family 5. Help available within family	Caregiving support
6. Multiple service usage 7. Variety and amount of formal and instrumental help 8. Use of information from professionals	Informational support
9. The availability and satisfaction of emotional support from significant others	Emotional support

Table 1.
Families Social Support Resources within the Framework of Ecocultural Theory.

children's own reading and writing ability and effort, and they were less confident with their children's abilities during the first grade [60]. They argued that mothers' beliefs about improvement of children's literacy skills decreased, and feelings of hopelessness increased during the first grade. It has been stated that mothers' lack of knowledge, and their own negative experiences about dyslexia lead to low motivation and negative attributions for success, which in turn linked with children's lower academic achievement [60]. Emphasizing the role of special education methods, effort and practice on the improvement of literacy skills can contribute to parents' awareness and supportive behaviors. Parents might be motivated to rearrange their home environment which can be sensitive to the needs of their children [54, 60]. Intervention programs also indicated that supporting parents in terms of guiding their children resulted in the improvement of children reading and writing skills [61].

Informational support is also linked with socio-emotional developmental outcomes of children. For example, it was found that children of parents who reported higher information support demonstrated less internalization problems [7]. Perceived informational support could help parents how to deal effectively with disability and to understand child's emotions related to failure. This may result in guiding the child about regulating their negative emotions and learning to express their feelings. In conclusion, it was mainly argued that information and support taken from professionals were generally inadequate [49, 59]. Getting informational support about diagnosis, prognosis and intervention strategies were especially emphasized to be beneficial for patents in dealing with behavioral, educational and emotional needs of the children [8, 53].

4.3.3.2 Caregiving support

Supplemental help for family (additional help in child care received from relatives or grandparents) and help available within family (availability of help received from husband or other children at home) are called as *caregiving support*. Studies indicated that caregiving support have a significant role for primary caregivers of children with LD [23]. School and educational workload make it difficult for caregivers to find enough time to meet their basic needs (e.g., visiting a doctor), which in turn associated with caregivers' feelings of burnout [52, 62, 63]. For example, full-time working parents experiencing a range of home-, work- and child-related difficulties have reported more concerns about their physical and psychological health and less interest in social activities [52]. When a caregiver shares the daily care burden with a significant other, this support might be protective for the psychological and physiological well-being. Since mothers are usually the primary caregiver in all over the world [64], mothers who are not receiving adequate caregiving support can be regarded as a risky group in terms of psychological and physical health. Social policies providing services for fulfilling mothers' physical and social needs can also support their participation in social life [63]. Researchers should elaborate on what kind of resources mothers of children with LD need or use in case of a lack of caregiving support in future studies.

4.3.3.3 Financial support

Nihira and colleagues [23] assessed socioeconomic status as income level and parent's occupation or employment status. However, instead of assessing only income level and parents' employment status, we have also evaluated families' perception and satisfaction of this support resource and its effect on child development. Experiencing economic difficulties or low financial support can influence child development directly or indirectly. It is important for families to access psychological, special education, and sometimes medical services to support their children's social, emotional, cognitive, and biological development. The access to these resources has a direct effect on child development; however, this can be costly for families. Financial support would create the chance for the child in attaining additional educational or psychological support services [23, 59]. Experiencing economic difficulties could have indirect influences on families and children by increasing family stress and certain parenting behaviors (e.g., strict discipline, low warmth). The elevated family stress negatively affects parents' involvement and investments in education of the children [29]. Also, children of mothers reporting low financial support demonstrated more problem behaviors such as externalizing problems [8, 65]. We can speculate that mothers might focus more on children's educational and socio-emotional needs, and cope better with the problems when they have low financial stress and chance to attain additional support services.

4.3.3.4 Intimate relations support

Connectedness of family, the quality of relationship between parents and father's help in child care are described as *intimate relations support*. Researchers claim that marital satisfaction spills over to parenting by increasing parents' self-efficacy, and reducing parenting stress and depression [66, 67]. In other words, a consistent and supportive close relationship supports both the well-being of the caregiver and parenting behaviors, which in turn linked to an increase in children's academic achievement and well-being [68, 69].

More broadly, studies involving the mothers of children with LD examined the marital relationship from a different perspective and indicated that this close relationship could be also affected by the diagnosis process [38, 62, 70]. In a qualitative study, parents reported that the disability had both positive and negative effects on their family relationships. While disability results in an increase in family harmony, awareness, and supporting each other in the majority of families, some families reported that blaming the child as a source of distress and difficulties in communication between family members negatively influenced the family system [38]. Researchers assessed deeply the causes of negative effects of disability on family relationship. Denial of the child's diagnosis, differences in parent's developmental expectations, inequalities in shared care arrangements, and financial problems lead to decrease in the quality of marital relationship [67]. Since parents of children with LD reported higher anxiety and depression levels compared to parents of children without any developmental disabilities [71], we can speculate that parental stress, economical handicaps and negative reactions to diagnosis would be negatively associated with marital quality in families of children with LD. According to family system theories, if the individual is the part of an organized family system, he or she is never truly independent and can be understood in the family context [72, 73]. Families are composed of subsystems such as marital subsystem, parent–child subsystem, male and female subsystems that are nested structures and influence each other. When one of the parents could not deal with a stressful condition, this parent would have difficulty in providing support to other family members in coping with their negative emotions. As a result, developing a new working mechanism of the family and connectedness of the family becomes even more significant for these families.

To summarize, although spousal or close relationship support is an important support mechanism for parents in dealing with disability, the quality of close relationship seems to be related to many factors such as reactions to diagnosis process. In future studies, researchers should examine why some families have such a positive experience while others do not. In other words, future works should focus on the role of individual and contextual factors in determining the nature of intimate relations support.

4.3.3.5 Emotional support

This support captures the availability and satisfaction of emotional support (e.g., sharing one's anxiety, feelings, happiness with someone) taken from close relatives and friends etc. Caregivers of children with LD reported mostly feelings of anger, anxiety, frustration, and helplessness [38, 53, 59]. Karande et al. [74] found that 75% of mothers of children with LD reported mild anxiety levels. Academic failure of children, uncertainty about the future and children behavioral problems resulted in a higher occurrence of anxiety in mothers. Caregivers reported that they generally suppress their negative emotions experienced during and after the diagnosis process, rather than sharing with their families, friends or relatives [38]. One of the reason was that their close environment was not willing to take enough time for listening to their problems [38, 52]. Also, parents clarified that their close environment could not understand themselves emotionally, even if they were able to provide caregiving or informational supports to them. If the mothers have the opportunity to share their negative emotions with their friends or relatives, they will be better in coping with the stress associated with the disability [52]. Receiving emotional support may lead parents to calm down or help them to regulate their negative feelings [75]. In turn, these mothers may deal with both their own and their children's unregulated emotions better and create a warm environment for their children [8].

5. The integrated model

In modern developmental theories, the ecological environment was defined as a set of nested structures, including proximal (e.g., family) and distal (e.g., culture) processes. The ecocultural theory is one of these new approaches that integrate family ecology, members, and culture into one ground [9, 11] and assumes that familial (e.g., specific support resources) and cultural factors (e.g., values) organize and shape family activities, routines, and resources. As mentioned before, researchers greatly increased our understanding of the role of cultural and family factors in determining child development [8, 23, 44]. Based on both findings of empirical studies and ecocultural perspective, we presented an integrated model including both proximal (family) and distal (culture) contextual factors for evaluating child development (see **Figure 1**).

Researchers discussed that children's and families' experiences should be examined with the context of social, economic, educational policies and welfare of the societies [51, 53]. In the cultural level, we included a range of ecological characteristics in predicting child development such as cultural values, education system, economical welfare, technological innovations, educational goals for children with LD, inclusion policy in education system, public knowledge and awareness about LD. To illustrate, a computerized training program implemented at primary schools of Finland has been found to be effective among children with dyslexia [61]. The program included enhancing the accuracy of processing for phonemic sounds and learning to connect phonemes, and this program was implemented with the help of special education teachers. Creating such an enriched environment for supporting children's learning process at homes and schools might also increase collaboration and interaction between parents and teachers [29]. Effective parental involvement in inclusive educational settings could increase their knowledge about interventions and quality of parental involvement in home-based learning situations. This would be one of the key factors that promote child's competence and development.

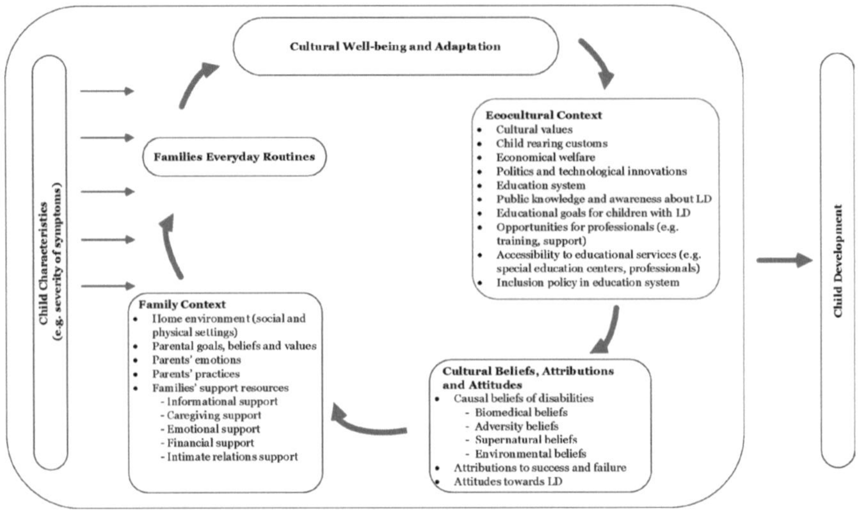

Figure 1.
An integrated model for evaluating the role of ecocultural and family context on child development in learning disabilities within the scope of ecocultural theory. Note. The model was formed by authors based on previous work of assessing child development [10] and disabilities [23, 48] with ecocultural perspective [9, 10, 22].

In addition, the model assumes that linkages between cultural values and family support resources may be traced back, at least to some extent, to the public beliefs about LD, attributions to success or failure, and attitudes towards families of children with LD. To illustrate, vertical collectivism negatively influences the interpretation and attributions of lay people about disability, which in turn linked with more negative attitudes towards families and children. The negative view of LD restricts the support resources and social networks of families in terms of access to professional, educational and social support services [44, 48]. Thus, negative attitudes and unrealistic beliefs about LD could be considered as risk factors for families and children [29, 53]. Inspection of these links would enhance our understanding of how families' support resources are processed by cultural values, beliefs and attributions in future studies.

In the family level, specific support resources have a significant role on the family system. In particular, each specific support resources compensate different requirements of the family. For example, while emotional support helps family members in dealing with their negative emotions, professional support provides information about diagnosis, treatment processes and formal services to motivate the family for change and adaptation. Future studies might benefit from examining differential role of specific support resources on families, and linkages between specific support resources and cultural factors. In addition, we included characteristics of home environment, parents' emotions and practices in the model to develop a comprehensive evaluation of family environment. For example, chaos and stress in family environment, and parents' unregulated negative emotions would have negative influences on family relationships, parenting behaviors (e.g. strict discipline) and child development. Further, Kağıtçıbaşı [32] argued that the values at the cultural level shapes individuals' actions and tendencies, but could not explain all individuals' behaviors and motivations. That's why parents' internalized values, beliefs and goals were included in the family context as determinants of behavior.

Recently, the child's influence on the family functioning and parenting have been so widely recognized by researchers [75]. According to modern developmental perspectives, children are active agents in constructing their environment and there is an interaction between children and environment [20]. Studies indicated that severity of symptoms of LD altered the effect of disabilities on the families and children such as parent–child relationships and child outcomes [8, 76, 77]. For example, it was observed that mothers' perceived emotional support had no significant effect on children externalizing problem behaviors when the severity of symptoms of children increased [8]. Since the severity of symptoms might be an important determinant in assessing development of children and functioning of families, we included the child characteristics (e.g. severity of symptoms) in the model. Future research might benefit including severity of LD when examining the relationship between family contextual variables and child developmental outcomes.

In all, the model presumes that the functioning of families and children are multiply determined, that source of contextual stress and support can directly or indirectly affect parents and children by influencing their family support resources. Assessing the relations with individual and contextual factors along with the interaction between individual-contextual factors would enable us to take different factors into account and help to capture a more comprehensive picture of families' and children's experiences. Since developmental interventions aim to change the links between predictors and outcomes [78], establishing a knowledge about precursors, mediators and/or moderators about families' experiences and resources would increase effectiveness of the future interventions.

6. Conclusion and implications for professionals

Inspection of the influence of contextual factors on beliefs, resources, and development of children provided unique preliminary findings on significant aspects of the experience of children with LD. These findings might guide the practices of the professionals and policies for interventions in this field in different ways. First, the Individualized Education Program (IEP) addresses educational goals for children with disabilities in various academic domains (e.g., mathematic, reading, etc.), and it guides professionals and families in terms of managing, monitoring, and organizing the children's special education process [79]. Researchers clarified that teachers and parents should work together on the development of a comprehensive understanding of the special educational needs of children [79].

IEP is one of the educational procedures in which parents, teachers, and children could meaningfully communicate for academic progress [80]. Parents and teachers seemed to have difficulties in communication with each other for IEP due to a variety of reasons such as parents' lack of knowledge and low motivation for effort and change, teachers' bias about the role of parents in the educational process, and lack of enough time, etc. [80]. Also, as we have stressed before, parents could hold diverse beliefs of disability depending on their cultural orientation, and in these circumstances, these beliefs might limit parents' or families' patterns of behaviors in attaining professional support. Despite a considerable amount of work on parents' beliefs about disability, assessment of teachers' beliefs and attributions have been overlooked in the literature. Even with an educational background, teachers could have contradictory beliefs of disabilities (both biological and environmental) at the same time and biases about the prognosis of disability based on their cultural background and experiences.

In order to increase collaboration between teachers and families, both families and teachers should gain a reflection about their own beliefs and assumptions about disabilities. To achieve this, training sessions and support services for professionals should include raising awareness about their own beliefs and attributions of disabilities, and the role of families' values and beliefs. Through these training programs, teachers might develop their own strategy and guideline for how to provide effective informational support to families. Also, teachers could improve the involvement of families in children educational program by taking actions in (1) acknowledging families' context, routines, beliefs, values and knowledge about disabilities, (2) improving parent's knowledge, awareness, and information about the disability and prognosis. If parents are able to understand the significance of IEP, they will be more willing to collaborate with teachers in order to monitor their children's progress and inclusion in education. Children should also be included in their IEP program meetings with their parents. Parents and children might be provided with an optimal environment that they can express their views, concerns, and emotions about the progress. Expressing themselves and providing motivation for change and effort to families in school context would spill over to families' experiences in home context such as increasing families coping, children motivation for achievement and doing homework [81].

Recently, based on an education support modeling, teachers, families, volunteers, and peers of children are coming together in social and educational activities to increase collaboration, to deal with learning barriers and communication problems [82]. Through such activities, school community could lead to an increase in their helping behaviors towards families. This participation and awareness might influence parent's perception and attainment to support resources positively, which in turn might also lead to a decrease in rejection, stigmatization, and stereotypes in the society.

In conclusion, ecocultural theory emphasizes the role of family support resources, cultural values and beliefs on families of children with LD. In particular, ecocultural understanding would support our knowledge about (1) the relationship between families' distal and proximal environments, (2) the influence of family and cultural factors on parenting and child development, (3) considering roles of children and families in shaping their environment, (4) guiding researchers in developing intervention programs more sensitive to individual, familial and cultural characteristics of children with LD, (5) developing educational and inclusion policies to increase professionals, school community and public awareness about causal beliefs, attributions and attitudes towards LD.

Author details

Suzan Cen-Yagiz* and Berna Aytac
Department of Psychology, Faculty of Letters, Hacettepe University, Turkey

*Address all correspondence to: suzancen@hacettepe.edu.tr

References

[1] American Psychiatric Association. Diagnostic and statistical manual of mental disorders 5th ed. Arlington, VA: American Psychiatric Publishing; 2013.

[2] Antshel K M, Joseph G R. Maternal stress in nonverbal learning disorder: A comparison with reading disorder. Journal of Learning Disabilities. 2006; 39(3): 194-205. doi:10.1177/0022219406 0390030101

[3] Lyytinen H, Ahonen T, Eklund K, Guttorm T K, Laakso M L, Leinonen, S., ... Viholainen H. Developmental pathways of children with and without familial risk for dyslexia during the first years of life. Developmental Neuropsychology. 2001; 20(2): 535-554.

[4] Keogh B K, Gallimore R, Weisner T. A sociocultural perspective on learning and learning disabilities. Learning Disabilities Research and Practice. 1997; 12(2): 107-113.

[5] Al-Yagon M, Mikulincer M. Socioemotional and academic adjustment among children with learning disorders: The mediational role of attachment-based factors. The Journal of Special Education. 2004; 38(2): 111-123.

[6] Dyson L L. Children with learning disabilities within the family context: A comparison with siblings in global self–concept, academic self–perception, and social competence. Learning Disabilities Research and Practice. 2003; 18(1): 1-9.

[7] Heiman T, Berger O. Parents of children with Asperger syndrome or with learning disabilities: Family environment and social support. Research in Developmental Disabilities. (2008): 29(4): 289. 300.

[8] Cen S, Aytac B. Ecocultural perspective in learning disability: Family support resources, values, child problem behaviors. Learning Disability Quarterly. 2017; 40(2): 114-127.

[9] Weisner T S. The ecocultural project of human development: Why ethnography and its findings matter. Ethos. 1997; 25(2): 177-190.

[10] Weisner T S. Ecocultural understanding of children developmental pathways. Human Development. 2002a; 45(4): 275-281.

[11] Weisner T S. Essay review making a good thing better: ways to strengthen sociocultural research in human development essay review of children's engagement in the world: Sociocultural perspectives by Artin Göncü. Human Development. 2002b; 45: 372-380.

[12] Bernheimer L P, Gallimore R, Weisner T S. Ecocultural theory as a context for the individual family service plan. Journal of Early Intervention. 1990; 14(3): 219-233.

[13] Kargin T, Guldenoglu B. Learning Disabilities Research and Practice in Turkey. Learning Disabilities -A Contemporary Journal. 2016; 14(1): 71-78.

[14] Bruck, M. Social and emotional adjustment of learning disabled children: A review of the issues. In Ceci S J, editor. Handbook of cognitive, social, and neuropsychological aspects of learning disabilities. Routledge, Taylor and Francis; 1986. p. 361-369.

[15] Al-Yagon M. Perceived close relationships with parents, teachers, and peers: Predictors of social, emotional, and behavioral features in adolescents with LD or comorbid LD and ADHD. Journal of Learning Disabilities. 2016; 49(6): 597-615.

[16] Greenham S L. Learning disabilities and psychosocial adjustment: A critical review. Child Neuropsychology. 1999; 5(3): 171-196.

[17] Rogoff B. The cultural nature of human development. New York, NY: Oxford University Press; (2003).

[18] Trommsdorff, G. An eco-cultural and interpersonal relations approach to development over the life span. Online readings in Psychology and Culture. 2002. Available from: http://kops.uni-konstanz.de/handle/123456789/11063 [Accessed: 2020-11-22]

[19] Worthman C M. The ecology of human development: Evolving models for cultural psychology. Journal of Cross-Cultural Psychology. 2010; 41(4): 546-562.

[20] Super C M. Harkness S. Culture structures the environment for development. Human Development. 2002; 45(4): 270-274.

[21] Bronfenbrenner U. Ecology of the family as a context for human development: Research perspectives. Developmental Psychology, 1986; 22(6): 723-742.

[22] Weisner T S. Human development, child well-being, and the cultural project of development. New Directions for Child Development. 1998; 81: 69-85.

[23] Nihira K, Weisner T S, Bernheimer L P. Ecocultural assessment in families of children with developmental delays: construct and concurrent validities. American Journal on Mental Retardation. 1994; 98: 551-566.

[24] Phenice L A, Griffore R J, Hakoyama M, Silvey L A. Ecocultural adaptive research: A synthesis of ecocultural theory, participatory research, and adaptive designs. Family and Consumer Sciences Research Journal. 2009; 37(3): 298-309.

[25] Skinner D, Weisner T S. Sociocultural studies of families of children with intellectual disabilities. Mental Retardation and Developmental Disabilities Research Reviews. 2007. DOI: 10.1002/mrdd.20170

[26] Daley T C, Weisner T S. "I speak a different dialect": Teen explanatory models of difference and disability. Medical Anthropology Quarterly. 2003; 17: 25-48.

[27] Kellegrew D H. Constructing daily routines: A qualitative examination of mothers with young children with disabilities. American Journal of Occupational Therapy. 2000; 54(3): 252-259.

[28] Bull L. The Use of Support groups by parents of children with dyslexia, early child development and care. 2003; 173 (2-3): 341-347.

[29] Yotyodying S, Wild E. Predictors of the quantity and different qualities of home-based parental involvement: Evidence from parents of children with learning disabilities. Learning and Individual Differences. 2016; 49: 74-84.

[30] Markus H R, Kitayama S. Culture and the self: Implications for cognition, emotion, and motivation. Psychological Review. 1991; 98(2), 224-253.

[31] Schwartz S. A theory of cultural values and some implications for work. Applied Psychology. 1999. DOI:10.1080/026999499377655

[32] Kağıtçıbaşı Ç. Family, self, and human development across cultures: Theory and applications. New Jersey, NJ: Psychology Press; 2009.

[33] Hampton N Z, Xiao F. Attitudes toward people with developmental disabilities in Chinese and American students: The role of cultural values, contact, and knowledge. Journal of Rehabilitation. 2007; 73(3): 23-32.

[34] Celinska D K. Narrative Voices of Early Adolescents: Influences of

Learning Disability and Cultural Background. International Journal of Special Education. 2009; 24(3): 150-172.

[35] Pestana C. A qualitative exploration of the life experiences of adults diagnosed with mild learning disabilities from minority ethnic communities. Tizard Learning Disability Review. 2011. DOI:10.1108/13595471111185701

[36] Scior K, Hamid A, Mahfoudhi A, Abdalla F. The relationship between awareness of intellectual disability, causal and intervention beliefs and social distance in Kuwait and the UK. Research in Developmental Disabilities. 2013; 34 (11): 3896-3905.

[37] Fatimilehin I A, Nadirshaw Z. A cross-cultural study of parental attitudes and beliefs about learning disability (mental handicap). Mental Handicap Research. 1994; 7(3): 202-227.

[38] Chang M Y, Hsu L L. The perceptions of Taiwanese families who have children with learning disability. Journal of Clinical Nursing. 2007; 16 (12): 2349-2356.

[39] Triandis H C. Collectivism and individualism as cultural syndromes. Cross-Cultural Research. 1993; 27 (3-4): 155-180.

[40] Stone-Mac Donald, A. Cultural beliefs about disability in practice: experiences at a special school in Tanzania. International Journal of Disability, Development and Education; 2012; 59(4): 393-407.

[41] Furnham A, Chan E. Lay theories of schizophrenia. Social Psychiatry and Psychiatric Epidemiology. 2004; 39(7): 543-552.

[42] Schwartz S H. Les valeurs de base de la personne: Théorie, mesures et applications [Basic human values: Theory, measurement, and applications]. Revue Française De Sociologie. 2006; 42: 249-288.

[43] Jorm A F. Mental health literacy: Public knowledge and beliefs about mental disorders. The British Journal of Psychiatry. 2000; 177(5): 396-401.

[44] O'Hara J. Learning disabilities and ethnicity: Achieving cultural competence. Advances in Psychiatric Treatment. 2003; 9(3): 166-174.

[45] Demirutku K. Parenting styles, internalization of values, and the self-concept. [thesis]. Ankara: Middle east Technical University; 2007.

[46] Österholm M. Beliefs: A theoretically unnecessary construct?. In Sixth Congress of the European Society for Research in Mathematics Education; January 28th-February 1st 2009, Lyon, France Institut National de Recherche Pédagogique; 2010. p. 154-163.

[47] Scior K, Furnham A. Development and validation of the Intellectual Disability Literacy Scale for assessment of knowledge, beliefs and attitudes to intellectual disability. Research in Developmental Disabilities. 2011; 32(5): 1530-1541.

[48] Harry B. Trends and issues in serving culturally diverse families of children with disabilities. The Journal of Special Education. 2002; 36(3): 132-140.

[49] Tews L, Merali N. Helping Chinese parents understand and support children with learning disabilities. Professional Psychology: Research and Practice. 2008; 39(2): 137-144.

[50] Jorm A F. Mental health literacy: Empowering the community to take action for better mental health. American Psychologist. 2012; 67(3): 231-243.

[51] Shifrer D. *stigma* and stratification limiting the math course progression of adolescents labeled with a learning disability. Learning and Instruction. 2016; 42: 47-57.

[52] Chien W T, Lee I Y. An exploratory study of parents' perceived educational needs for parenting a child with learning disabilities. Asian Nursing Research. 2013; 7(1): 16-25.

[53] Katchergin O. Between negative stigma (cultural deprivation) and positive stigma (learning disability): the historical development of two special education tracks. Culture, Medicine, and Psychiatry. 2012; 36(4): 679-711.

[54] Blundell R, Das R, Potts H, Scior K. The association between contact and intellectual disability literacy, causal attributions and stigma. Journal of Intellectual Disability Research. 2016; 60(3): 218-227

[55] Lancaster P E. Parenting children with learning disabilities. In: Fine M J, Lee S W, editors. Handbook of Diversity in Parent Education. 2001. p. 231-252. DOI:10.1016/ B978-012256483- 3/50012-5

[56] Hastings R P. Parental stress and behaviour problems of children with developmental disability. Journal of Intellectual and Developmental Disability. 2002; 27(3): 149-160.

[57] Cantwell J, Muldoon O T, Gallagher S. Social support and mastery influence the association between stress and poor physical health in parents caring for children with developmental disabilities. Research in Developmental Disabilities. 2014; 35(9): 2215-2223.

[58] Chukwu N E, Okoye U O, Onyeneho N G, Okeibunor J C. Coping strategies of families of persons with learning disability in Imo state of Nigeria. Journal of Health, Population and Nutrition. 2019; 38(1): 1-9.

[59] Sandy P T, Kgole J C. Mavundla T R. Support needs of caregivers: Case studies in South Africa. International Nursing Review. 2013; 60(3): 344-350.

[60] Natale K, Aunola K, Nurmi J E, Poikkeus A M, Lyytinen P, Lyytinen H. Mothers' causal attributions concerning the reading achievement of their children with and without familial risk for dyslexia. Journal of Learning Disabilities. 2008; 41(3): 274-285.

[61] Hintikka S, Aro M, Lyytinen H. Computerized training of the correspondences between phonological and orthographic units. Written Language and Literacy. 2005; 8(2): 79-102.

[62] Ciğerli Ö, Topsever P, Alvur T M, Görpelioğlu S. Engelli çocuğu olan anne-babaların tanı anından itibaren ebeveynlik deneyimleri: Farklılığı kabullenmek. Turkish Journal of Family Medicine and Primary Care. 2014; 8(3): 75-81.

[63] Milliken A, Mahoney E K, Mahoney K J, Mignosa K, Rodriguez I, Cuchetti C, Inoue M. “I'm just trying to cope for both of us”: Challenges and supports of family caregivers in participant- directed programs. Journal of Gerontological Social Work. 2019; 62(2): 149-171.

[64] Edwards P C, Ren L, Brown J. Early contexts of learning: family and community socialization during infancy and toddlerhood. In: Jensen L A, editor. The Oxford handbook of human development and culture: An interdisciplinary perspective. New York: Oxford University Press. 2015. p. 165-184.

[65] Flouri E, Midouhas E, Ruddy A, Moulton V. The role of socio-economic disadvantage in the development of comorbid emotional and conduct problems in children with ADHD. European Child and Adolescent Psychiatry. 2017; 26(6): 723-732.

[66] Kersh J, Hedvat T T, Hauser-Cram P, Warfield M E. The contribution of marital quality to the well-being of parents of children with developmental disabilities. Journal of Intellectual Disability Research. 2006; 50 (12): 883-893.

[67] Abd Rauf A A, Akmar Ismail M, Balakrishnan V, Cheong L S, Admodisastro N I, Haruna K. Analysis of support for parents in raising children with dyslexia. Journal of Family Issues. 2020. DOI: 0192513X20948925.

[68] Cohen S R, Holloway S D, Domínguez-Pareto I, Kuppermann M. Support and self-efficacy among Latino and White parents of children with ID. American Journal on Intellectual and Developmental Disabilities. 2015; 120(1): 16-31.

[69] Taderera C, Hall H. Challenges faced by parents of children with learning disabilities in Opuwo, Namibia. African Journal of Disability. 2017; 6(1): 1-10.

[70] Kanbir A E. Engelli çocuğa sahip ailelerde evlilik doyumu: Niteliksel bir çalışma. [thesis]. İstanbul: Maltepe University; 2018.

[71] Bonifacci P, Montuschi M, Lami L, Snowling M J. Parents of children with dyslexia: Cognitive, emotional and behavioural profile. Dyslexia. 2014; 20(2): 175-190.

[72] Mandak K, O'Neill T, Light J, Fosco G M. Bridging the gap from values to actions: a family systems framework for family-centered AAC services. Augmentative and Alternative Communication. 2017; 33(1): 32-41.

[73] Minuchin P. Families and individual development: Provocations from the field of family therapy. Child Development. 1985; 289-302.

[74] Karande S, Bhosrekar K, Kulkarni M, Thakker A. Health-related quality of life of children with newly diagnosed specific learning disability. Journal of Tropical Pediatrics. 2009; 55(3): 160-169.

[75] Belsky J. The determinants of parenting: A process model. Child Development. 1984; 83-96.

[76] Cen-Yagiz S, Aytac B. A Multi-Informant Study: Mother–Child relationship and children with learning disability. International Journal of Disability, Development and Education. 2019; 1-16.

[77] Capozzi F, Casini M P, Romani M, De Gennaro L, Nicolais G, Solano L Psychiatric comorbidity in learning disorder: Analysis of family variables. Child Psychiatry and Human Development. 2008; 39(1): 101-110.

[78] Weisz J R, Sandler I N, Durlak J. A, Anton B S. Promoting and protecting youth mental health through evidence-based prevention and treatment. American Psychologist. 2005; 60(6): 628-648.

[79] Connor D J, Cavendi sh W. Sharing power with parent s: Improving educational decision making for student s with learning disabilities. Learning Disability Quarterly. 2018; 41(2):79-84.

[80] Lalvani P. Disability, stigma and otherness: Perspectives of parents and teachers. International Journal of Disability, Development and Education. (2015); 62(4): 379-393.

[81] Hagger M S, Sultan S, Hardcastle S J, Chatzisarantis N L. Perceived autonomy support and autonomous motivation toward mathematics activities in educational and out-of- school contexts is related to mathematics homework behavior and attainment. Contemporary Educational Psychology. 2015; 41: 111-123.

[82] Gómez-Zepeda G, Petreñas C, Sabando D, Puigdellívol I. The role of the Support and Attention to Diversity Teacher (SADT) from a community-based perspective: Promoting educational success and educational inclusion for all. Teaching and Teacher Education. 2017; 64: 127-138.

Chapter 11

Eye Tracking Using Nonverbal Tasks Could Contribute to Diagnostics of Developmental Dyslexia and Developmental Language Disorder

Zuzana Bilkova, Martin Dobias, Jaromir Dolezal, Vratislav Fabian, Helena Havlisova, Jiri Jost and Olga Malinovska

Abstract

There are not many studies dealing with a comparison of the eye movements of individuals with dyslexia and developmental language disorder (DLD). The aim of this study is to compare the eye movements in the two most common language disorders, dyslexia and DLD and to consider their contribution to diagnostics. In the research the oculomotor test was administered to 60 children with the clinical diagnosis of dyslexia or DLD and 58 typically developing children (controls). The test included a prosaccadic task, antisaccadic task and a nonverbal sequential task with self regulation of the pace. Controls could be singled out from other two clinical groups by means of the oculomotor imaging. Both of the clinical groups in comparison with the controls were characterized by worse overall performance. Through the employment of the oculomotor it was possible to differentiate between both of the clinical groups. The dyslexics had an overall worse oculomotor performance than the DLD group. The results of the study show that the oculomotor test has the potential to contribute to diagnostics of dyslexia and DLD and the screening of these disorders at pre-school age.

Keywords: saccade, antisaccade, dyslexia, developmental language disorder, orthographic complexity

1. Introduction

Developmental language disorder (DLD, also called specific language impairment or developmental dysphasia) is characterized by difficulties in the acquisition and the use of language with a co-existing absence of any clear etiology – hearing impairment, intellectual disability, neurological or psychiatric findings and insufficient language stimuli. Difficulties include a delayed start and slower acquisition of lexical and grammatical forms, smaller vocabulary as well as difficulties with receptive and expressive language skills. Individuals with DLD acquire the meaning of new words and new meaning of already acquired words with difficulty and they also need more time to identify familiar words. Developmental dyslexia (further dyslexia) is usually associated with problems of writing and reading language. In the diagnostic process, as well with DLD, sense defects, intellectual disability, neurological or psychiatric findings and poor learning opportunities must be excluded [1].

DLD is the most commonly studied disorder of the oral language while dyslexia is the most commonly studied disorder of the literary language. In both cases, these are language disorders that are often associated with each other. Individuals with DLD may also meet the criteria for dyslexia whereas the appearance of dyslexics in DLD population is significantly higher than in the normal, non-DLD population. This is similar with the occurrence of individuals with DLD in the dyslexic population. The comorbid occurrence of both disorders is estimated to be approximately twice as common as isolated occurrence [2]. Researchers therefore ask whether their relationship can be characterized as sisterly or whether one is a mother and the second is the child, or possibly if they are independent of each other. Tallal [3, 4] suggested a simple deficit model, according to which dyslexia and DLD are different manifestations of one and the same disorder. The common cause is the deficiency in phonological processing, accurately in distinguishing of fine acoustic sequences occurring in the order of tens of milliseconds. This deficiency gains a various depth. If it is deep, the individual has problems with reading as well as in the oral language. As a consequence, comorbidity of both disorders appears. If the deficit is not so deep, then the individual has problems in reading and only to a limited extend struggles in oral language. Tallal is aware that not all individuals with DLD have a problem in rapid auditory processing, and further that not all individuals with a deficiency of rapid auditory processing develops DLD. The aforementioned experience is difficult to explain using her model, although the author contends that there are methodological disadvantages regarding the present tests of rapid auditory processing which may not be sensitive enough and may therefore offer false negative results.

Bishop and Snowling [5] made a proposal of a model which expands the phonological aspect by means of the semantic-syntactical aspect. Individuals with dyslexia and DLD have in common problems in phonological processing. Unlike the Tallal's model, the degree of the phonological difficulties is roughly the same in both disorders. Both disorders differ in their respective semantic-syntactic aspect: individuals with DLD, unlike the individuals with dyslexia, have significant semantic-syntactic difficulties. Some individuals are difficult to classify in this model. Hence, the authors mark them as "poor comprehenders." Although they have good phonological abilities and are able to decode written text very well, they have difficulties to fill in its meaning.

Both of the aforesaid models perceive the deficiency in the phonological processing as the main factor contributing to dyslexia. Therefore dyslexia is regarded as a language disorder. Neurobiologically-oriented authors perceive dyslexia also as non-language disorder (for example [6–8]) with nonverbal symptoms as dyschronism, dysbalance, sensorismotor dyscoordination or a disturbance of orientation in place as well as space. Initially, language disorder thus had for this reason a new dimension built into a multidimensional model [9, 10]. The model works at four levels: etiological, neural, cognitive and behavioral. The model recognizes that many factors are involved in the etiopathogenesis of the disorder; some are risky, others protective; some are genetics while others are environmental. Their interaction forms neural structures necessary for cognitive functions, so deviations in cognitive functioning produce behavioral symptoms generating a particular picture of the neurodevelopmental disorder. According to the model for the beginning and the subsequent development of the disorder, a simple etiological factor is insufficient; there are indeed many factors involved on the disorder. If there are etiology and cognitive deficiencies, collectively shared by several disorders, comorbidity is to be expected. The model accesses the dynamic nature of the neurodevelopmental disorders and their development and to the high plasticity of the brain. The model allows for a better understanding of why, for example, in the Bakker's treatment of dyslexia, the change of poles happens of the L-type to the P-type or vice versa [11], and why remedial efforts on the behavioral level can produce structural improvements in neuronal networks associated with phonological processing and reading ([12] for review), and why phonological type of dyslexia ("deep" type) changes in the visual type ("surface" type) [13], as well as why dyslexia is associated with ADHD or DLD.

1.1 Eye movements of individuals with dyslexia

The oculomotor studies in dyslexics may be divided into two groups: in the first group we include studies on eye movements during reading and in the second group studies concerning eye movements in non-reading tasks. The studies of the first group agree, that while reading the eye movements of individuals with dyslexia differ significantly from the control group ([14]; newer [15, 16]). They are characterized by a larger number of fixations and a longer period of their duration, by larger number of saccades, from which a large part falls on regressions. The regressions of dyslexics are often shorter than by the control group and move within the frame of one word (the so-called innerword regressions) in an attempt to identify it, whereas regressions of the control group are more often between words. Their function is to contribute to the understanding of links between the passages of the text. These findings are independent of language region, for example in English-speaking countries [14], German-speaking countries [17] and China [18]. Any interpretation of these findings in terms of causes and consequences is very difficult, for a difficult question must be addressed. Are the nonfunctional eye movements the cause of the poor reading or is the poor reading the cause of the poor eye movements? To clear up that question, the researchers use non-reading tasks free of language influences which at the same time demanding of the subject under examination the identical or very similar regime of eye movements as occur during a real reading.

Non-reading tasks are possible to classify according to which particular kind of eye movements is stimulated. During so-called fixation task, the subject's duty is to observe a stationary point and for a certain time not to let it go out of eye sight. This task tests the so-called fixation stability that means the ability to keep the picture of a stationary object on command. Pavlidis [19] is one of the first to point out a worsening of the fixation stability by individuals with dyslexia in a non-reading task. Eden et al. [20] also included into their testing battery a fixation task by which they managed to distinguish dyslexics from the control group. More recently this difference was confirmed by Tiadi, et al. [21] and by Vagge et al. [22]. The fixation instability is considered as a sign of distinguishing dyslexics from the control group. However, these findings are not always consistent. The causes may be found in varieties of demands on the subject of the fixation task, differences in the time of its duration and eventually different degrees and types of the dyslexic disorder. Fischer and Hartnegg [23] point out two kinds of fixation instability, which are to some extent independent of each other and whose substitution contributes to the lower consistency of the findings.

In the so-called standard saccadic task the subject is required to move his/her eyes from one fixation position to another. The changes of the positions generally take place in the horizontal plane, in which his/her eyes are also moving according to the lines of the text – therefore we speak of the horizontal saccades. Regarding measurement, the saccadic reaction time is used, also the saccadic velocity and duration, the saccadic amplitude, the main sequence relationship, i.e. peak velocity or duration as a function of amplitude, and accuracy. The majority of studies do not find any difference between individuals with dyslexia and the control group (see review study Rommelse et al. [24]; more recently Vagge et al. [22]). From previous findings it appears that the standard saccadic task (1) has restricted potential to discriminate dyslexics from typically-developing readers and (2) it shows a normal function of cerebral circuits in/by dyslexics, which control reflexive, subcortical level of saccadic eye movements. Its submission in the testing battery corresponds to the exclusive nature of dyslexia diagnostics, i.e. excluding among other ailments neurological disorders.

The so-called antisaccadic task holds a privileged position. While undergoing the test, the subject's duty is again to follow up the changing position of the point to which the subjects fixes his/her eyes. However, in contrast to the standard saccadic task, he/she must transfer to the opposite direction. For example, the point which the subject is supposed to follow up actually appears on the left side of the screen. However, the subject's task is to look exactly at the opposite side. The antisaccadic task tests the voluntary component of the eye movements. His/her reaction to change to the left is based on automatically triggered reflexive mechanisms which must at first be suppressed by his/her will. Not until then it is possible to program a new direction of the movement, in our case, to the right. The antisaccadic task is therefore considered as an inhibitory capability test. It is correspondingly called neurological for the test of the frontal dysfunction [25]. The antisaccades were in case of the dyslexics systematically researched by the team of B. Fischer [26–28] who observed significant escalation in the directional mistakes in contrast with the control group. More recently this finding was confirmed by Bucci et al. [29] or Lukasova et al. [30].

The nonverbal sequential task was applied in dyslexics by Pavlidis [19, 31]. The task of the subject was to watch a set of horizontally arranged lights, which turned on and off in sequence. These lights were turned on and off, always from the left to the right and again when the last light in the line went out, a new cycle of observation began from left to right. There was always one single light on in the line. The subject followed up with a number of such cycles, respectively lines. However, for diagnostics, Pavlidis used only the first cycle, which he considered to be the most valuable. In contrast to the simple fixation task or the standard saccadic task, this task was testing more complex oculomotor behavior, which included fixation stability as well as saccadic movements with an automatic and voluntary component. By means of this task Pavlidis managed to find significant differences between dyslexics and the control group and especially to facilitate the researcher's interest in the relationship between eye movements and dyslexia. However, a number of authors replicated Pavlidis' research with different results. Some authors agreed [32], while others did not confirm his findings [22]. The causes can be understood due to a different methods (differently formulated sophistication of the task, different experimental procedure, different number of parameters used for the evaluation of the eye movements, differently sensitive devices for eye movements registration), in the selection of the participants and the typology of dyslexics and inaccuracies or inconsistencies of their descriptions.

1.2 Eye movements in individuals with DLD

The eye movements in the conditions of non-verbal tasks are rarely studied in individuals with DLD, unlike persons with dyslexia. Children with DLD are given language tasks accompanied with picture illustrations. During that time, eye movements are being scanned (for example, Andreu et al. [33]). In these studies eye movements are understood as a supportive method which should appropriately support the primary language examination, and not be understood as a biological marker of the disorder. Less frequent are oculomotor studies, where individuals with DLD are administered non-language tasks. These include Kelly et al. [34] studies, who administered the fixation task, the standard saccadic task and the antisaccadic task to different groups of children: to high-functional autistic children with language disorder, high-functional autistic children without language disorder, and finally to the individuals with DLD and control group. Persons with language disorder (whether with combination of autism or not) were characterized by fixation instability and by a significantly higher proportion of directional errors in the antisaccadic task. On the other hand, in a standard saccadic task their performance was comparable with the control group. The study showed that the basic level of oculomotor system controlled by the lower cerebral levels is intact for those individuals with DLD as well as in high-functioning individuals with autism. The study also showed that the deficit of the voluntary control of the eye movement is not exclusive for individuals with autism, but is connected to the language status, that means a presence versus an absence of a language disorder. Language is an important mediator of the executive control. For example, language can be helpful in supporting the children to reflect and realize in a clear way the conditions of the task (explicit verbalization of a type "if a point appears on one side of the screen, do not look at it, but on the opposite side"). The voluntary control deficit manifests itself with difficulties to suppress the reflexive reactions and to maintain the fixation stability. A similar finding is mentioned also by Norbury [35].

Studies which were engaged in comparing eye movements in individuals with dyslexia and individuals with DLD, are probably not so numerous. In databases like (PubMed, PsychINFO, ScienceDirect, Scopus, SpringerLink employing such key words as dyslexia, developmental language disorder, eye movement, saccade) we were not successful in finding such any study. Therefore we have decided to research their relationship and to verify the diagnostic contributions of the oculomotor examination of both disorders in non-language tasks.

2. Method

2.1 Participants

The clinical group (N = 60) constituted pupils with diagnosed dyslexia (n = 27) and DLD (n = 33) with an average age of 121 months, a standard deviation of 8 months and a range of 108–140 months. The pupils attended altogether six elementary schools in Prague specializing in children with special educational needs. An official governmental agency handles diagnostics and follow-up care for children with neurodevelopmental disorders in the Czech Republic. The government agency follows this work according to DSM-5 or a similar norm ICD-10. The diagnosis is a result of a team work of a psychologist, a special education teacher, a social worker and further a pediatrician, a speech therapist, a hearing doctor, eventually a child neurologist or another specialist. From standardized testing methods for example for testing IQ the WISC-III is used, re-standardized for the Czech population. For testing reading and writing, tests made and standardized are being used which had been produced by the team of the late Zdenek Matejcek, the vice president of IARLD (International Academy for Research in Learning Disabilities). For testing of the language skills, Heidelberg's test of the language development by J. Grimm and P. Schöler (HSET) is used, re-standardized for the Czech language. Phonological tests (test of the phoneme awareness and spoonerisms and the test of the auditory analysis and synthesis proposed and standardized by Czech authors). For testing of self-esteem of pupils with the special needs, SPAS test (Student's Perception of Ability Scale by F. J. Boersma and J. W. Chapman) is used, again re-standardized for the Czech population. For identification of at-risk children between the age of 6–8 years, children's screening from Kline, Graham, King, and Wringley is used. For checking language and literary deprivation of the child and the stable functioning of its family, the test of the family background from M. J. Herbert is used, re-standardized for the Czech environment, as well as the test ADOR (Adolescent about himself and parents) designed and standardized by the team of the aforementioned Zdenek Matejcek.

The control group ($N = 56$, average age 119 months, standard deviation 7 months, ranging from 108 to 136 months) is composed of pupils attending elementary school. The criteria for selection were better grades than average in both Czech language as the mother tongue and mathematics, non-problematic behavior without pathological pediatric finding and finally parental agreement with oculomotor examination. For all children, both the clinical and control group intellectual disorders were excluded or any disorders of the autistic spectrum, any psychiatric or neurological disorders, emotional deprivation, sensory defects (eye defects were corrected) or any serious pediatric complications. The pediatric evaluation conclusion was always a healthy condition. The families of children were rated as functional, i.e. none of them was monitored by the social welfare authorities. All children were of Czech nationality and their mother tongue was Czech – as with both their parents. None of the children came from a bilingual family or an immigrant family. The average age difference of both groups was insignificant ($t = 1.046$, $p = 0.297$).

2.2 Oculomotor test

The oculomotor test consisted of three tasks: standard saccadic, antisaccadic and non-verbal sequential tasks with self-regulation of the speed. All the tasks tested eye movements in horizontal plane. In the standard or "classic" saccadic task, the examined subject at first always had to fix his/her eyes at the point in the middle of the screen for 1000 ms. Afterwards a saccadic stimulus, the point appeared randomly left or right in a horizontal plane, always at a constant distance of 9 degrees of the visual angle (dva) from the center and always at the time of 700 ms. The point was black on a white background and had a diameter of 5 mm. The examined subject was instructed to move his/her eyes as quickly as possible to the saccadic stimulus. The task contained 20 attempts; 10 attempts oriented to the left, 10 to the right and the order was random. The time interval between the ending of the fixation point and the start of the saccadic stimulus was zero (sometimes called the "null" condition). As to oculomotor measurements, we have used the number of dysmetric saccades in relation with the number of attempts in the test and average size of their amplitude from the target amplitude. Because almost all the dysmetric saccades were hypometric, we have taken into consideration only the hypometric saccades (sometimes called "undershoots"). Both measurements characterize the accuracy of the saccadic movement. Among other things, the accuracy of the saccadic movement is dependent, on the quality of the neural circuits controlling the saccades. Normometry is a sign of the normal, healthy functioning of the saccadic system. One of the possible causes of dysmetria is cerebellum dysfunctions [25]. The value of this finding, i.e. dysmetria, results from a cerebellum theory of dyslexia [6, 8, 36]. This theory operates with a narrow relationship between cerebellum dysfunction and dyslexia. Directional errors in this task were extremely rare and, therefore, are not under consideration.

During antisaccadic task, the examined subject was to fix his/her eyes at the point of the center of the screen at first (the time of its duration was constant = 1000 ms) and then, afterwards, when the saccadic stimulus appeared – randomly on the left or right, but always at a constant distance of 9 degrees of the visual angle from the center and always for the time of 1000 ms. According to the instruction a saccadic movement was to be executed (so-called antisaccade) on the opposite side into the spot situated approximately as far as possible from the fixation point. The task consisted of 20 attempts; 10 attempts oriented to the left, 10 to the right, and the order was again performed randomly. The time interval between ending of the fixation point and the start of the saccadic stimulus was zero. For oculomotor measurements, we have employed (1) the number of correct reactions (antisaccades); (2) the number of saccades during the time of the fixation of the central point – this parameter is characterized as the fixation in/stability, the basis of which could be an increased arousal, which the antisaccadic task provoked in the participants and led to an increased saccadic activity; and (3) the ratio of correct antisaccades to prosaccades, i.e. directional errors. The standard saccadic task tested cerebral mechanisms associated with a lower level of control, whereas antisaccadic task tested mechanisms connected with higher, executive level of control [25].

Non-verbal sequential task with self-regulation of the speed (further the "self-pacing task") is submitted to the subject as six lines of dots after six dots in a row. The points were black on a white background and had a diameter of 5 mm. The angular dimensions of the entire picture equaled to ca 12° horizontally and ca 7.7° vertically. The distance between the dots in the line was always constant and equaled to ca 2.4°; between the lines ca 1.5°. The task of the subject was to "jump" with his/her eyes to all dots in every line, always in the direction from left to right and down from the top, thereby keeping to the comparable regime as one does while reading. At the same time, the examined person was not allowed to assist with his/her finger. When the participant reached to the last dot of the last line, he said "stop." It differs from the classical sequential non-reading task that Pavlidis worked with, whereby the subject alone sets the speed of his/her advancement. It also, hypothetically, sets higher demands on voluntary eye motor control than the task of Pavlidis. However, to verify this hypothesis, a neuroimaging study is probably necessary. The self-pacing task was proposed and already used by dyslexics earlier [37], where it has proven itself effective. We have not come across this task by any other authors. We are now upgrading it through an examination of saccades in the standard saccadic task and antisaccadic task. For oculomotor dimensions we have used (1) a number of forward saccades, (2) the number of regressive saccades, (3) the number of transition fixations from going over from one line to the other, and (4) the ratio between the fixation time in the first half and second half of the task. Using these parameters, we measure the fixation stability, voluntary control over saccades, the equability of the oculomotor performance in time and the efficiency of the visual orientation in the surface.

2.3 Registration of the eye movements

We have used a device technically labeled I4Tracking produced by Medicton Group, Ltd., Czech Republic in cooperation with the Technical University in Prague. The device works on the principle of video-oculography and facilitates contactless, distant scanning of eye movements. It offers to the examined subject an examination at a high comfort; the subject sits in front of the screen of the monitor on which the task is projected, without him/her being attached to the device, without the scanning part of the device being attached to the subject's head. We appreciate this attribute especially for children as well as anxious people who are more likely to be reluctant to cooperate. The disadvantage of this otherwise highly valued technology is a difficult on-line control. A chin rest was deployed to minimize head movements and stabilize the viewing distance at approx. 130 cm. Stimuli were visually presented on a 22-inch monitor with a resolution of 1920 x 1080. The sampling frequency equaled to 80 pictures per second.

2.4 Procedure

We motivated the subjects at first by an "astronaut" instruction which had already proved itself to be effective once before. Subjects heard the following: "Just imagine you are an astronaut and on the screen in your spaceship you are watching the universe. There are planets and stars moving and your task is to watch every planet or star and not let your eyes off of it." In the first examination phase, we administered a standard saccadic task. In the second phase we administered anti-saccadic task and in the third phase the self-pacing task. There were short breaks between the phases, when we instructed the subject about the new upcoming task. Each examination phase was preceded by a 9-point calibration. The total examination time approximated 10 minutes.

2.5 Data processing

The oculometric data obtained on-line we have further processed off-line in the Mathlab setting. For processing of the measured data we used the programming packet Eye Movements Signal Analysis (EMSA, further only "toolbox") developed at the Technical University in Prague. Scanned signals representing the view coordinates on the monitor were at first preprocessed, specifically the detection of the biological artifacts was done (blinking, unwilling head movements) and of the technical artifacts (incorrect detection) and their follow-up correction by interpolation. All data records were visually checked and records that were not of a high quality were not included into further processing. Afterwards the aforementioned basic parameters of the eye movements were calculated; in general we can say that the designated parameters are quantifying the temporo-spatial deviations from the ideal course of the eye movements.

We linked together all subjects in the first phase of the analysis into one group characterized by a "general" disorder (see further **Table 1**). We will refer to this group as "clinical". In the second phase we attempted to differentiate the clinical group more clearly for one part with the prevalence of dyslexia and part with prevalence of DLD (see **Table 2**).

		Classification of participants according to eye movements		
		CL	**TD**	**N**
Classification of participants according to clinical diagnosis	CL	55 (91.67%)	5 (8.33%)	60
	TD	5 (8.62%)	53 (91.38%)	58
				118

Note. TD = typically developing group; CL = clinical group (participants with dyslexia, DLD or comorbidity). Percent correctly classified: (55 + 53) / 118 → 91.53%.

Table 1.
Discriminant analysis, whereby the clinical group was not differentiated any further.

		Classification of participants according to eye movements		
		DD	DLD	N
Classification of participants according to clinical diagnosis	DD	23 (85.19%)	4 (14.84%)	27
	DLD	4 (12.12%)	29 (87.88%)	33
				60

Note. DD = developmental dyslexia group; DLD = developmental language disorder group;
Percent correctly classified: (23 + 29) / 60 → 86.67%.

Table 2.
Discriminant analysis, whereby the clinical group was differentiated according to the prevalence of dyslexia or DLD.

We processed the data with the help of discriminant analysis, into which we inserted the oculomotor measures of the participants and their membership to a group of typically developing, clinical group or group of participants with dyslexia or DLD. The question was whether the oculomotor measures would be discriminating the sample of participants satisfyingly with regard to their membership in groups. Furthermore, we condensed the oculomotor measurements using factor analysis (varimax rotation), in order to construct profiles of the eye movements from the extracted factors for individual groups.

3. Results

Table 3 presents the descriptive statistics of the oculomotor measures. The typically developing group had a tendency to achieve a better oculomotor performance than others; the group of individuals with dyslexia had a tendency to achieve a worse oculomotor performance than others.

By rotating (varimax method) we found a total of 3 factors which explained approximately 65% of the total variance.

The Factor F1 had its Eigenvalue 3.452 and explained 38.4% of the total variance. F1 is the factor of the oculomotor stability, characterized by confidence from going from one line to the other (this certainty was indexed by the number of transition fixations) and by the certainty of the movement in the line characterized through minimal regressions. The subject perfectly adapts to the conditions of the task and is able to move flawlessly in the task. The growth of the factor signals a worsening oculomotor performance in the self-pacing task, i.e. the number of transition fixations increases as well as the number of regressions in the lines and the number of forward saccades decreases.

Factor F2 had its Eigenvalue of 1.297 and explained 14.4% of the total variance. F2 is the factor of the basic dynamics of the saccades. As F2 grows, the proportion of undershoots in the prosaccadic task increases, the size of the undershoots increases, and the proportion of corrected errors in the antisaccadic task decreases. As the factor increases, it may be concluded that the subject has an impaired ability to focus on the target, its distance and accordingly determine the magnitude of the saccadic movement. Because it also correlates with the antisaccadic task, frontal dysfunction may be inferred, specifically the impaired ability to correct erroneous prepotent responses.

Factor F3 had its Eigenvalue of 1.097 and explained 12.2% of the total variance. Growth of F3 indicates a decreasing proportion of correct antisaccades and an increasing proportion of prosaccadic errors, an increasing proportion of saccadic

Oculomotor measure	Mean			Contrast		
	TD[a]	DD[b]	DLD[c]	TDxDD	TDxDLD	DDxDLD
Prosac: The number of hypometric saccades[d]/ number of attempts	0.560	0.856	0.741	*ns*	*ns*	*ns*
Prosac: the size of difference between normometric saccade and hypometric saccade (px)	37.225	73.438	62.457	*	*	*
Antisac: the number of correct antisaccades	11.706	6.888	6.878	*	*	*ns*
Antisac: the number of saccades at the time of fixations of the central point	4.603	8.185	5.363	*	*ns*	*ns*
Antisac: the ratio of correct antisaccades to prosaccades (directional errors)	2.70	2.17	1.95	*ns*	*ns*	*ns*
Self-pacing: the number of progressive saccades falling on the saccadic stimulus on average	0.763	0.665	0.716	*ns*	*ns*	*ns*
Self-pacing: the number of regressive saccades falling on the saccadic stimulus on average	0.078	0.171	0.111	*ns*	*ns*	*ns*
Self-pacing: the number of transition fixations falling on movement from one line to the next on average	1.310	3.0	2.545	*ns*	*ns*	*ns*
Self-pacing: time in the first half/time in the second half	0.506	0.514	0.523	*ns*	*ns*	*ns*

Note. Prosac = prosaccadic task; Antisac = antisaccadic task; Self-pacing = nonverbal sequential task with self-pacing; TD = typically developing group; DD = developmental dyslexia group; DLD = developmental language disorder group.
*ns = not statistically significant; *denotes a statistically significant difference (ANOVA: F = 204.6, Df = 1061, p = .000).*
[a]n = 58.
[b]n = 27.
[c]n = 33
[d]Difference between target amplitude and saccadic amplitude >20 px.

Table 3.
Descriptive Statistics.

intrusions at the time of central point fixation, and an increasing imbalance between the time the subject goes through the first vs. the second half of the self-pacing task. Frontal dysfunction may be inferred; specifically debilitated inhibition and a lowered ability to suppress prepotent responses.

Based on these factors, we have generated profiles of the oculomotor performances for the individual groups (see **Figure 1**).

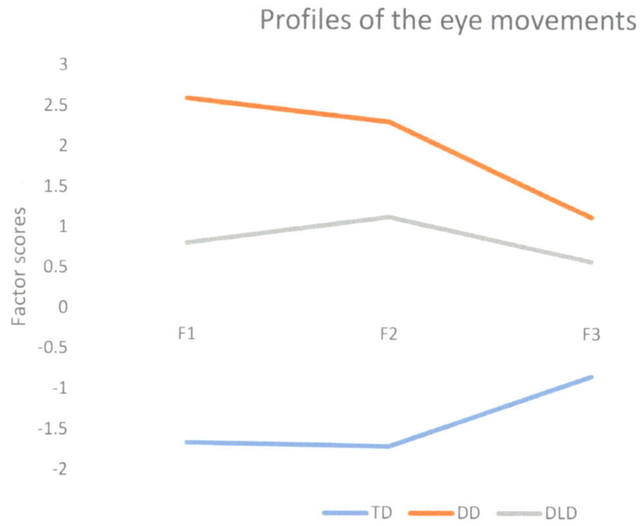

Figure 1.
Profiles of the eye movements. On the horizontal axis factors F1 up to F3 are marked, and on the vertical axis the averages of the factor scores are marked for individual groups. TD = typically developing, DD = developmental dyslexia, DLD = developmental language disorder.

ANOVA (F = 37.43, df = 353, p = 0.000) showed significant differences between the control group and both clinical groups (dyslexic and DLD) in all three factors. Compared to the control group, both clinical groups showed an overall poorer oculomotor performance; in the self-pacing task they did more transitional fixations, more regressions, and less regular saccades; in the prosaccadic task they made more undershots; in the antisaccadic task they made more directional mistakes. The difference between the dyslexic and DLD group was significant for factors F1 and F2; for F3 factor it did not reach statistical significance, although for dyslexics it was leading towards worse performance. The dyslexic group had an overall worse oculomotor performance than the DLD group.

4. Discussion

The conformity of the classification according to eye movements with the classification according to the clinical diagnosis reached 91%, see **Table 1**. This may be partially comparable with the study of Benfatto et al. [15]. However, its authors employed eye tracking while reading a short natural passage of text. Their participants were – when compared with ours – pupils of the third grade of elementary school (age 9–10 years) and were assessed as poor readers or as typically developing readers. Using statistical cross-validation techniques, they achieved a classification accuracy of nearly 96%. Benfatto et al. concluded that eye tracking has the potential to become an objective and accurate screening method useful for identifying school children at risk of dyslexia. A comparable conclusion was also reached by Smyrnakis et al. [16] in a similar study. Our finding supports the screening assumption of Benfatto et al. and also Smyrnakis et al. related to dyslexia but our finding further extends it to DLD. Additionally, we have used non-reading tasks in our study, in contrast to Benfatto et al. and Smyrnakis et al. Therefore, we can transfer the issue regarding screening to the pre-school age. Hypothetically, eye tracking has the potential to contribute to an early identification of children who may be at risk of dyslexia and/or DLD before the child even enters school.

4.1 Discrepancies between oculomotor and clinical classification

The agreement of the classification according to the oculomotor test with the classification according to the clinical finding depended on the type of clinical diagnosis, i.e. dyslexia or DLD. More often, DLD problems of dyslexics were more frequently ignored in the clinical trial from the point of view of the oculomotor test than dyslexic problems of DLD patients (14.84% vs. 12.12%, **Table 2**). Specifically, in 4 subjects with clinically-diagnosed dyslexia, the oculomotor test showed DLD symptoms. The DLD symptoms in those children were most probably secondary in the clinical picture of the disorder and therefore were left without notice by the clinician. In clinical practice, we have encountered individuals diagnosed with DLD in their pre-school age, with whom the DLD disorder had faded out but then while attending school, dyslexic difficulties had come to the forefront. Obviously dyslexic difficulties are evaluated as more serious so the child was examined with the diagnosis "dyslexia." In fact, these 4 participants could be classified as a mixed disorder/comorbidity of dyslexia and DLD.

The 23 participants with the diagnosis of dyslexia (**Table 2**), in which the oculomotor test did not indicate other DLD-type problems, represented on the other hand "pure" dyslexics. In the DLD group (see **Table 2**), the oculomotor test showed 4 participants with a clinical diagnosis of DLD whose difficulties could also have been caused by dyslexia. These individuals could be classified as a mixed disorder of DLD and dyslexia with the dominance of DLD. In those 29 participants where the conformity between the oculomotor finding and the clinical was attained, the so-called "pure DLD" was substantiated.

4.2 Influence of language milieu

Just like English, Czech is also a morphophonemic language. The spelling system utilizes sound units (phonemes) and semantic units (morphemes). Although English is characterized as a non-transparent language which places high phonological demands on the reader, Czech with its high consistency is "phonologically friendly" – the letter corresponds to the sound, which is written as it is pronounced. While English is said to be morphologically simple, Czech is the opposite. Thanks to phonological transparency, Czech 1st graders read coherent texts fluently and with comprehension in the first half of the 1st grade. Owing to the nature of the Czech language and the relatively rapid development of reading skills in a typically developing child, reading tests are not just lists of words, but coherent texts that are administered in the first half of the 1st grade [38]. Because of the grammatical (morphological, syntactic) complexity of Czech language, Czech pupils acquire Czech grammar throughout their schooling, i.e. for 9 years, and even then many of them do not master it perfectly. In the described linguistic environment of the Czech language, reading difficulties become eminent much more easily, while language difficulties (morphological, syntactic) recede into the background. DLD-type difficulties, especially of a milder degree, are easy to become less noticeable among the widespread grammatical difficulties of Czech pupils and can be more easily overlooked diagnostically, in contrast to dyslexic difficulties. Within the grammatically demanding environment of the Czech language, DLD-type difficulties seem to be masked, while reading difficulties are highlighted. With this effect of the Czech language environment, we explain why in the observed confusions the clinical approach preferred the diagnosis of dyslexia and neglected the DLD-type difficulties of the dyslexic group.

4.3 Dual-stream model

Johansson [39] and more recently Specht [40, 41] or Rastle [42] in their studies present the growing evidence for the validity of the dual-stream model of the speech perception and speech comprehension. The ventral stream serves speech comprehension (semantic-syntactic function). It closely interacts with the dorsal stream which plays the strategic role in speech production and likewise serves the auditory-motor integration. The model structurally includes the areas of the temporal, parietal and frontal cortex and probably also other brain areas which were not included in the model at the time. According to Specht, it belongs to other areas which do not have specific language functions, but also serves other non-language functions. For our purpose, motor functions and relevant motor areas of the cortex are interesting. Hypothetically, the dysfunction of the dorsal path could adversely affect oculomotor behavior. This fits in well for children with dyslexia and DLD, where we observed corresponding clinical and oculomotor findings. With just a smaller number of children with dyslexia or DLD ($N = 5$, **Table 1**) where we found standard eye movements, we may assume, according to the dual modal, a normal function of the dorsal path and a malfunction of the ventral path, which clinical examinations have determined. In contrast, we found subnormal eye movements in five typically-developing children (**Table 1**). Hypothetically, we could infer a malfunction of the dorsal path and the normal function of the ventral path. In both of these groups of children, a comparison of clinical and oculomotor findings could suggest an isolated occurrence of the disorder (either in one or the other path). The reasoning behind this interpretation is merely hypothetical and a confirmation would demand an application of neuro-imaging methods.

4.4 Antisaccadic task and executive functions

The antisaccadic task is widely regarded to be one of the tests of executive functions [43]. Executive functions represent a broader construct, to which planning, generativity, inhibition, set-shifting, working memory and attentional control are usually integrated [44]. The antisaccadic task is used to investigate especially cognitive flexibility and response inhibition [25].

Our study showed deterioration of antisaccadic performance in both clinical groups, dyslexic and DLD group. Both clinical groups made fewer correct antisaccadic reactions and more directional errors than the control group. At the same time, the differences between the two clinical groups were insignificant (**Table 3**). The antisaccadic task did not require language/reading skills. Poor performance in the antisaccadic task in our clinical groups can therefore not be explained by a deficit in language/reading, but by a deficit in executive processing. There is no doubt that in our antisaccadic task, inner speech as a language tool could help facilitate the antisaccadic performance, but it was probably not the sole source of antisaccadic difficulties because the antisaccadic task did not require inner speech to perform well. The problems of dyslexic and DLD subjects in the antisaccadic task were also observed by other authors, cited in the Introduction (subchapters 1.2 and 1.3). We found fewer published studies of eye movements in DLD subjects in the antisaccadic task – most likely because language is perceived as a qualitatively different function from sensorimotor functions, which include eye movements. Dyslexics need visuo-spacial processing for reading with which eye movements correlate. However, mutual comparisons of antisaccadic performance of subjects with dyslexia and DLD are probably rare; hence we cannot verify the results of our study from studies by other authors.

4.5 Oculomotor tasks vs. differential diagnostics

Based on our finding that both language disorders (dyslexia, DLD) were reflected in the non-linguistic oculomotor tasks, we conclude that brain networks, which are the basis of all language functions, are connected to the networks that control eye movements. Because antisaccades specifically activate the dorsolateral prefrontal cortex [25], the antisaccadic task is a useful tool for investigating frontal dysfunction and volitional processes. However, the antisaccadic task is unlikely to be useful for any differential diagnostics between dyslexia and DLD, because the same mistakes in the antisaccadic task are made by schizophrenics or neurological patients [25]. A more specific test for language/reading in comparison with the antisaccadic task seems to us to be the self-pacing task. In addition to volitional processes, this task also requires hierarchical sequencing which is the core component of syntactic processing. The task is not limited only to language stimuli and is not demanding on the working memory. In line with the review fMRI studies of language [45, 46] we believe that the performance in the self-pacing task will be more connected with the involvement of the left dorsal pars opercularis, which also serves non-linguistic syntax, and that the performance of the self-pacing task is less connected with the involvement of the left ventral pars opercularis, which serves working memory and sequencing of articulatory events. The left ventral pars opercularis is therefore a more specific language area than dorsal pars opercularis.

4.6 Are dyslexia and DLD being distinctive disorders?

Researchers ask whether their relationship can be characterized as sisterly or whether one is a mother and the second is the child, or possibly if they are independent of each other [44]. Various models have been proposed to address this issue, and we regard the multidimensional model to be the most appropriate one [9, 10], see Introduction. We would classify the oculomotor finding at the behavioral level. Therefore, we do not expect the oculomotor examination to provide a comprehensive answer to this question. However, it can enrich it with a new aspect. In our oculomotor test, the profiles of DLD subjects were similar and differed only in the degree of deviation; in dyslexics, the deviations from the controls were greater, see **Figure 1**. Oculomotorically, both disorders appear to us to be close. Although they are studied under the classification of linguistic disorders, we can also characterize them with a common non-linguistic symptomatology, specifically the oculomotor. According to our study, the oculomotor (non-linguistic) accompaniment of both disorders is the rule rather than the exception and makes them, at the symptomatology level, to a large extent also non-linguistic disorders. From our study's perspective, the causal relationship between the linguistic nature of both disorders and eye movements remains unclear: is a language disorder the cause of the deviant eye movements or are the deviant eye movements the cause of a language disorder? Or do both deviations, linguistic and oculomotor, have a common cause?

4.7 Implications of the study

We currently see the benefits of our study in the research dimension. It would be premature to talk about the transfer of this method based on the measurement of eye movements into the clinical practice of child psychologists, special needs teachers/speech therapists, pedopsychiatrists or others. The study showed the promising potencies of this method for the diagnostics of dyslexia and developmental language disorder. However, it pointed out a number of issues that will need to be resolved before the method can be transferred to the field. First, eye movements as a manifestation of brain activity contain a lot of information about various mental functions; we can now register by far not all the information and that we can register is difficult to differentiate diagnostically. Second, the oculomotor tasks used in the examination of eye movements are, in fact, the questions we ask the examined subject-a child in oculomotor language. The child answers us, again in oculomotor language. To get a valid and reliable answer, we must also ask a high quality question. This area of oculomotor tasks therefore requires further research efforts. Third: the child is highly teachable and their brain is highly plastic and dynamically evolving. This characteristic is reflected in the oculomotor performance. When, at what stage of development is it possible to identify impending pathological dispositions, such as dyslexic or DLD-dispositions or schizophrenic dispositions, and to differentiate them from developmentally normal fluctuations and also from each other? How can all these peculiarities, developmentally normal and developmentally abnormal, be embodied in the standards of oculomotor performance? What will we consider in oculomotor performance defined by different tasks as a norm, as a broader norm, as a borderline finding, as a pathology? Fourth: in the diagnostic use of eye movements, we work with measurement parameters at the level of units of milliseconds and angular minutes. Is this a sufficient sensitivity or will it be necessary to register finer differences?

5. Conclusion

Both language disorders, dyslexia and DLD, are also characterized by non-linguistic manifestations, specifically by eye movements that have been tested using non-linguistic tasks. Oculomotorically, we were able to differentiate (a) a group of children with dyslexia and/or DLD from a group of children typically developing; (b) a group of children with dyslexia from a group of children with DLD. According to our results, the cognitive basis of these differences is a result of an altered executive processing, the neural substrate of which is regarded to be the prefrontal cortex. Executive processing in dyslexics seems to us to be worse in comparison with DLD subjects in the conditions of the employed oculomotor tasks.

We interpret the discrepancies between the clinical and oculomotor classification by the peculiarities of the language environment. The morphologically demanding Czech environment conceals the milder degrees of DLD, while the dyslexic difficulties penetrate more easily to the forefront of clinical attention. Hypothetically, the location of the disorder may also be involved in the discrepancies. According to the dual model, the dorsal stream is suspected to induce oculomotor problems as well as ventral stream semantic problems.

From these findings we conclude that the oculomotor examination in the conditions of non-verbal tasks may contribute to (a) the diagnostics of the neurodevelopmental disorders of the linguistic type, dyslexia and DLD; (b) the differential diagnostics of these disorders. The oculomotor examination under the conditions of non-verbal tasks appears to us as a screening method with good prospects for these disorders in the pre-school population.

The study indicated that the oculomotor examination under the conditions of non-verbal tasks has a promising potential for diagnostics. However, much research effort is likely to be required before this method, as sufficiently valid and reliable, can be transferred into the clinical practice.

Conflict of interest

Martin Dobias, Jaromir Dolezal and Vratislav Fabian have received research grant Number TA01011138 from the Technological Agency of the Czech Republic.

The funding agency had no role in the design and conduct of the study; collection, management, analysis, and interpretation of the data; preparation, review, or approval of the manuscript; nor the decision to submit the manuscript for publication. Zuzana Bilkova, Helena Havlisova, Jiri Jost and Olga Malinovska did not receive any specific grant from funding agencies in the public, commercial, or not-for-profit sectors and declare that they have no conflicts of interests to report.

Ethical Standards and informed consent

All procedures followed were in accordance with the ethical standards of the responsible committee on human experimentation (institutional and national) and with the Helsinki Declaration of 1975, as revized in 2000. Informed consent was obtained from all participants for being included in the study.

Author details

Zuzana Bilkova[1], Martin Dobias[2], Jaromir Dolezal[3], Vratislav Fabian[2], Helena Havlisova[1], Jiri Jost[1] and Olga Malinovska[1*]

1 Faculty of Education, University of South Bohemia, Czech Republic

2 Faculty of Electrical Engineering, Czech Technical University in Prague, Prague, Czech Republic

3 Czech Institute of Informatics, Robotics and Cybernetics, Czech Technical University in Prague, Czech Republic

*Address all correspondence to: omalinovska@pf.jcu.cz

References

[1] American Psychiatric Association: Diagnostic and Statistical Manual of Mental Disorders, Fifth Edition. Arlington, VA, American Psychiatric Association, 2013.

[2] Catts, H. W., Adlof, S. M., Hogan, T., & Weismer, S. E. (2005). Are Specific Language Impairment and Dyslexia Distinct Disorders? J Speech Lang Hear Res., *48*(6), 1378-1396.

[3] Tallal, P. (1991). The neuropathology of developmental dysphasia: behavioral, morphological, and physiological evidence for a pervasive temporal processing disorder. Reading and Writing, *3*(3-4), 363-377.

[4] Tallal, P. (2012). Of bats and men. J Neurophysiol, *108*, 1545-1547.

[5] Bishop, D. V. M., & Snowling, M. J. (2004). Developmental dyslexia and specific language impairment: same or different? Psychol Bull, *130*, 858-886.

[6] Nicolson, R. I., Fawcett, A. J., & Dean, P. (2001). Developmental dyslexia: The cerebellar deficit hypothesis. Trends in Neurosciences, *24*, 508-511.

[7] Stein, J. (2019). The current status of the magnocellular theory of developmental dyslexia. Neuropsychologia, 130, 66-77.

[8] Stoodley, D. J. & Stein, J. F. (2013). Cerebellar Function in Developmental Dyslexia. Cerebellum, *12*, 267-276.

[9] Pennington, B. R. (2006). From single to multiple deficit models of developmental disorders. *Cognition, 101*, 385-413.

[10] Ramus, F., Marshall, Ch. R., Rosen, S., & van der Lely, H. K. J. (2013). Phonological deficits in specific language impairment and developmental dyslexia: towards a multidimensional model. Brain, *136*, 630-645.

[11] Dryer, R., Beale, I. L., & Lambert, A. J. (1999). The Balance Model of Dyslexia and Remedial Training. Journal of Learning Disabilities, *32*(2), 174-186.

[12] Kershner, J. R. (2016). Network dynamics in dyslexia: Review and implications for remediation. Research in Developmental Disabilities, *59*, 24-34.

[13] Thompson, M. E. (1999). Subtypes of Dyslexia: A Teaching Artefact? Dyslexia, *5*, 127-137.

[14] Rayner, K. (1998). Eye Movements in Reading and Information Processing: 20 Years of Research. Psychological Bulletin, *124*(3), 372-422.

[15] Benfatto, M. N., Seimyr, G. O., Ygge, J., Pansell, T., Rydberg, A., & Jacobson, Ch. (2016). Screening for Dyslexia Using Eye Tracking during Reading. PLoS ONE, 11(12), 1-16.

[16] Smyrnakis, I., Andreadakis, V., Selimis, V., Kalaitzakis, M., Bachourou, T., Kaloutsakis, G., Kymionis, G. D., Smirnakis, S., Aslanides, I. M. (2017). RADAR: A novel fast-screening method for reading difficulties with special focus on dyslexia. PLoS ONE *12*(8): e0182597. https://doi.org/ 10.1371/ journal.pone.0182597

[17] Hutzler, F., & Wimmer, H. (2004). Eye movements of dyslexic children when reading in a regular orthography. Brain and Language, *89*, 235-242.

[18] Pan, J., Yan, M., Laubrock, J., Shu, H., & Kliegl, R. (2014). Saccade-target selection of dyslexic children when reading Chinese. Vision Res, *97*, 24-30.

[19] Pavlidis, G. Th. (1981). Do Eye Movements Hold the Key to Dyslexia? Neuropsychologia, *19*, 57-64.

[20] Eden, G. F., Stein, J. F., Wood, H. M., & Wood, F. B. (1994). Differences in eye movements and reading problems in dyslexics and normal children. Vision Research, *34*(10), 1345-1358.

[21] Tiadi, A., Gérard, C., Peyre, H., Bui-Quoc, E., & Bucci, M. P. (2016) Immaturity of Visual Fixations in Dyslexic Children. Front. Hum. Neurosci, *10*, Article 58, 1-7.

[22] Vagge, A. Cavanna, M., Traverso, C. E., & Iester, M. (2015). Evaluation of ocular movements in patients with dyslexia. Ann. of Dyslexia, *65*, 24-32.

[23] Fischer, B., & Hartnegg. K. (2009). Instability of Fixation in Dyslexia: Development – Deficits – Training. Optometry & Vision Development, *40*(4), 221-228.

[24] Rommelse, N. J., Van der Stigchel, S., Sergeant, J. A. (2008). A review on eye movement studies in childhood and adolescent psychiatry. Brain and Cognition, *68*, 391-414.

[25] Leigh, R. J., & Zee, D. S. (2015). *The Neurology of Eye Movements*. Philadelphia, PA.: Oxford University Press.

[26] Biscaldi, M., Fischer, B., & Aiple, F. (1994). Saccadic eye movements of dyslexic and normal reading children. Perception, *23*, 45-64.

[27] Biscaldi, M., Fischer, B., & Hartnegg, K. (2000). Voluntary saccadic control in dyslexia. Perception, *29*, 509-521.

[28] Biscaldi, M., Gezeck, S., & Stuhr, V. (1998). Poor saccadic control correlates with dyslexia. Neuropsychologia, *36*(11), 1189-1202.

[29] Bucci, M. P., Mélithe, D., Ajrezo, L., Bui-Quoc, E., & Gérard, C. L. (2014). The influence of oculomotor tasks on postural control in dyslexic children. Frontiers in Human *Neuroscience, 8*, Article 981, 1-10.

[30] Lukasova, K., Silva, I. P., & Macedo, E. C. (2016) Impaired Oculomotor Behavior of Children with Developmental Dyslexia in Antisaccades and Predictive Saccades Tasks. Front. Psychol, *7*:987. doi: 10.3389/fpsyg.2016.00987.

[31] Pavlidis, G. Th. (1983). The „Dyslexia Syndrome" and Its Objective Diagnosis by Erratic Eye Movements. In K. Rayner (Ed.), *Eye Movements in Reading: Perceptual and Language Processes* (pp. 441-464). New York: AP.

[32] Martos, F. J., & Vila, J. (1990). Differences in Eye Movements Control Among Dyslexic, Retarded and Normal Readers in the Spanish Population. Reading and Writting: An Interdisciplinary Journal, *2*, 175-188.

[33] Andreu, L., Sanz-Torrent, M., Olmos, J. G., & MacWhinney, B. (2013). The formulation of argument structure in SLI: an eye-movement study. Clin Linguist Phon, *27*(2), 111-133.

[34] Kelly, D. J, Walker, R., & Norbury, C. F. (2013). Deficits in volitional oculomotor control align with language status in autism spectrum disorders. Developmental Science, *16*, 56-66.

[35] Norbury, C. F. (2014). Sources of variation in developmental language disorders: evidence from eye-tracking studies of sentence production. Phil. Trans. R. Soc. B, *369*, 20120393.

[36] Freedman, E. G., Molholm, S., Gray, M. J., Belyusar, D., & Foxe, J. J. (2017). Saccade adaptation deficits in developmental dyslexia suggest disruption of cerebellar-dependent learning. Journal of

Neurodevelopmental Disorders, *9*, 36-43.

[37] Jost, J. (2009). *Oční pohyby, čtení a dyslexie* [Eye Movements, Reading and Dyslexia] Prague: Fortuna [in Czech].

[38] Matejcek, Z. (1998). Reading in Czech. Part I: Test of Reading in a Phoneticallly Higly Consistent Spelling System. Dyslexia, *4*, 145-154.

[39] Johansson, B. B. (2006): Cultural and Linguistic Influence on Brain Organization for Language and Possible Consequences for Dyslexia: A Review. Annals of Dyslexia, *56*(1), 13-50.

[40] Chang, E. F., Raygor, K. P., & Berger, M. S. (2015). Contemporary model of language organization: an overview for neurosurgeons. J Neurosurg, *122*, 250-261.

[41] Specht, K. (2014). Neuronal basis of speech comprehension. Hearing Research, *307*, 121-135.

[42] Rastle, K. (2019). The place of morphology in learning to read in English. Cortex, 116, 45-54.

[43] Aichert, D. S., Wöstmann, N. M., Cost, A., Macare, Ch., Wenig, J. R., Möller, R., & Ettinger, U. (2012). Associations between trait impulsivity and prepotent response inhibition. J *Clin Exp Neuropsychol, 34*(10), 1016-1032.

[44] Bishop, D. V. M., Nation, K., & Patterson, K. (2014). When words fail us: insights into language processing from developmental and acquired disorders. Philos. Trans. R. Soc. B *369*: 20120403.

[45] Price, C. J. (2010). The anatomy of language: a review of 100 fMRI studies published in 2009. Ann. N.Y. Acad. Sci. *1191*, 62-88.

[46] Price, C. J. (2012). A review and synthesis of the first 20 years of PET and fMRI studies of heard speech, spoken language and reading. NeuroImage, *62*, 816-847.